Jinxin Liu, Xiaoping Tang (Eds.)
Atlas of AIDS Co-infection

Atlas of AIDS Co-infection

Edited by
Jinxin Liu, Xiaoping Tang

DE GRUYTER

清華大学出版社
TSINGHUA UNIVERSITY PRESS

This work is co-published by Tsinghua University Press and Walter de Gruyter GmbH.

Contributors Committee

Chief Editors: Jinxin Liu, Xiaoping Tang
Subeditors: Weiping Cai, Chibiao Yin, Fuchun Zhang, Chunliang Lei
Reviewers: Daqing Ma, Yiai Lin
Editor committee: Chibiao Yin, Songfeng Jiang, Jinxin Liu, Wanshan Chen, Bihua Chen,
                   Xiejie Chen, Haolan Hw, Lieguang Zhang, Fuchun Zhang, Xiaofeng Guo,
                   Xiaoping Tang, Chunliang Lei, Weiping Cai, Wanhua Guan, Deyang Huang,
                   Zhiping Zhang, Qingxin Gan, Yi Liang, Yan Ding, Zhoukun Ling, Tianli Hu

ISBN 978-3-11-057989-5
e-ISBN 978-3-11-035394-5
e-ISBN (EPUB) 978-3-11-038790-2

Library of Congress Cataloging-in-Publication data
A CIP catalog record for this book has been applied for at the Library of Congress.

Bibliographic information published by the Deutsche Nationalbibliothek
The Deutsche Nationalbibliothek lists this publication in the Deutsche Nationalbibliografie;
detailed bibliographic data are available in the Internet at http://dnb.dnb.de.

© 2016 Walter de Gruyter GmbH, Berlin/Boston and Tsinghua University Press, Beijing
This volume is text- and page-identical with the hardback published in 2016.
Typesetting: metamedien | Werbung und Mediendienstleistungen, Burgau
Printing and binding: Hubert & Co. GmbH & Co. KG, Göttingen

♾ Printed on acid-free paper
Printed in Germany

www.degruyter.com

Foreword

In recent years, HIV/AIDS-related opportunistic infections have drawn worldwide attention only due to their escalating prevalence and their complexity in etiology. From their onsets to their progress in the course, opportunistic infections vary in terms of different stages and different immunosuppression of hosts. In the advanced stage of AIDS, they may lead to multiple complications simultaneously. As a result, they present varying unspecific manifestations in imaging so that to make an affirmative diagnosis we depend more on the clinical observations and laboratory data, especially the results from bacterial culturing and pathological analyses. But the particularity of AIDS allows few chances for us to obtain the specimen for biopsy. Favorably, the radiological examinations on the AIDS-related infections have the advantage of non-invasiveness, accurate location of lesions, full scale of observation and repeatability, which no doubt to say makes imaging diagnoses so valuable for the detection, diagnosis, treatment and prognosis of AIDS-induced opportunistic infections.

Guangzhou No. 8 Hospital is a government-run hospital, only designated by the local government to service the AIDS patients in South China. In the past twenty years, we have attained fair knowledge and rich experience in prevention and treatment of AIDS-related opportunistic infections. In the context, the two experts, Prof. Jinxin Liu and Prof. Xiaoping Tang from the hospital, co-worked hard to compile the book, An Atlas of Thoracic and Abdominal Images of AIDS Patients, which I believe is of significance for clinical reference.

The book contains 15 chapters and has collected in it more than 101 cases of AIDS-related infections and over 1,000 radiographic and CT images with rich legends, which is a general summary of clinical studies on AIDS-related opportunistic infections in recent years. Therefore, I wish that this book would play a role in promoting the clinical diagnosis and treatment of AIDS patients.

May 1, 2010
Academician of Chinese Engineering Academy
Fuwai Hospital of Chinese Academy of Medical Sciences

Preface

AIDS (acquired immunodeficiency syndrome) is a severe clinical immunosuppressive syndrome caused by human immunodeficiency virus (HIV) infection. By severely suppressing human T lymphocyte immune function, HIV may induce various malignant tumors and all kinds of opportunistic infections. The opportunistic infections are commonly caused by fungi, bacteria and viruses, and clinically show the manifestations of fever, weight loss and systemic lymphadenopathy.

Epidemically, AIDS has spread rapidly worldwide since the first AIDS case was detected in America in 1981. According to UNAIDS Report on the Global AIDS Epidemic 2009 and 2010 Prospects in Prevention and Care of AIDS, at least 60 million people were infected by HIV and 25 million of them died of AIDS-related diseases. In 2008, comparatively, only 33.4 million were HIV-infected including 2.7 million new victims and 2 million died of AIDS.

The similar situation happens in China for the rapid increase of HIV cases. By the end of October 2009, 319,877 HIV/AIDS patients were reported and documented. Of them 102,323 were AIDS patients and 46,845 died. Comparatively, the prevalence of AIDS epidemic was so late that the majority of medical imageologists in China are green hands in terms of full-scale and systematic investigations in AIDS imageology. At this point, it is essential for medical doctors to familiarize themselves with clinical and imaging manifestations of AIDS.

Clinically, imageological examinations can present the lesions caused mainly by opportunistic infections and partly by HIV infections. The imaging manifestations of AIDS with opportunistic infections are characterized by complexity and non-specificity only because AIDS patients can contract various different opportunistic infections due to individual immunosuppression at the different stages of AIDS. In this case, the diagnoses of opportunistic infections in AIDS patients are dependent on clinical symptoms, imaging data, experimental results and most importantly, bacterial identification and pathological analyses. Therefore, specimen collections and biopsies become essential and fundamental for the diagnoses. But the particularity of AIDS makes clinical diagnosis tricky in China. Luckily, the imaging examinations are advantageous for its noninvasiveness, repeatability, accurate location and full-scale observation, which together contribute the great value to the identification, assessment of curative effect and prognosis of AIDS.

Opportunistic infections most commonly involve the thoracic and abdominal organs and tissues, which are most available for specimen collection and biopsy for the sake of affirmative diagnoses. For recent years, we have undertaken a number of imaging diagnoses of typical opportunistic infections in AIDS patients in Guangzhou No. 8 People's Hospital. Therefore, we would like to share our experience in imaging diagnoses of the opportunistic infections with peers as well as other clinical doctors by gathering, compiling and publishing the imaging findings from our clinical practice. The atlas is a collection of images on AIDS patients together with respective legends.

It elaborates not only the imaging features of AIDS patients by dynamically presenting the thoracoabdominal images and depicting the onset and progress of each AIDS case, but the onset, progress, treatment and improvement of AIDS-induced opportunistic infections of all kinds as well by integrating the clinical data of each case. From this point of view, the book is a complete summary of thoracoabdominal diagnostic imaging and treatment of AIDS patients and therefore is of great value for the clinical diagnosis and treatment of AIDS.

Thanks to the hard work of all other compilers, the atlas is successfully completed. We would like to thank the leaders of Guangzhou No. 8 People's Hospital. It could not be so smooth and successful without their support. Moreover, we really wish to express our gratitude to Prof. Yuqing Liu, academician of the Chinese Academy of Engineering, who wrote the preface for the atlas. Finally, we are strongly hopeful that the peer experts as well as the readers in this discipline would not bother to dedicate their critics on this book only because there may be some mistakes in it for the sake of our limited clinical experience and the rapid development of imaging technology.

LIU Jin-xin, TANG Xiao-ping
March 15, 2010

Preface of second edition

As time flies, it has been over three years since the publishing of An Atlas of Thoracic and Abdominal Images of AIDS Patients. Happily, a few doctors or researchers have still asked me for the book until yesterday, indicating that it is still valuable to a certain extent though it needs further supplementing and perfecting.

I can't help feel his hardship when I have been pondering over the words by Prof. Yanhao Li in the preface of the third edition of his works: "Writing is hard, but writing with your heart is harder" since I submitted the first edition of manuscript in 2010. This empathy pushed me for my preliminary and major principles for my passion to compile this book: 1. Authenticity of the data for the atlas is predominant, with fewer textual descriptions as well as our own insights; 2. After it comes familiarity, e.g., We should compile in it what we have studied and mastered; 3. The book needs constant enrichments by accumulating latest scientific findings.

Nowadays, sources for solving problems are always available on line by 'surfing' in and "downloading" from the Internet. However, they are controversial when it comes to their authenticity. Only the authentic first-hand image data are of great value for the scientific research.

Currently, the cases of AIDS still remain relatively rare in most hospitals in China. More importantly, a lot of my peers just hold an incomplete picture of it from the prospective of its imaging manifestations. This status certainly arouses our interest in the compilation of the atlas. Therefore, we gathered the first-hand image data based on our long-term experience in 2010, in hopes that these collected data could facilitate the readers with a comprehensive understanding of AIDS-related opportunistic infections from the future perspective.

The second edition of the atlas come out with new cases by differential diagnosis and more importantly latest achievements we have harvested through these years, which hopefully could be referential and helpful for our peers.

Writing is always a matter of regret. Therefore, we are strongly hopeful that the peer experts would not bother to dedicate their critics on this book only because there may be some mistakes in it for the sake of our limited clinical knowledge.

LIU Jin-xin
May 1, 2014

Contents

1 Imaging findings of bacterial pneumonia in AIDS

1.1 Introduction

The incidence of AIDS patients with opportunistic infections is related with the virulence of pathogenic bacteria and the patient's immune level. The level of CD4+ cell in the peripheral blood (Table 1.1) is the best reflection of the immune status, many opportunistic infections will arise when CD4+ cell counts declines. The incidence of pulmonary infection is the highest in the opportunistic bacterial infections. AIDS with bacterial pneumonia accounted for more than 30% of HIV/AIDS with pulmonary infection. It can be occurred at each stage, especially in the early stage (i.e. the count of CD4+ is relatively high). The incidence of AIDS patients with pulmonary bacterial infections is five times that of HIV-negative people. The *Staphylococcus* is the main pathogens, followed by *Streptococcus pneumniae*, *Haemophilus influenzae*, *Pseudomonas aeruginosa* and so on.

The main clinical features are recurrent fever, cough, expectoration, fatigue and weight loss, and some patients with chest pain, diarrhea and superficial lymph nodes enlargement.

Table 1.1: HIV infection classification and AIDS diagnostic criteria revised by U.S. Centers for Disease Control in 1993

CD4+ T cell number	HIV infection Classification	Clinical classification		
		A asymptomatic and acute HIV infection or PGL	B people who have symptoms, but different from A or C	C disease which has AIDS features
≤500/μl		A1	B1	C1
200–499/μl		A2	B2	C2
<200/μl (T cell which has AIDS indications)		A3	B3	C3

PGL: persistent generalized lymphadenopathy.

1.2 Imaging findings

Case 1.1 (Fig. 1.1 a–g)

A 25-year-old male patient. Fever occurred two weeks ago before hospitalized, up to 40 °C no obvious chills, cough, expectoration or sore throat. Lumbago occurred one week ago and gradually get worse, accompanied by the generalized muscle aches. Admission body temperature was 38.8 °C. Pharynx mild congestive, bilateral tonsil no enlargement. Bilateral lung breath sounds coarse, no dry or moist rales. Left lower extremity showed multiple 0.5×0.5 cm pustules. Superficial lymph nodes no enlargement. CD4+ cell count was 28/µl. Bronchoalveolar lavage fluid (BALF), blood, marrow and pustular fluid culture: *Staphylococcus aureus* positive. The diagnosis was AIDS with *Staphylococcus aureus* pneumonia.

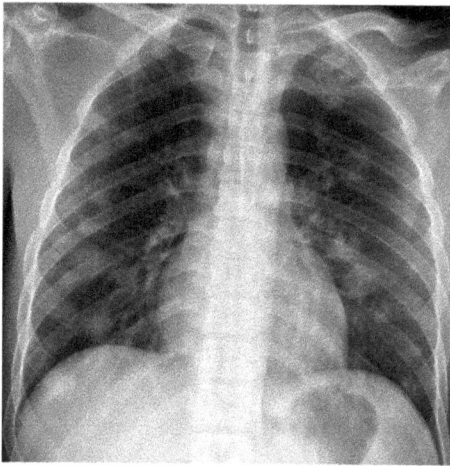
(a)

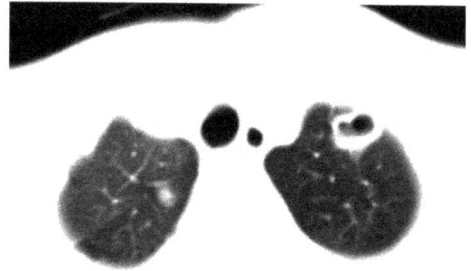
(b)

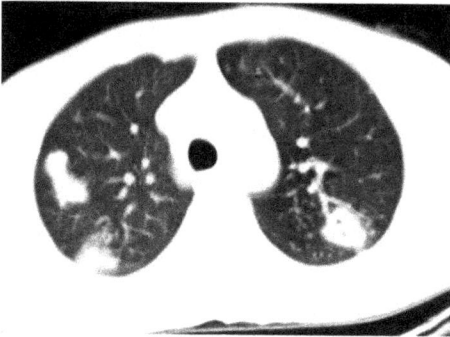
(c)

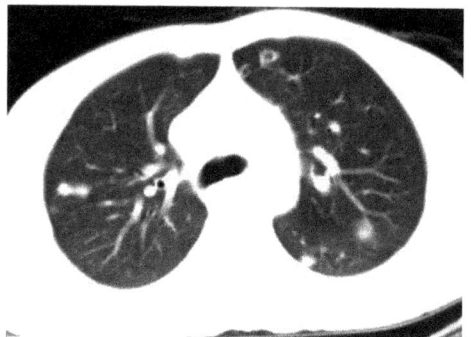
(d)

Fig. 1.1 a–g: *Staphylococcus aureus* pneumonia.

(e)

(f)

(g)

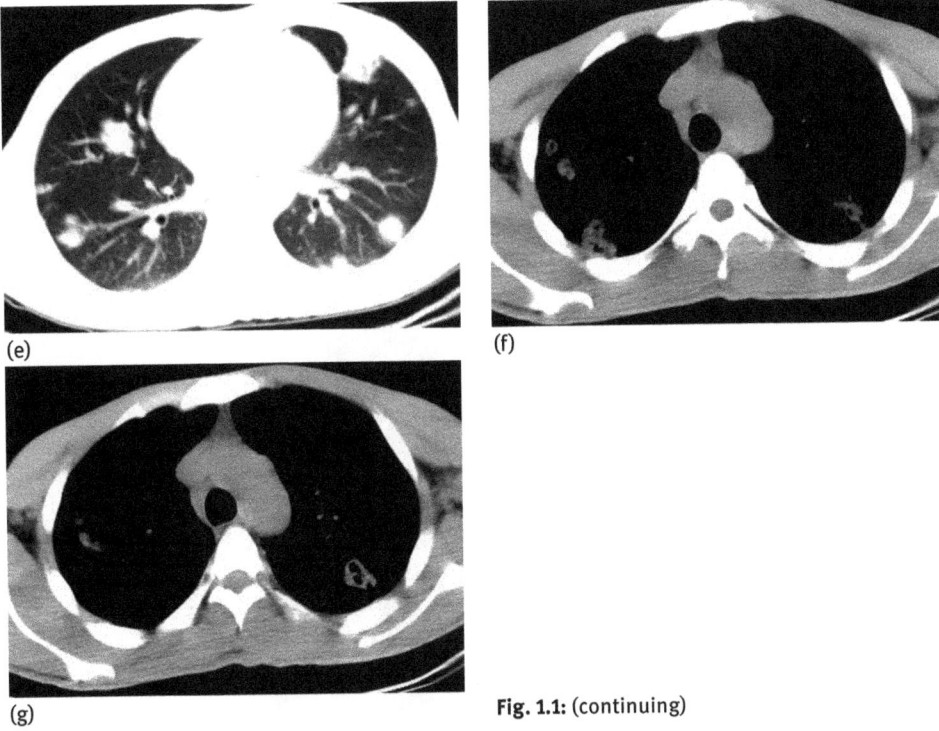

Fig. 1.1: (continuing)

Chest X-ray showed multiple and various size of nodules in bilateral lung, with blurring edge, and low-density area was seen in some lesions (a). CT showed multiple nodules in bilateral lung, mainly located in subpleural area, edge blur, cavity can be seen in most nodule lesions, with uneven thickness cavity wall, and air-fluid level was seen in some cavities (b–g).

Case 1.2 (Fig. 1.2 a–g)

A 25-year-old male patient. Fever and chill occurred two months ago, highest body temperature up to 40.0 °C, accompanied by cough and expectoration with some blood stained sputum, getting worse for a month. Admission body temperature was 37.2 °C. Physician examination: throat congestion, no tonsil enlargement. Dry rales were heard at expiratory in bilateral lung. The scattered rash was seen in the whole body, and with some ulcer and eschar. No superficial lymph nodes enlargement. CD4+ cell count was 4/μl. Bronchoalveolar lavage fluid (BALF), blood and marrow culture: *Staphylococcus aureus* positive. The diagnosis was AIDS (C3) accompanied by *Staphylococcus aureus* pneumonia and septicemia.

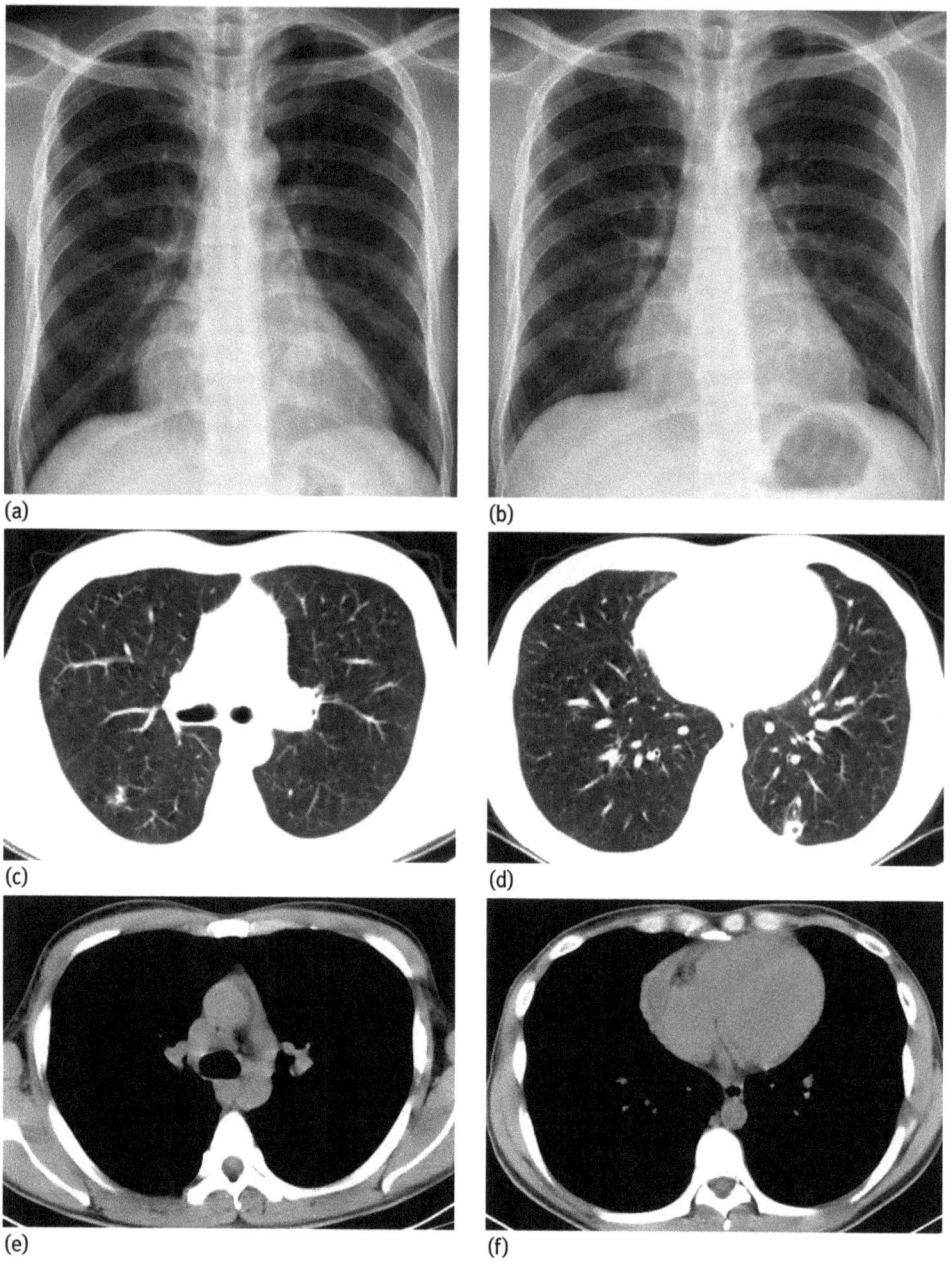

Fig. 1.2 a–g: *Staphylococcus aureus* pneumonia.

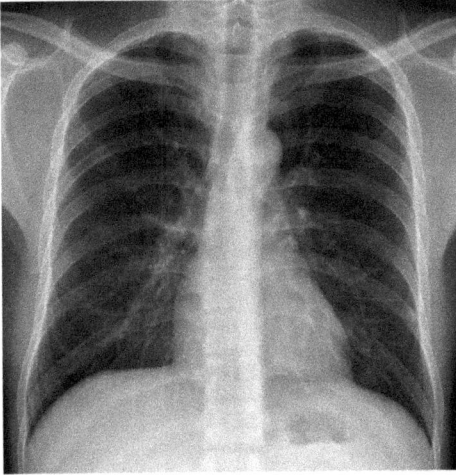

(g)

Fig. 1.2: (continuing)

The chest radiograph showed multiple small cystic lesions with thin walls in the right upper lung, the nodular opacity in the left lower lung and the heart shadow extending flask-shaped (a). After 15 days treatment, the lesions were absorbed in the right lung and the nodules shrank in the right lower lung and heart postzone as showed in the chest radiograph (b). Chest CT scans with lung window showed multiple nodules in bilateral lung and small cavity in the left lower lung lesions (c, d). The CT scans with mediastinal window showed mediastinal lymph node enlargement (e) and pericardial effusion (f). After 25 days treatment, lesions were absorbed in the bilateral lung, and normal heart shadow was showed in the chest radiograph (g).

Case 1.3 (Fig. 1.3 a–j)
A 42-year-old male patient. Persistent fever occurred one week ago, body temperature fluctuated at 38–39 °C, accompanied by cough with a little yellow white thick phlegm and slight chills. The symptoms got worse two day ago, with severe obvious cough. Admission body temperature was 37.8 °C. Respiratory smooth, bilateral lung breath sounds coarse, a little moist rale could be heard. The scattered rash was seen in the whole body skin, and with some ulcer and eschar. No superficial lymph nodes enlargement. CD4+ cell count was 388/μl. Bronchoalveolar lavage fluid (BALF), and blood culture: *Staphylococcus aureus* positive. The diagnosis was AIDS (B2) accompanied by *Staphylococcus aureus* pneumonia and septicemia.

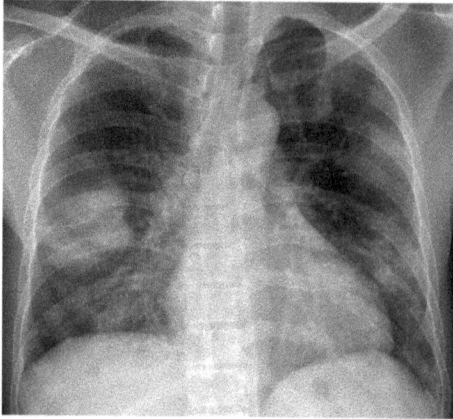
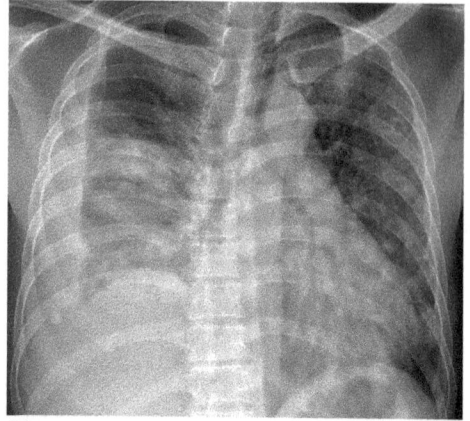

(a)
(b)

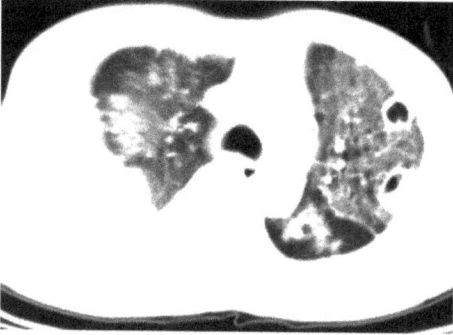
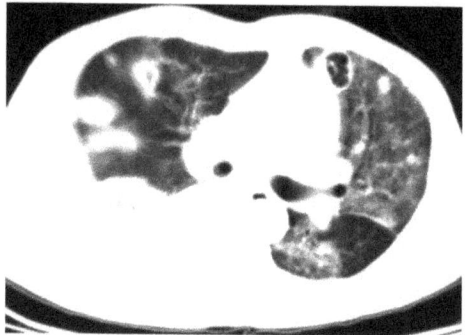

(c)
(d)

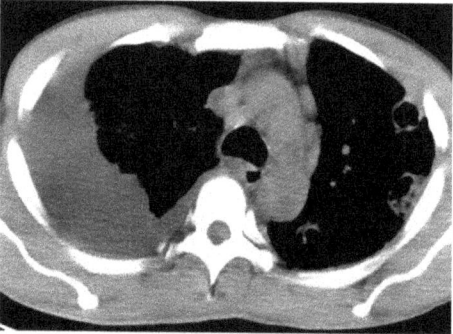
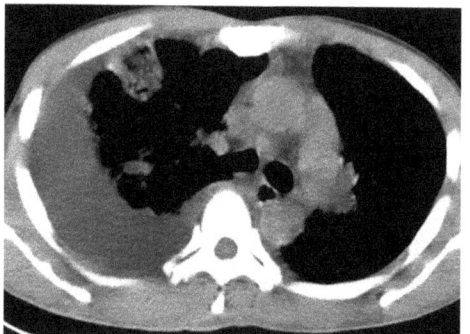

(e)
(f)

Fig. 1.3 a–j: *Staphylococcus aureus* pneumonia.

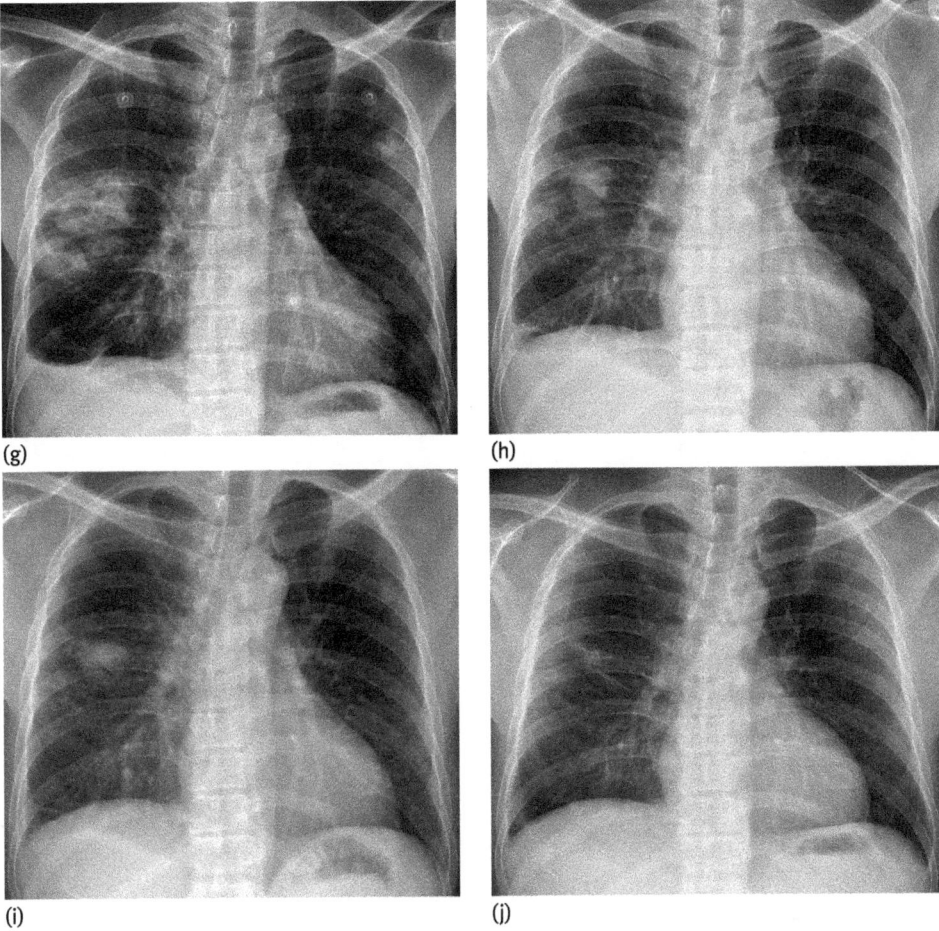

(g)

(h)

(i)

(j)

Fig. 1.3: (continuing)

The chest radiograph showed multiple lumpy and patchy high-density opacities of various sizes, blurring edges, and thickened fuzzy lung-markings in the bilateral lung (a). After 4 days treatment, the lesions were worsened with many small cavities in them and moderate pleural effusions in the right side as showed in the chest radiographs (b). The CT scans with lung window showed multiple nodules of various sizes in bilateral lung, with cavities in some nodules, and the ground-glass-like image in the bilateral upper lobes (c, d). The CT scans with mediastinal window showed multiple opacities in some nodules, pleural effusion in the right lung and mediastinal lymph nodes enlargement (e, f). After 17, 29, 38, 73 days treatment, lesions in the both lungs and pleural effusion in the right lung were gradually absorbed as showed in the chest radiographs (g–j).

Case 1.4 (Fig. 1.4 a–b)

A 59-year-old male patient. Fever occurred one week ago, body temperature fluctuated at 38–39 °C, persistent fever, accompanied by cough with a little yellow white thick phlegm and slight chills. The symptoms got worse two day ago, with obvious cough. Admission body temperature was 36.3 °C. Respiratory smooth, bilateral lung breath sounds clear, no dry or moist rales. Enlarged bilateral cervical and supraclavicular lymph nodes can be touched. CD4+ cell count was 39/μl. Bronchoalveolar lavage fluid (BALF) culture: *Staphylococcus epidermidis* positive. The diagnosis was AIDS (C3) accompanied by *Staphylococcus epidermidis* pneumonia.

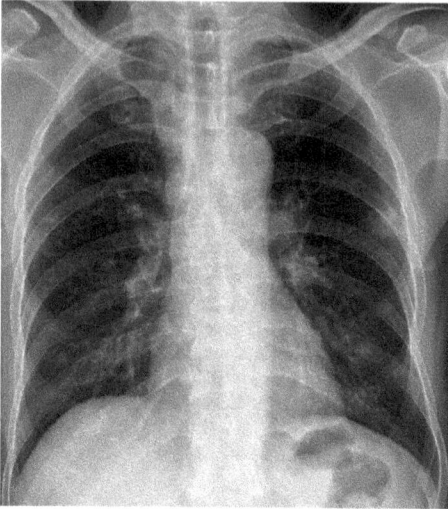 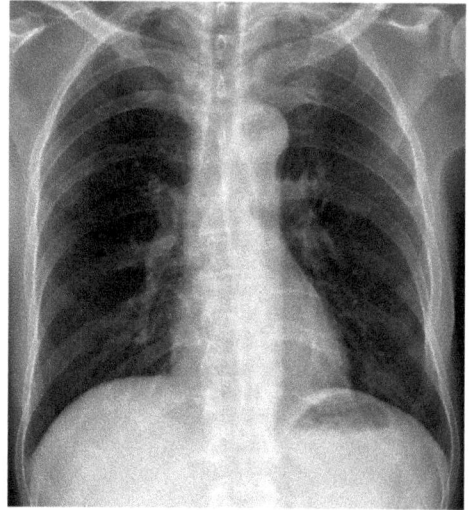

(a) (b)

Fig. 1.4 a–b: *Staphylococcus epidermidis* pneumonia.

The chest radiograph showed the scattered small patchy and blotchy high-density opacity in the bilateral lung, with blurring edge (a). After 58 days treatment, the chest radiograph showed the evidently absorbed lesions in the bilateral lung (b).

Case 1.5 (Fig. 1.5 a–b)

A 16-year-old male patient. Recurrent fever, cough and expectoration, accompanied by weight loss for 6 months. Admission body temperature was 36.5 °C. A little wheezing rales and moist rales were heard in left lower lung. The bilateral buccal visible red rash, which can fade after pressing. Soybeans size lymph nodes in submandibular and cervical can be touched. CD4+ cell count was 13/μl. Sputum culture: *Streptococcus pneumoniae* positive. The diagnosis was AIDS (C3) accompanied by *Streptococcus pneumoniae*.

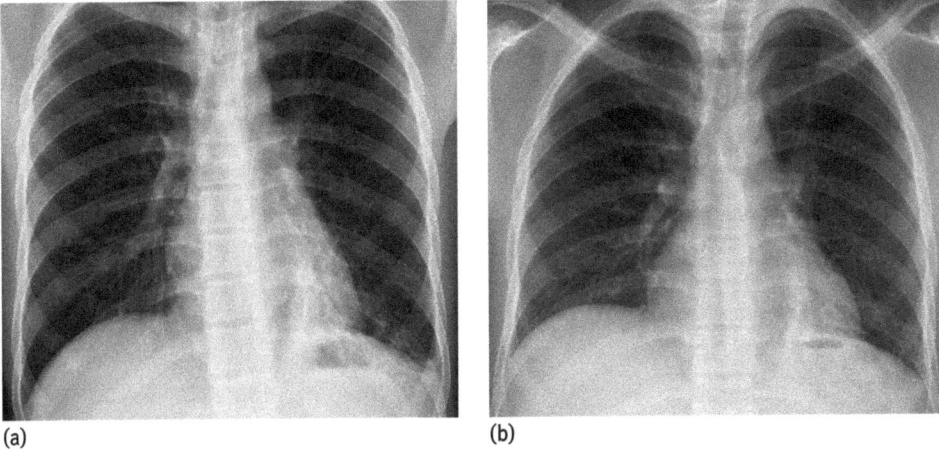

(a)

(b)

Fig. 1.5 a–b: Streptococcus pneumonia.

The chest radiograph showed the high-density inhomogeneous opacities and the blurring edge in the left lower lung (a). After 21 days treatment, the lesions were evidently absorbed in the left lower lung as showed in the chest radiograph (b).

Case 1.6 (Fig. 1.6 a–b)

A 29-year-old male patient. Cough without obvious incentive occurred two months ago before admission, with a little white thin sputum. Fever occurred six days ago, body temperature up to 39 °C, cough and expectoration got worse. Admission body temperature was 37.6 °C. Lung breath sounded weaken, no dry or moist rales. Enlarged lymph nodes in submandibular and bilateral axillary and inguinal can be touched. CD4+ cell count was 3/μl. Sputum culture: *Pseudomonas aeruginosa* positive. The diagnosis was AIDS (C3) accompanied by *Pseudomonas aeruginosa* pneumonia.

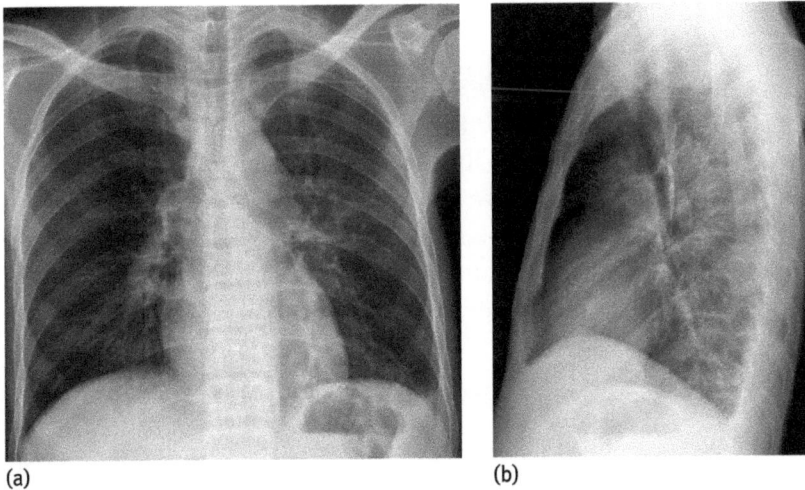

(a)

(b)

Fig. 1.6 a–b: *Pseudomonas aeruginosa* pneumonia.

The chest radiographs showed the patchy high-density opacity with the blurring edge in the heart postzone of the left lower lung and around the left porta pulmonis (a, b).

Case 1.7 (Fig. 1.7)
A 37-year-old male patient. Fever occurred one month ago before admission, body temperature fluctuated at 37–39 °C, accompanied by cough and a little yellow white thin sputum and slight chills. Admission body temperature was 37.5 °C. The bilateral lower lung percussion was dullness, bilateral lung breath sounds coarse, bilateral lower lung breath sounds weaken, no dry or moist rales. Superficial lymph nodes no enlargement. CD4+ cell count was 52/μl. Bronchoalveolar lavage fluid (BALF), blood and marrow culture: *Pseudomonas aeruginosa* positive. The diagnosis was AIDS (B3) accompanied by *Pseudomonas aeruginosa* pneumonia.

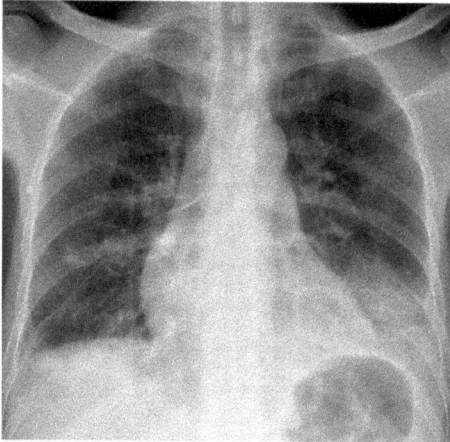

Fig. 1.7: *Pseudomonas aeruginosa* pneumonia.

The chest radiograph showed the multiple patchy opacities with blurring edge in the bilateral lower lung.

Case 1.8 (Fig. 1.8 a–d)
A 51-year-old male patient. Fever occurred five days ago, body temperature up to 42 °C, accompanied by chills, cough and a little yellow thick phlegm. Admission body temperature was 38 °C. Bilateral lung breath sounded weaken, the tiny moist rales can be heard in right lower lung. Superficial lymph nodes no enlargement. CD4+ cell count was 1/μl. Sputum culture: *Pseudomonas aeruginosa* positive. The diagnosis was AIDS (C3) accompanied by *Pseudomonas aeruginosa* pneumonia.

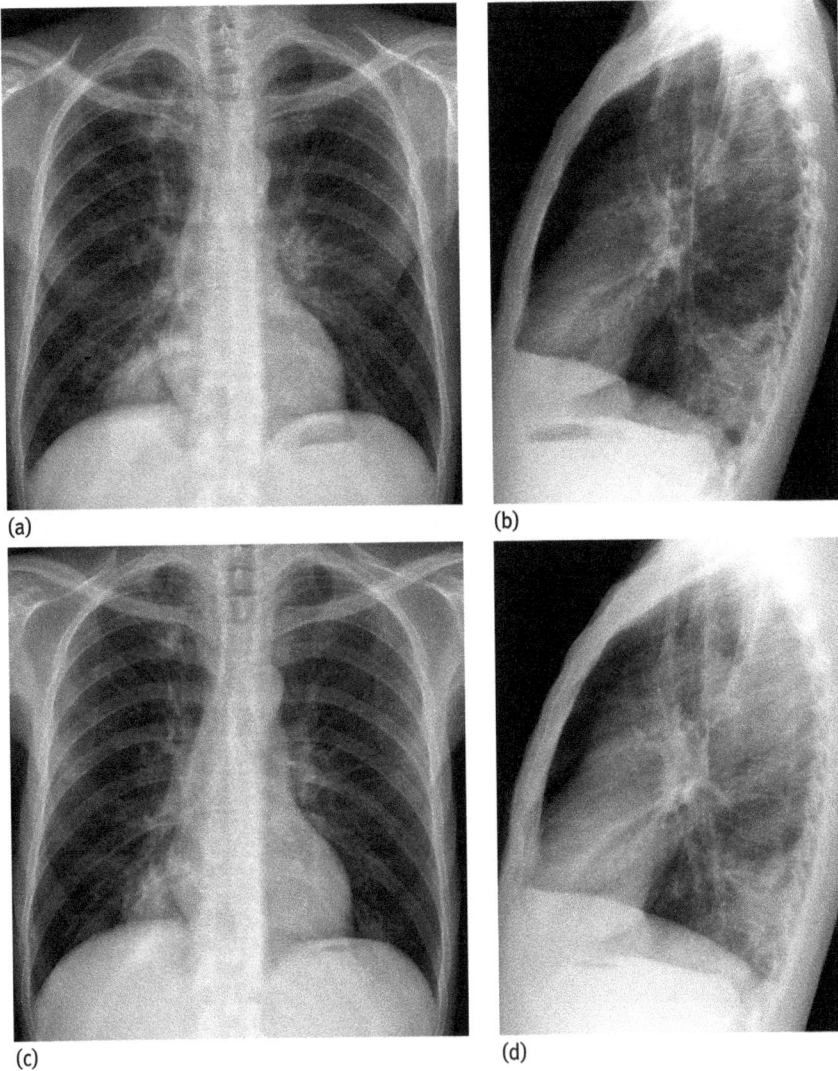

Fig. 1.8 a–d: *Pseudomonas aeruginosa* pneumonia.

The chest radiographs showed the multiple high-density patchy opacities of various size in the right lung and the blurring edge (a, b). After 8 days treatment, the lesions were partially absorbed in the right lung as showed in the chest radiographs (c, d).

Imaging features

Focal consolidation is the most common pulmonary manifestation of AIDS complicated by bacterial pneumonia, and typically it is distributed in the lobes or segments. Imageologically, it presents with high-density multiple patchy opacities. Notably, pulmonary cavitary lesions are another common manifestation of AIDS with bacterial pneumonia.

The characteristic imaging manifestations of *Staphylococcus aureus* pneumonia in AIDS patient include: the little patches grow fast into larger size of opacities and in the center are honeycomb opacities or emphysema, and pleural effusion or bullae. The primary *Staphylococcus aureus* pneumonia presents with its focal consolidations in the lobe or segment and by imaging study it manifests with patchy opacities with visible opacities in them. The hematogenous *Staphylococcus aureus* pneumonia present with pulmonary multiple nodules in the bilateral lung, mainly located in pulmonary peripheral or subpleural areas, with cavities of different sizes and even some air-liquid interfaces. The most common complication is empyema, pneumothorax secondly.

The typical features of AIDS with *Pseudomonas aeruginosa* pneumonia present with bilateral multiple scattered patchy opacities or nodules, which grow fast into larger patchy and fuzzy opacities.

AIDS complicated with bacterial infections may be at high risk of being concomitant with other pathogens. For the affirmative diagnosis, therefore, it is suggestive to take other etiological tests by way of cultures of blood, alveolar wash fluid and sputum and even fiberoptic bronchoscopy biopsy, if necessary.

Editors: Songfeng Jiang, Haolan He, Xiaoping Tang,Yi Liang

2 Imaging findings of AIDS with pulmonary *Rhodococcus equi* disease

2.1 Introduction

Rhodococcus equi (Color Figure 2.0), called *Corynebacterium equi,* is a Gram stain positive bacteria. The case of human with *Rhodococcus equi* infection was first reported in 1967. It mainly affects immunocompromised patients, especially the AIDS patients. The *Rhodococcus equi* secondary infection in AIDS patients is a severe complication. *Rhodococcus equi,* commonly considered as a pathogen only to horses, pigs and cattle, can often reside in nasal passages, throats, external auditory canals, eye conjunctiva, vulva and skin of humans and animals. *Rhodococcus equi* infection in human is rarely reported. In recent years, however, the cases of human respiratory diseases and septicemia caused by *Rhodococcus equi* grow in number due to the increase of AIDS patients. *Rhodococcus equi* infection, anyway, remains to be a rare opportunistic infection.

Rhodococcus equi grows slow, produces orange-red pigment and never breaks down any sugar or alcohol. In most cases, it is catalase positive, and oval and club-like in shape, but polymorphic sometimes. As an intracellular facultative parasite, the in vitro infectivity is restricted in the monocyte-macrophage lineage. It is pathogenic seemingly due to its sustained destroy to the alveolar macrophages by way of its fusing with lysosomes to result in the absence of pahgosome. Its pathogenic capacity may depend on the host and microbes. In addition, acid ester of sugar contained in the cell wall of is also associated with its virulence.

When AIDS complicated with pulmonary *Rhodococcus equi* infection always manifests with subacute pneumonia and bacteremia. It was reported that pathogen diffusion in the lung was slow in the early infection stage, and its infection presents with mild fever which may distract physician's attention, therefore, makes the early diagnosis very difficult. Early clinical symptoms usually present a low-grade fever which often does not attract attention. When it progresses to pneumonia, it presents with such obvious clinical symptoms as fever, cough, expectoration and chest pain. The CD4+ lymphocyte count of AIDS patients with pulmonary *Rhodococcus equi* infection is often less than 50/μl.

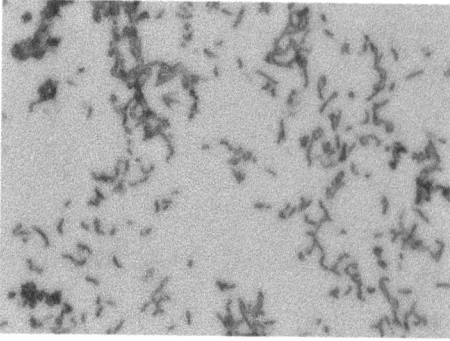

Fig. 2.0: *Rhodococcus equi* (pure culture), Gram stain,×400.

2.2 Imaging findings

Case 2.1 (Fig. 2.1 a–j)

A 41-year-old male patient. Cough and hemoptysis occurred three months ago, occasional fever. Admission body temperature was 38.3 °C. The dry and moist rales can be heard in right lung at the bottom. The superficial lymph nodes showed no enlargement. CD4+ cell count was 77/μl. BALF and blood culture: *Rhodococcus equi* positive. The diagnosis was AIDS (C3) accompanied by *Rhodococcus equi* pneumonia).

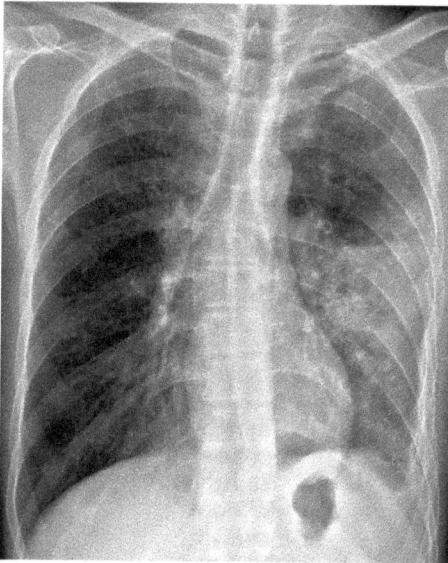

(a)

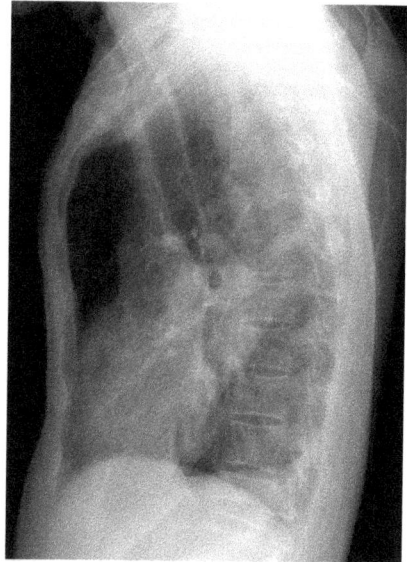

(b)

Fig. 2.1 a–j: *Rhodococcus equi* pneumonia in the lingular segment of left upper lobe.

(c)

(d)

(e)

(f)

(g)

(h)

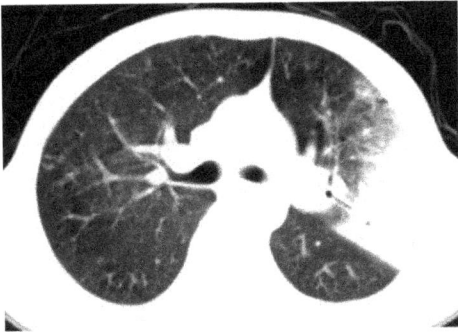

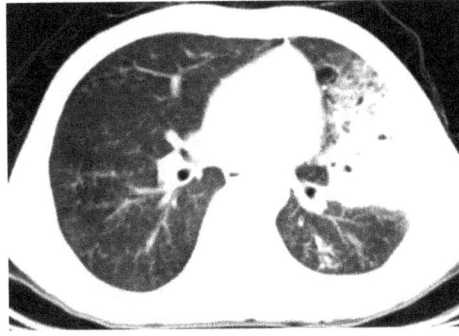

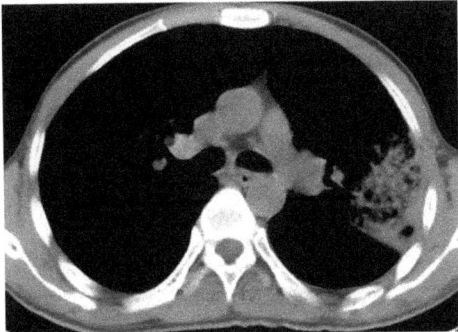

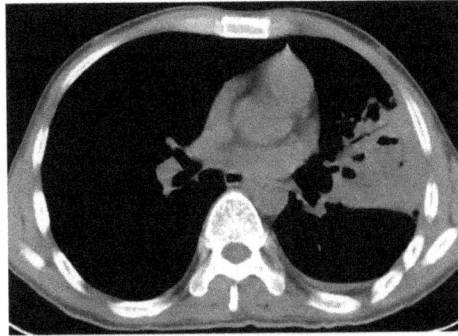

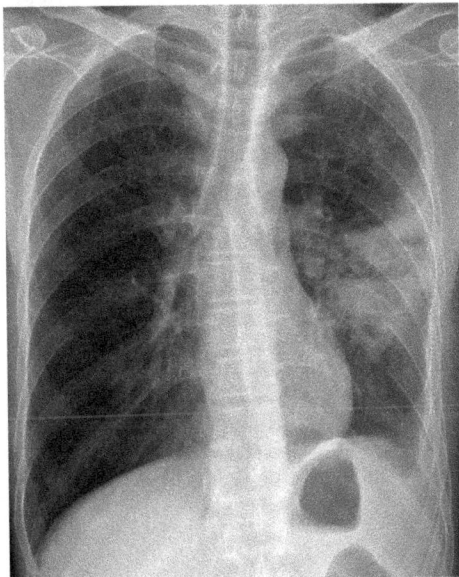

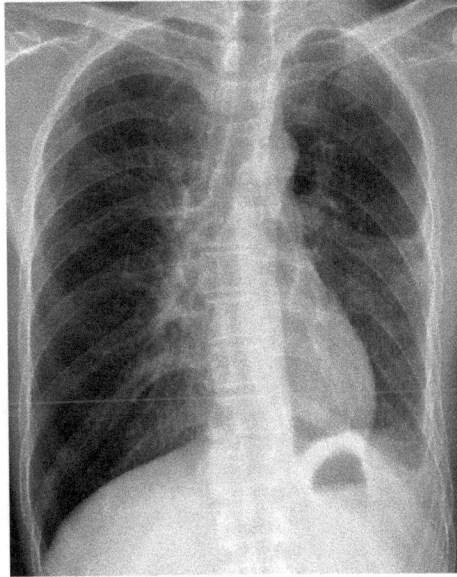

Fig. 2.1: (continuing)

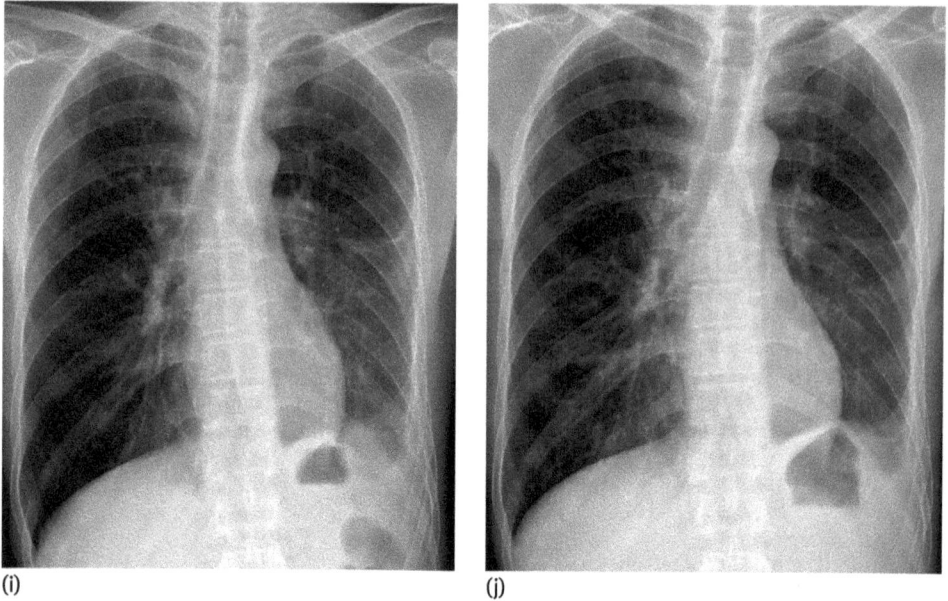

(i) (j)

Fig. 2.1: (continuing)

The chest radiographs showed the high-density patchy opacity in the lingular segment of left upper lobe the blurring edge, the small low-density uneven-distributed patchy areas in the lesions, and the thickened left pleura (a, b). The CT scans confirm consolidated opacities in the lingular segment of left upper lobe along the lung segment, the low-densitypatchy opacities and the small cavities in the lesions, and the high-density spotty opacities in the left lower lobe (c–f). After 13 days treatment, the left lung lesions was significantly reduced, with sharp edge and the spread low-density areas in the lesions as showed in the chest radiograph (g). After 5.6 months, the lesions in left lung were further absorbed and the funicular high-density opacity was seen in the localities as showed in the chest radiographs (h, i). After 10 months, the lesions in the left lung were radically absorbed and a little funicular high-density opacity with sharp edge was still seen in the localities, as showed in the radiographs (j).

Case 2.2 (Fig. 2.2 a–r)

A 28-year-old male patient. Fever with no obvious incentive occurred four months ago. Cough occurred one month ago, and a white thick phlegm with blood streak. Accompanied by back pain. Diarrhea occurred seven days ago, with nausea and vomit. Admission body temperature was 36.9 °C. Bilateral lung breath sounded coarse, no dry or moist rales. The superficial lymph nodes showed no enlargement. CD4+ cell count was 6/μl. Bone marrow culture: *Rhodococcus equi* positive. BALF culture: *Rhodococcus equi* and non-tuberculous mycobacteria positive. The diagnosis was AIDS (C3) accompanied by *Rhodococcus equi* pneumonia and non-tuberculous mycobacteria lung disease.

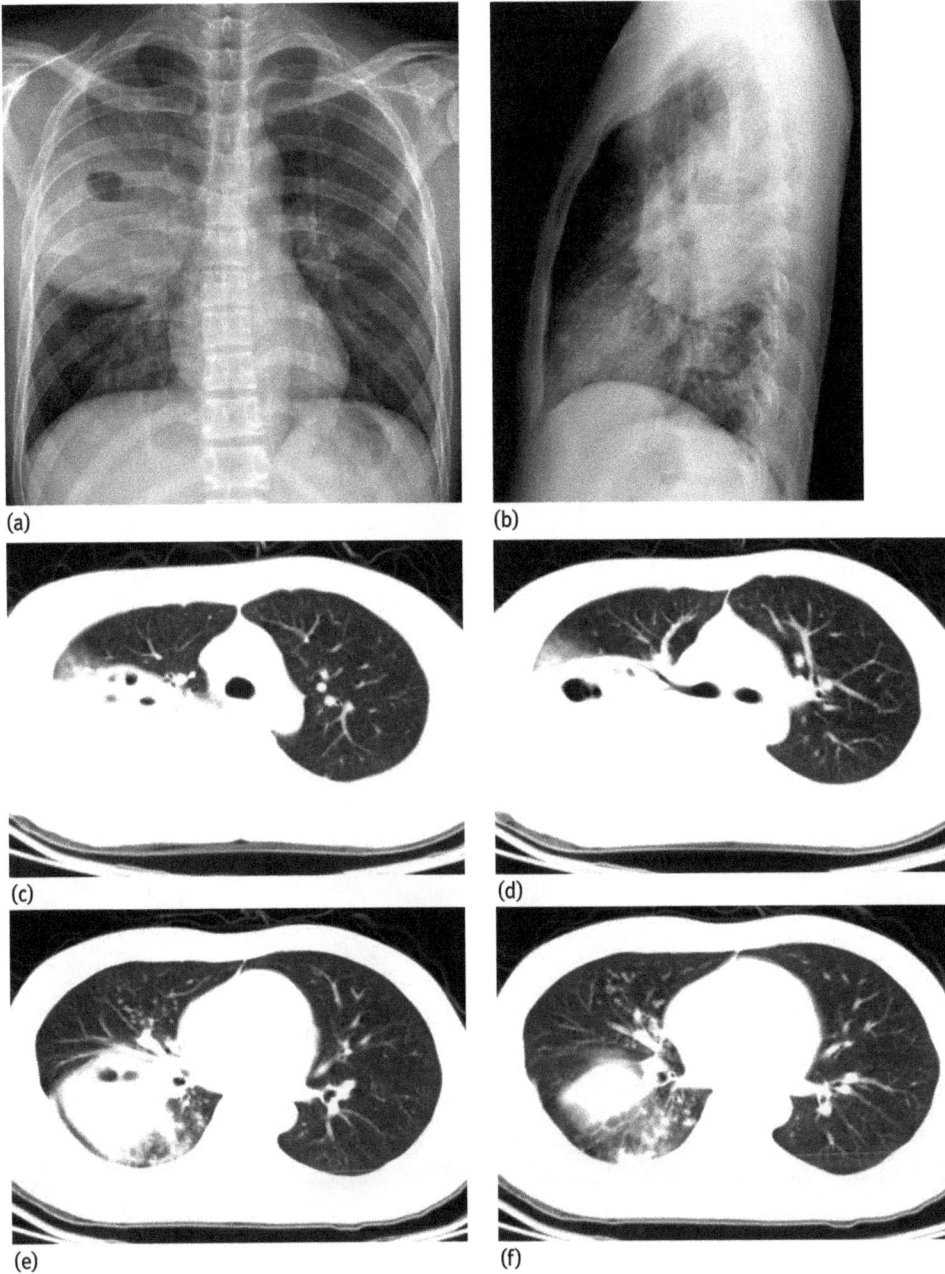

Fig. 2.2 a–r: *Rhodococcus equi* pneumonia and non-tuberculous mycobacteria pulmonary disease in the right lung.

The chest radiographs showed a huge rounded opacity in the right lung, with sharp edge and cavity with liquid-air interface in the lesion, the high-density patchy opacity with blurring edges around the lesion and thickened markings of the bilateral lung

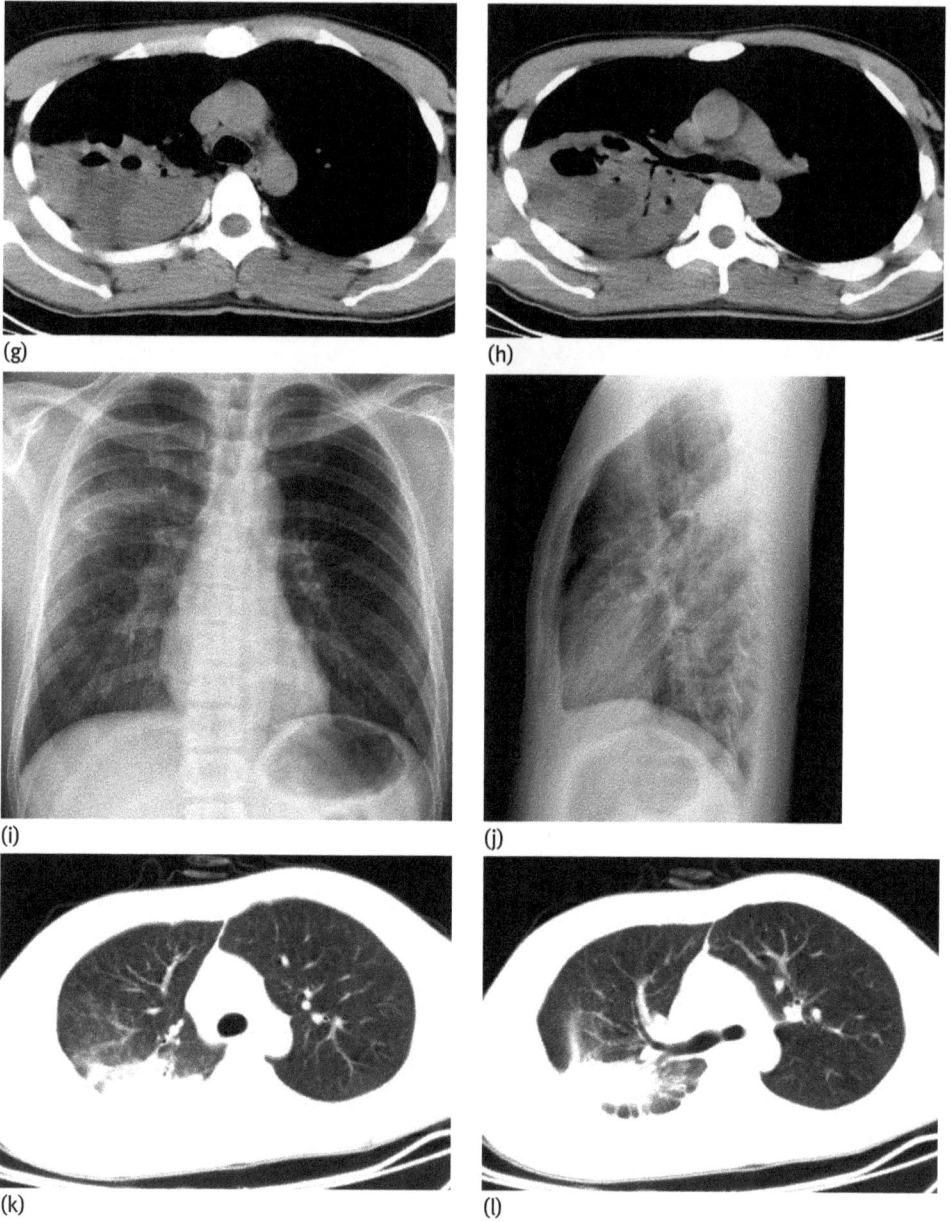

Fig. 2.2: (continuing)

(a, b). The CT scans with the lung window showed a huge high-density opacity in the posterior segment of upper lobe and the dorsal segment of lower lobe in the right lung with many cavities inside the lesion, and the small high-density spotty or patchy opacities with blurring edge around the lesion (c–f). The CT scans with mediastinal window showed a huge opacity in the right lung with low-density patchy lesions and cavities with liquid-air interfaces and bronchial air sign inside the lesion (g, h).

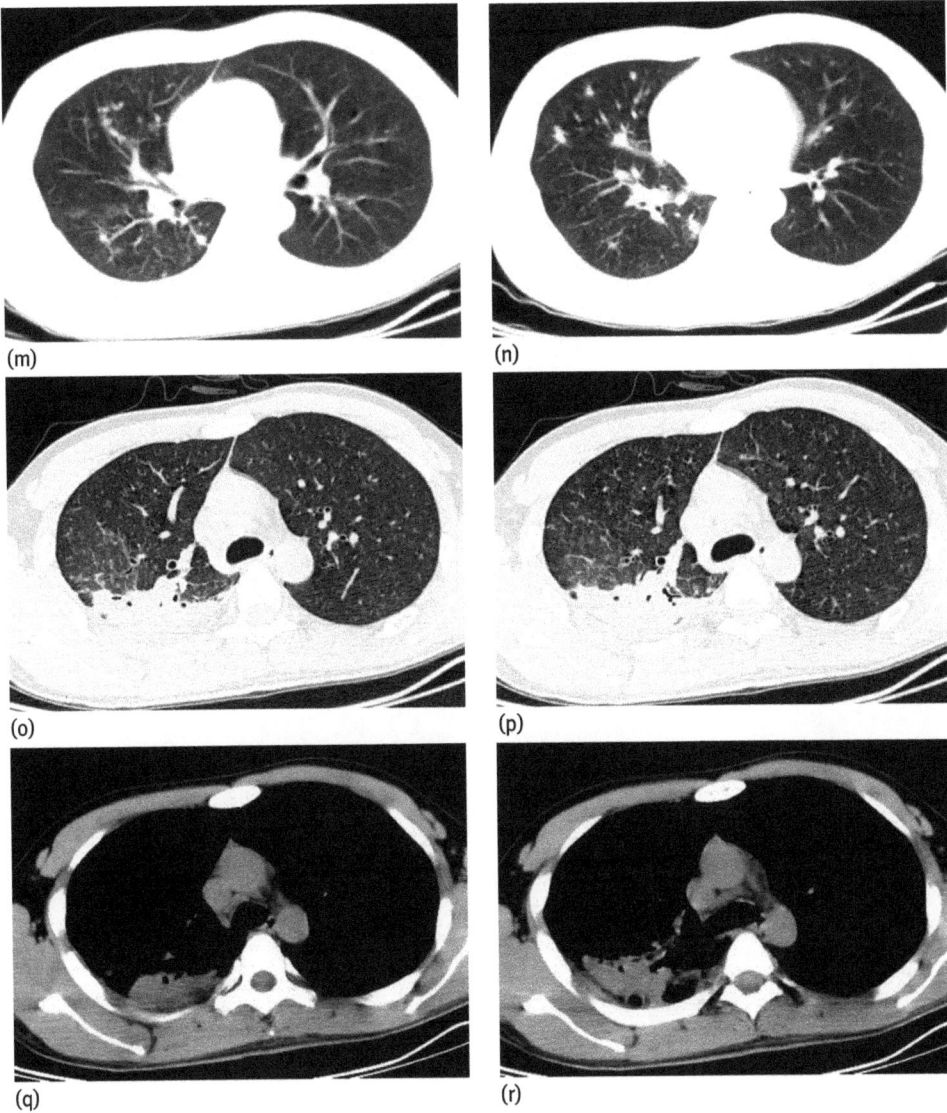

(m)

(n)

(o)

(p)

(q)

(r)

Fig. 2.2: (continuing)

After 6 months treatment, the lesions were mostly absorbed in the right lung and the high-density patchy opacities in the posterior segment posterior segment of right lobe with blurring edge, and high-density spotty opacities around the lesion were seen as showed in the chest radiographs (i, j). The CT scans of the chest with lung window show the high-density patchy opacity in the posterior segment of right lobe with glitches around it, and scattered small nodules in the middle and upper lobe (k–n). HRCT scans showed the small bronchiectasis in the posterior segment of right upper lobe (o, p). The CT scans with mediastinal window showed thickened pleurae with adhesion, but no enlargement in the mediastinal lymph nodes (q, r).

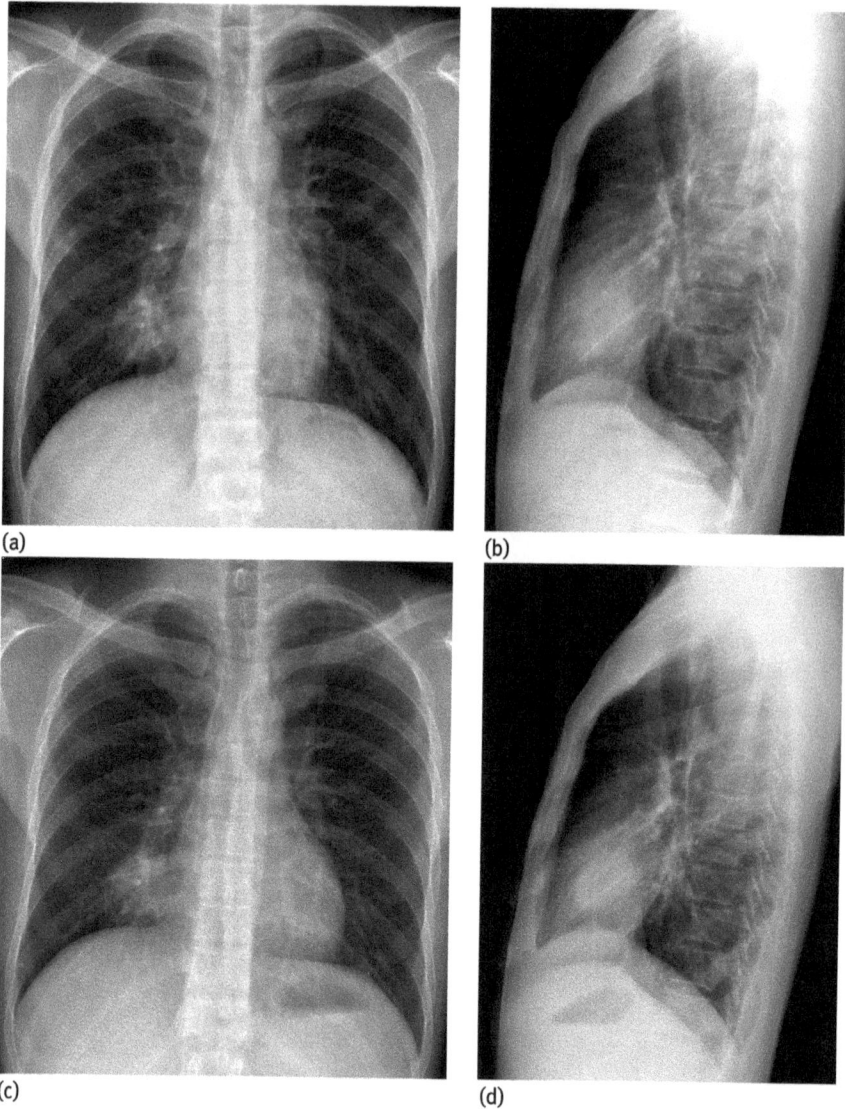

Fig. 2.3 a–d: *Rhodococcus equi* pneumonia

Case 2.3 (Fig. 2.3 a–d)

A 31-year-old male patient. Cough with no obvious incentive occurred three months ago, with a white thin phlegm. Fever occurred one month ago, body temperature at 38.39 °C, and become obvious afternoon, accompanied by sweating and blood streak phlegm. Gasp occurred two weeks ago. Admission body temperature was 37 °C. The tofu-like objects was seen on the surface of tongue. The hairy leukoplakia was seen in the side of tongue. The right lower lung breath sounded slightly weaken. No dry or moist rales. The superficial lymph nodes showed no enlargement. CD4+ cell count was 27/μl. BALF culture: *Rhodococcus equi* positive. The diagnosis was AIDS (B3) accompanied by *Rhodococcus equi* pneumonia.

The chest radiographs showed the high-density nodular opacity with uneven density and blurring edge on the right middle lobe and the scattered high-density patchy opacity on bilateral middle-upper lung, with blurring edges and multiple lesions in the right lung (a, b). After 28 days treatment, the lesions shrank in the right upper lobe, with sharper edge and the lesions in the bilateral middle-upper lung were completely absorbed (c, d).

2.3 Imaging features

Pulmonary infiltrative consolidation and cavity (single or multiple) are the main imaging features, and some cases are multi-lobe involvement, and a few cases may present pleural effusion and mediastinal lymph nodes enlargement.

Based on the dynamic imaging observations AIDS patients with *Rhodococcus equi* pneumonia in our hospital, the pulmonary infiltrative consolidations and cavities were evidently absorbed or dissipated by way of definite etiological diagnosis and effective treatment.

It is difficult to identify the imaging manifestation between AIDS with *Rhodococcus equi* pneumonia and AIDS with non-tuberculous mycobacteria lung disease at the early infection stage, for mixed infections may present in some cases, such as patient of figure 2.2, showed the right pulmonary infiltrative consolidation, accompanied by the cavity and the scattered nodules before treatment and the comparatively-reduced bronchiectasis inside the small patchy consolidated opacity in the patient after six months treatment. The radiologic findings of AIDS with non-tuberculous mycobacteria pulmonary disease together with literature review are evident that there is a higher chance that small bronchiectasis may present in AIDS patients with non-tuberculous mycobacteria lung disease, which is helpful for the differential diagnosis of the AIDS patients with *Rhodococcus equi* pneumonia from those with non-tuberculous mycobacteria pulmonary disease.

Editors: Haolan He, Songfeng Jiang, Fuchun Zhang, Yi Liang

3 Imaging manifestation of pulmonary candidiasis in AIDS

3.1 Introduction

Pulmonary candidiasis is one kind of common lung fungal infection, caused by endogenic infection, rarely from environment, which is different from other fungus. Common infection routes include inhalation and hematogenous infection.

Candida belongs to fungi blastomyces steel ball candida yeast division, cain for yeast fungus, has more than 300 species totally as a whole, but only a few are pathogenic to human, such as candida albicans and Candida tropicalis. Generally, candida is a kind of opportunistic pathogen and it widely resides in the nature environment and human oral cavity, nasopharynx tract, upper respiratory tract, gastrointestinal tract, vagina and skin. But when human immunity is weakened candidiasis may present.

Anatomically, candidiasis can be classified as superficical infection and deep-organ infection. The superficical infection of candidiasis can be subdivided into cutaneous and subcutaneous infections; and the deep-organ infection of candidiasis include pulmonary candidiasis, gastroenteritis, endocarditis, meningitis, mediastinitis and candidal septicaemia. Lung is most susceptible to it. Based on different involved organs and developing stages of disease, the histopathology of candidiasis shows pattern of inflammatory infiltration (such as skin lung), purulent infiltration (like kidney, lung and brain and granulomatous infiltration (like skin).

There are risk factors that may predispose candida infections: 1. AIDS; 2. preterm babies, newborns, malnutrition children and sick children; 3. chronicwastingdisease; 4. malignant haematological disease; 5. metabolism disorder disease; 6. long-term Immunosuppressive therapy (corticosteroids); 7. congenital immunodeficiency; 8. long-term broad-spectrum antibiotic therapy; 9. iatrogenicinfections as a result of long-term use of various catheters.

According to literature, invasive candidiasis caused by AIDS accounts for 47.4 % of the entire deep-organ fungal infections, which are caused mainly by candida, aspergillus, cryptococcus, mucor and penicillium. Currently, approximately 42 % of the fungal pneumonias in immunocompromised patients are caused by *Candida albicans* species.

The symptoms, signs and radiographic imaging manifestations of the pulmonary candidasis are nonspecific. Based on the clinical features, there are three types:
1. bronchitis: the lesion located in the bronchus, presenting slight symptoms such as cough (non-productive sputum);
2. hypersensitivity pneumonitis: dyspnea, rhinocnesmus, sneezing and nasal discharge, andwheezing in bilateral lung;

3. pneumonia: most common in AIDS and extremely-sick patients presenting with acute pulmonitis or sepsis, with chill, fever, cough, white thick phlegm mucus or purulent sputum frequentlywith blood streak and necrotic tissue,hemoptysis and even dyspnea, audible dry wet lung sounds.

The diagnosis of pulmonary candidiasis can be confirmed if candida spores and hyphae from specimens and lung tissues collected by pollution prevention bush and bronchscopy from lower respiratory tract are detected (Color Figure 3.1) or if the lung specimens, pleural fluid culture, or blood culture is positive.

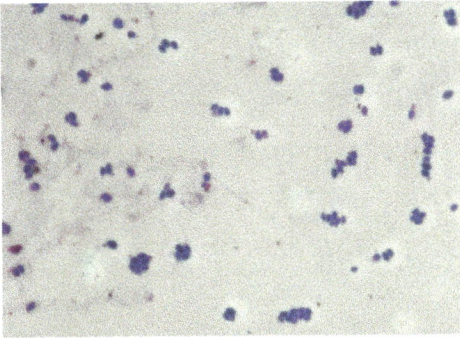

Fig. 3.0: Candida (pure culture), gram stain, original magnification ×400.

3.2 Imaging findings

Case 3.1 (Figure3.1 a–i)

Pulmonary candidiasis in a 41-year-old man of AIDS (C3) Complained of prolonged fever without any incentive for five months, the highest temperature up to 39 °C, accompanied with chilly and fatigue, without shivering or cough/sputum, body check found several small lymph nodes which have soft touching and smooth edge, can be moved without pain (haphagesia), located in retroauricular, neck, armpit, bilateral groins and infraclavicula. The right lung breath sound enhanced while the left lung breath sound diminished, especially the lower segment, the CD4+ cell count was 44/ul, CD4+/CD8: 0.01, BALF culture: *Candida albicans* positive.

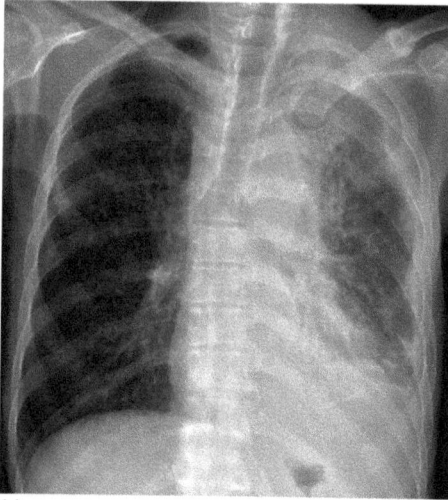

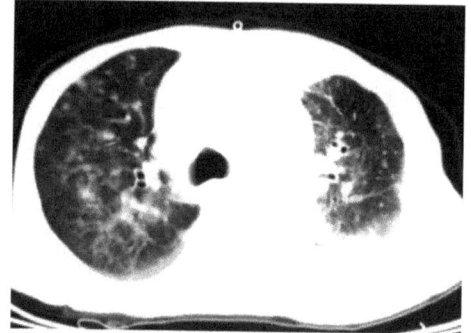

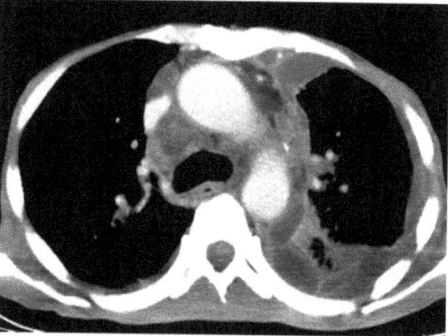

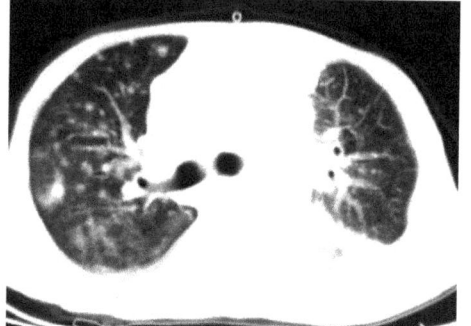

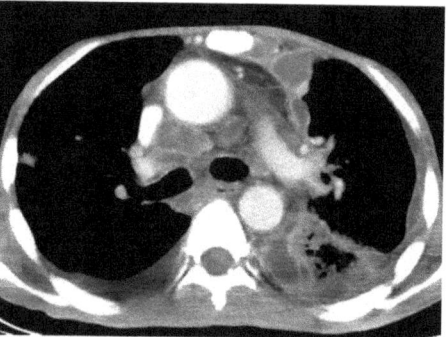

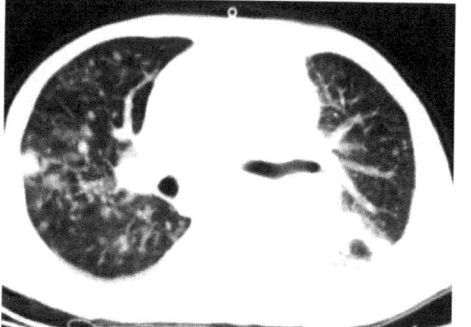

Fig. 3.1 a–i: Pulmonary candidiasis.

(g)

(h)

(i)

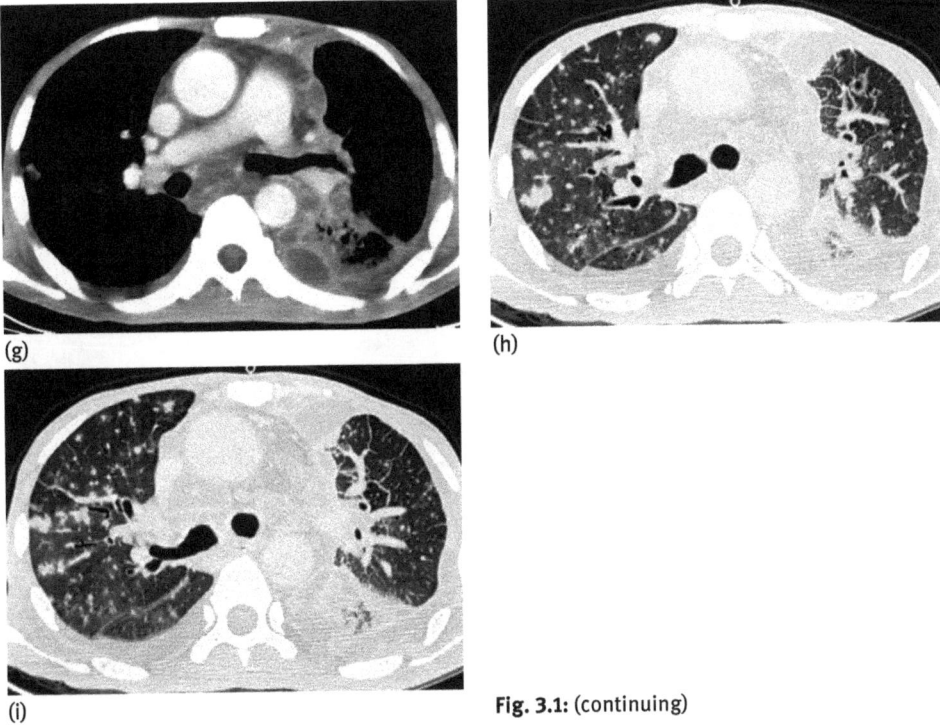

Fig. 3.1: (continuing)

The chest radiograph showed multiple small nodules and patchy opacities with blurring edges on the bilateral lung, pleural thickening in the left lower lung and mediastinal widening and shifting to the left side (a). The enhanced CT scans with lung window showed small diffusive nodules with blurring edges in the bilateral lung some fusing into patches (b, c). The CT scans with mediastinal window showed enlarged lymph nodes with ring-enhancement in the mediastinum and bilateral hilum, multiple encapsulated pleural effusions in the left thoracic cavity, a little pleural effusion in the right and atelectasis in the left lower lobe (d–g). HRCT demonstrated diffusive small nodules of both lungs clearly (h, i).

Case 3.2 (Figure3.2 a–l):
Medical History: Pulmonary candidiasis in a 41-year-old man of AIDS (C2) presented with fever, chilly and shivering five day ago before hospitalized, the fever pattern involved especially high fever in night and recovered to normal body temperature in daytime, the highest temperature was up to 40.0 °C, accompanied with cough and white mucus. A small mung bean-sized lymph node can be touched in the left neck, which had smooth edge and can be moved easily without haphalgesia. Body check: bilateral breath sound were rough , moist rale can be heard in the right lung, the CD4+ cell count was 479/ul, CD4+/CD8: 0.45, BALF culture: *Candida albicans* positive.

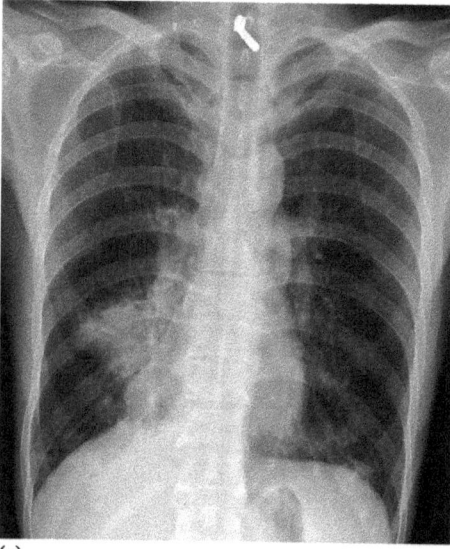

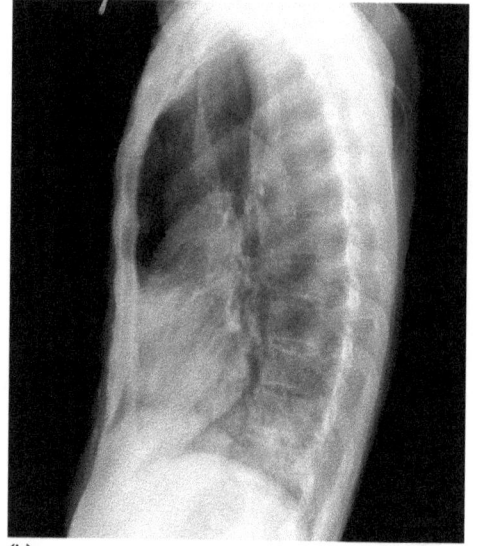

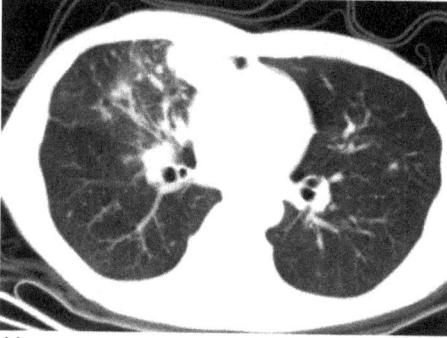

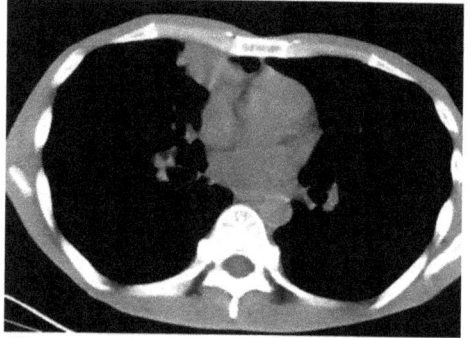

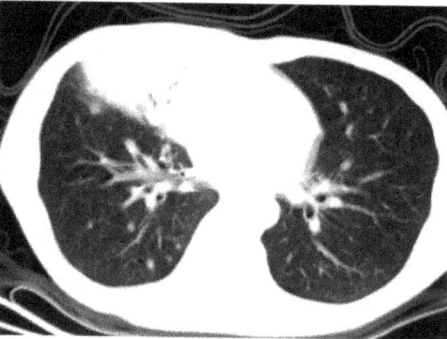

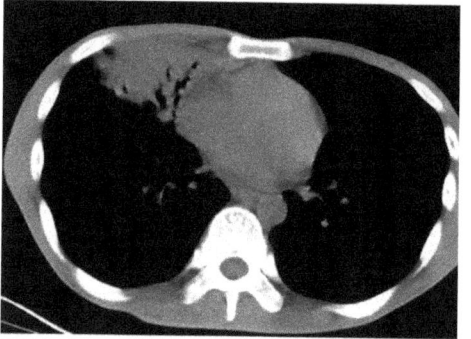

Fig. 3.2 a–l: Pulmonary candidiasis.

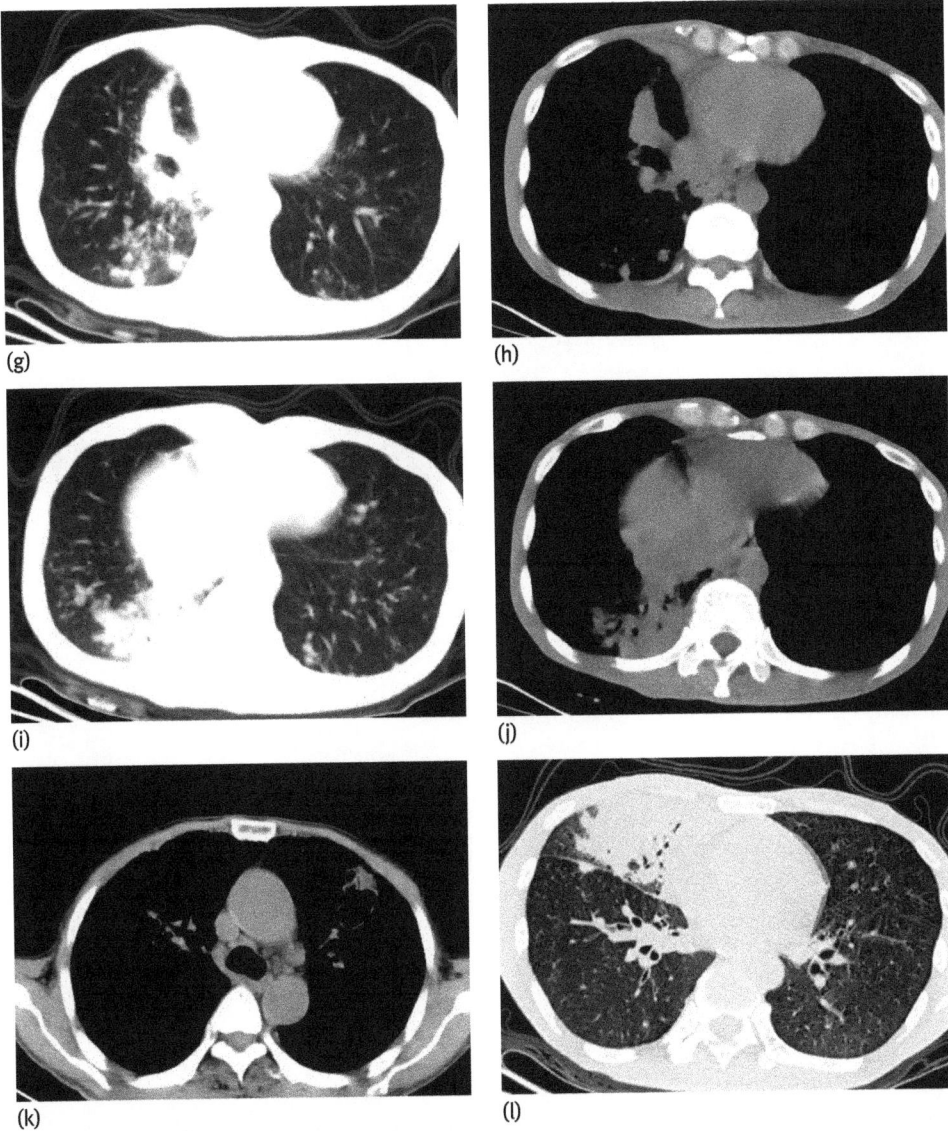

(g)

(h)

(i)

(j)

(k)

(l)

Fig. 3.2: (continuing)

The chest radiograph showed ill-edged clouding opacities located in middle lobe and posterior basal segment in the right lung (a, b). The CT scan with lung window showed multiple small nodules and patchy consolidation which has the trends of fusing, air bronchogram sign in the middle lobe and posterior basal segment in the right lung, but no obviously enlarged lymph nodes in mediastinum and bilateral hilar (c–j). HRCT scans show more evident bronchiectasis in right middle lobe (k–l).

Case 3.3 (Figure 3.3 a–k)

A 56-year-old man presented with fever productive white phlegm cough and short of breath a month ago before hospitalized. The body temperature fluctuated between 38.40 °C, without any features. Physician examination found coarse and rough breath sound in both lungs wet rales can be heard in left lower lung. CD4+ cell count was

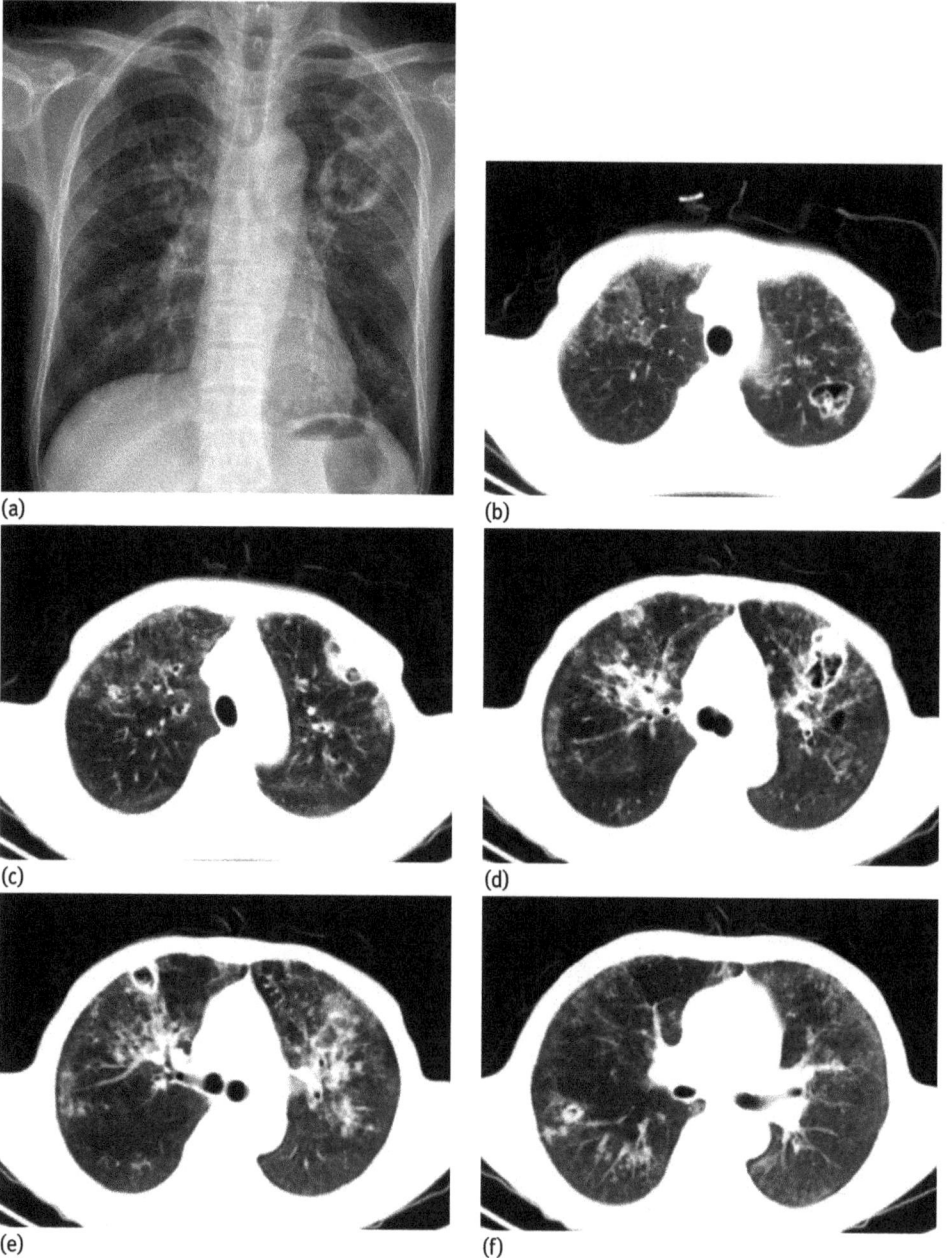

Fig. 3.3 a–k: Pulmonary candidiasis.

2/µl CD4+/CD8: 0.45. Bronchoalveolar lavage fluid (BALF) grew *Candida albicans*. The diagnosis was AIDS (C3) with pulmonary candidiasis.

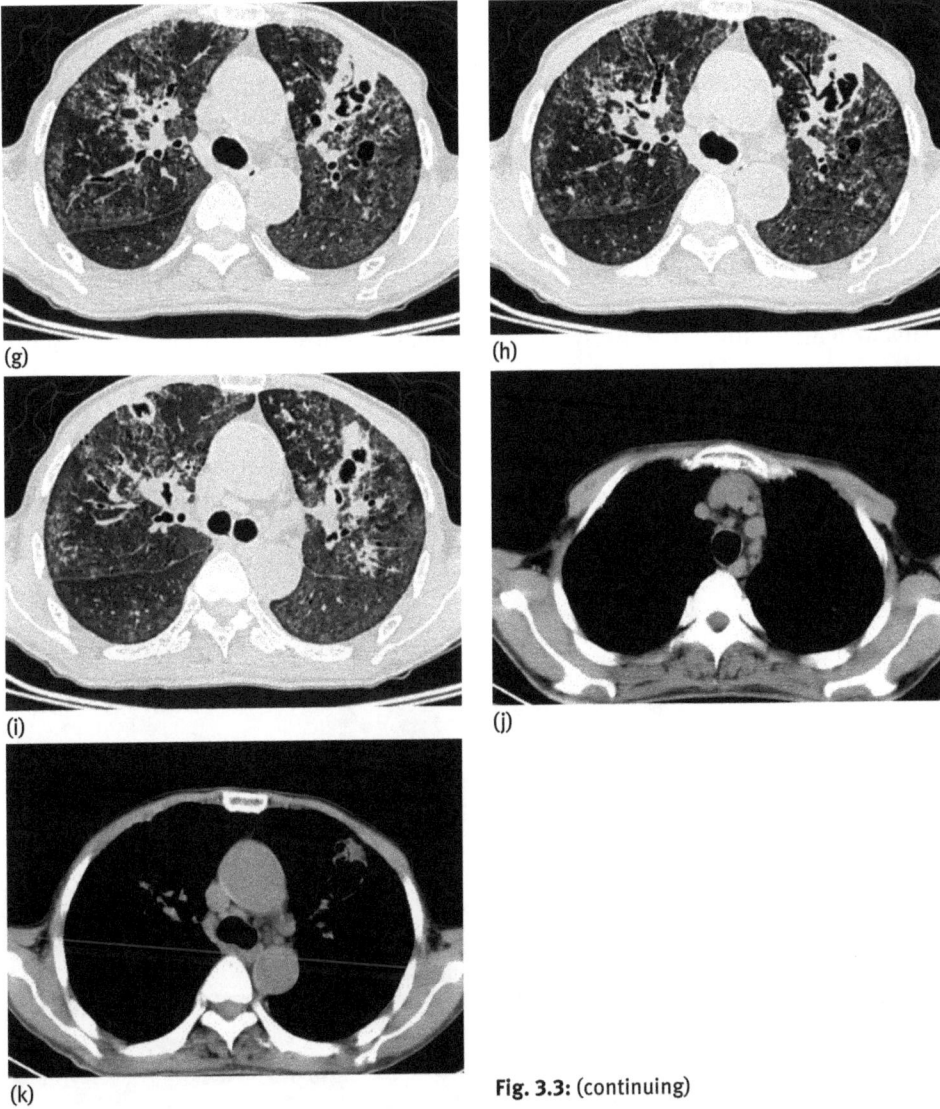

(g)

(h)

(i)

(j)

(k)

Fig. 3.3: (continuing)

The chest radiograph shows multiple high-density patchy opacities with blurring edge and ground-glass appearance in the bilateral lung, and cavitary opacities of different sizes on the upper lungs (a). The CT scans with lung window show high-density diffusethin patchy opacity with blurring edge in the bilateral lungs as well as multiple cavitary opacities of various sizes in it (b–f). HRCT scans show multiple gravel road sign, hollow cavities, funicularshadows and brochiectasis (g–i). CT scans with mediastinal window showed several small lymph nodes in the mediastinum (j, k).

Case 3.4 (Figure 3.4 a–j)

A 51-year-old man presented with fever, up to39 °C before hospitalized 20 days ago, accompanied with chilly, no shivering, short of breath while activities, occasional cough with little white phlegm. Physician examination found scattered old-performed maculopapule and pigmentation spots on extremity skin. No enlarged superficial lymph node can be palpated. Both breath sound weaken, no dry or wet rales. CD4+ cell count was 6/μl, CD4+/CD8: 0.01. Bronchoalveolar lavage fluid (BALF) grew *Candida albicans*. The diagnosis was AIDS (C3) with pulmonary candidiasis.

The chest radiograph showed multiple high-density patchy opacities with blurring edge and ground-glass appearance in the bilateral lung as well as more coarsened and messymarkings (a). After one month treatment, the lesions were significantly absorbed in the bilateral lung as showed in the chest radiograph (b). The CT scans with lung windows show lightly-ground-glass diffuse change and centrilobular emphysema in the bilateral lung, more coarsened lung-markings and interlobular

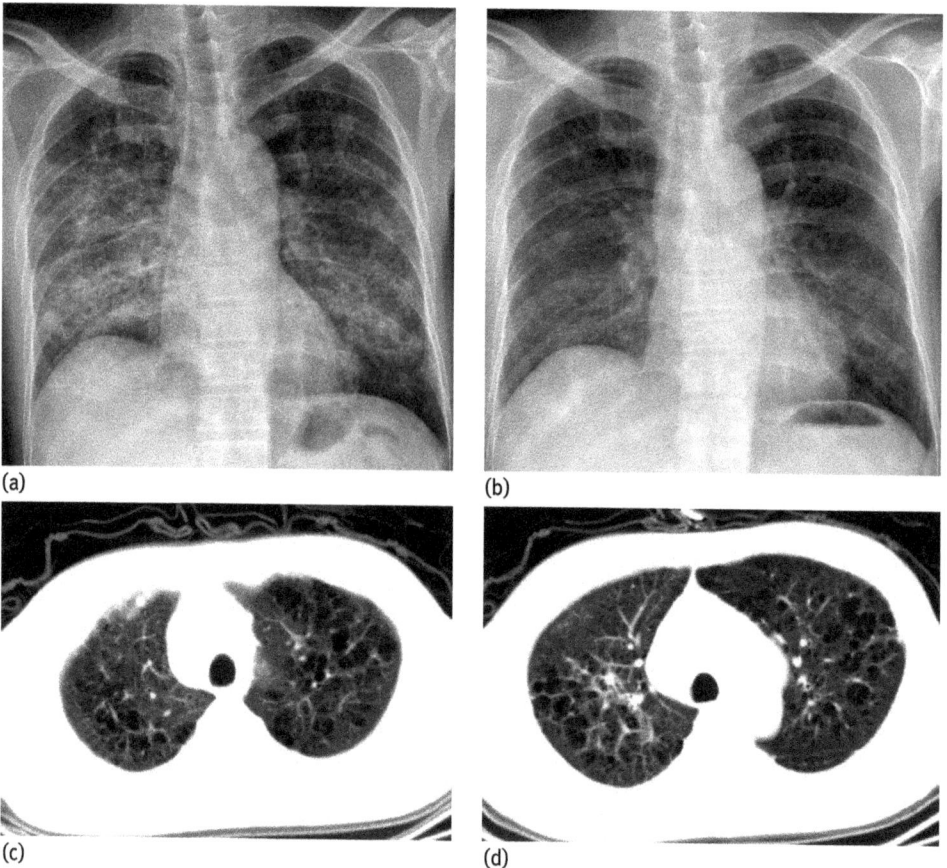

(a)

(b)

(c)

(d)

Fig. 3.4 a–j: Pulmonary candidiasis.

septal thickening (c–f). HRCT scans showed multiple coarsened lung-markings and centrilobular emphysema (g, h). The CT scans with mediastinal window show multiple enlarged mediastinal lymph nodes (i, j).

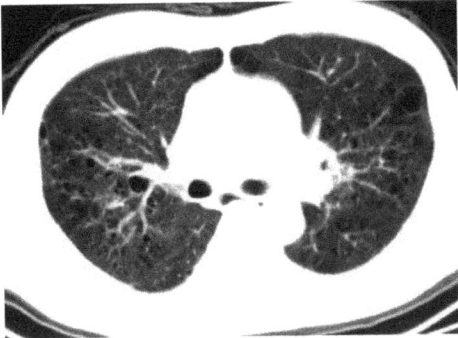
(e)

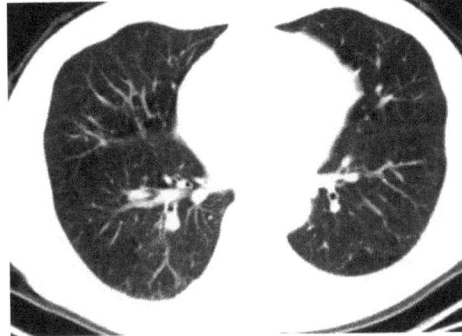
(f)

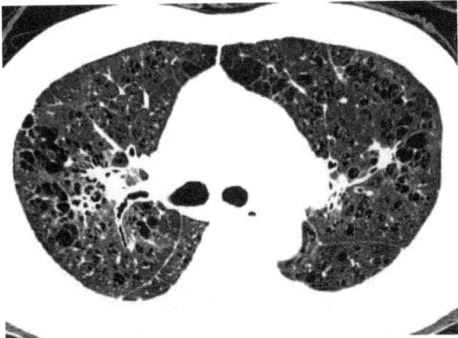
(g)

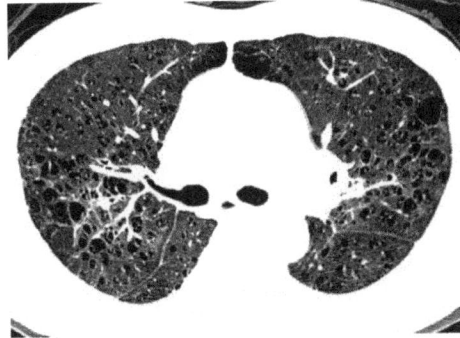
(h)

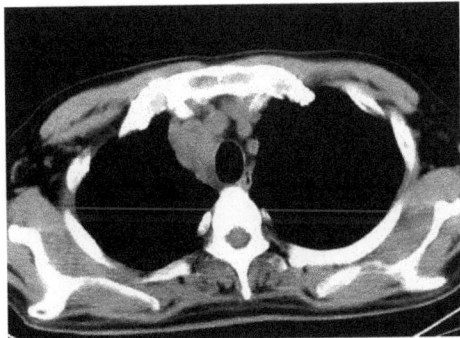
(i)

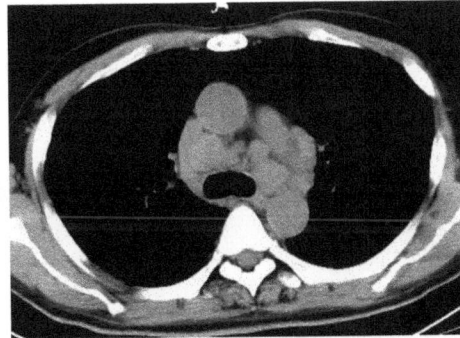
(j)

Fig. 3.4: (continuing)

3.3 Imaging features

The imaging features include:
1. focal inhomogeneous density patchy opacity or consolidation of lung segment, more often in lower lungs and partly with cavity in it;
2. mediastinum lymph nodes enlargement and;
3. varieties in disease patterns and rapid development (sharp change in short time).
4. The image manifestations of pulmonary candidiasis with AIDS are nonspecific, so the final definite diagnosis depends on the lung biopsy pathology and sputum testing and culture.

Editors: Xiejie Chen, Lieguang Zhang, Chunliang Lei,Yan Ding

4 Imaging findings of pulmonary aspergillosis in AIDS

4.1 Introduction

Pulmonary aspergillosis (PA) is a kind of infectious, progressive and allergic disease caused by Aspergillus species. Aspergilli are ubiquitous in nature and can be found in water, soil, food, air and decomposing organisms. The common pathogenic species are Aspergillus fumigatus, Aspergillus flavus and Aspergillus niger. Aspergillus is a kind of opportunistic pathogen that may cause diseases in the condition of host immunosuppressed status of the host or comprehensive invasion of a large number of hyphae in the host. The population at the high risk of PA includes those who have the long-term low leukocyte count, such like the patients with AIDS, leukemia, terminal cancer and organ transplantation. The histologic, clinical and imaging manifestations of PA are associated with the bacterial virulence and host immunoreaction.

PA is classified into three categories in clinical practice as follows:

1. Saprophytism of PA, known as aspergilloma, forms when PA grows in a pre-existing pulmonary cavity, or in the pulmonary cavitary lesions. Radiologic findings show the individual size of approximately 3–4 cm in diameter and solid round dense shadows within cavitary lung lesions. Clinically, aspergiloma can be stagnant in size for many years.

2. Allergic bronchopulmonary aspergillosis (ABPA), known as a kind of hypersensitive reaction, occurs when bronchi become colonized with Aspergillus. Wandering pulmonary infiltrations and central bronchiectasis on radiographic imaging are considered specific in PA.

3. Invasive pulmonary aspergillosis (IPA): IPA is on set opportunistically when a huge number of aspergilli invade into the lung in short term. As the most invasive disease, it occurs more commonly in patients with severe immunodeficiency, especially in AIDS patients. Compared with the others, IPA presents with more severe symptoms clinically. Literature reports it has the highest mortality of 56%–76%. Histopathologically, it manifests to be a pulmonary affection because aspergilli invade into small blood vessels or bronchioles and block the pulmonary blood vessels, causing first pulmonary infarction locally and then necrosis and cavetary formation in the pulmonary parenchyma. The patients presents with the main clinical symptoms like dry cough, mucual sputum or bloody sputum, dyspnea, fever, and chest pain. Hemoptysis and chest pain are typical of affected pulmonary blood vessels.

4. The diagnosis of pulmonary aspergillosis in AIDS patients is based on the comprehensive considerations of clinical symptoms, imaging manifestations, fungi testing and histopathological examinations. Anyway, aspergilluos hyphae positive under microscope and Aspergillus culture from biopsy is the gold standard for

its affirmative diagnosis (Color Figure 4.0). However, the pathological biopsies are dependent on the successful performances of bronchoscopy and bronchoalvcolar lavage, which is actually confined to the patient status and specificity of advanced AIDS. Therefore, it makes it difficult to diagnose PA. Therefore, radiographs and CT scans can be contributive in significant ways to the PA diagnosis in imageology.

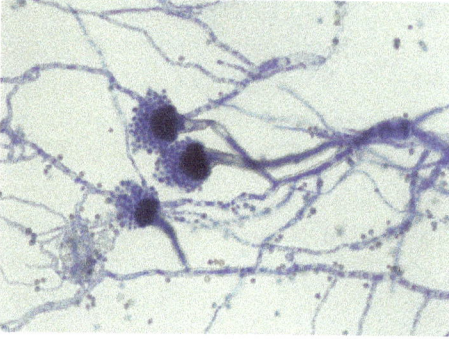

Fig. 4.0: Aspergillus, cotton blue stain, original magnification×400.

4.2 Imaging findings

Case 4.1 (Fig. 4.1 a–e)

Medical history: Pulmonary aspergillosis in a 41-year-old man with AIDS (C3), complained of recurrent fever and cough for 4 months, got worsen for 1 month before hospitalized, the CD4+ count was 97/μl, CD4+/CD8: 0.01, BALF culture: Aspergillus positive.

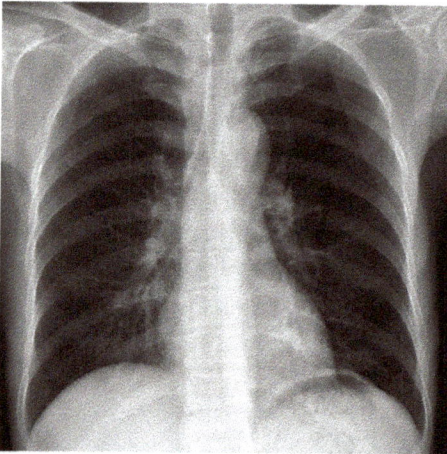

(a)

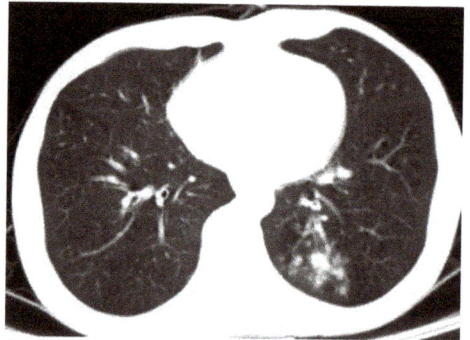

(b)

Fig. 4.1 a–e: Pulmonary aspergillosis.

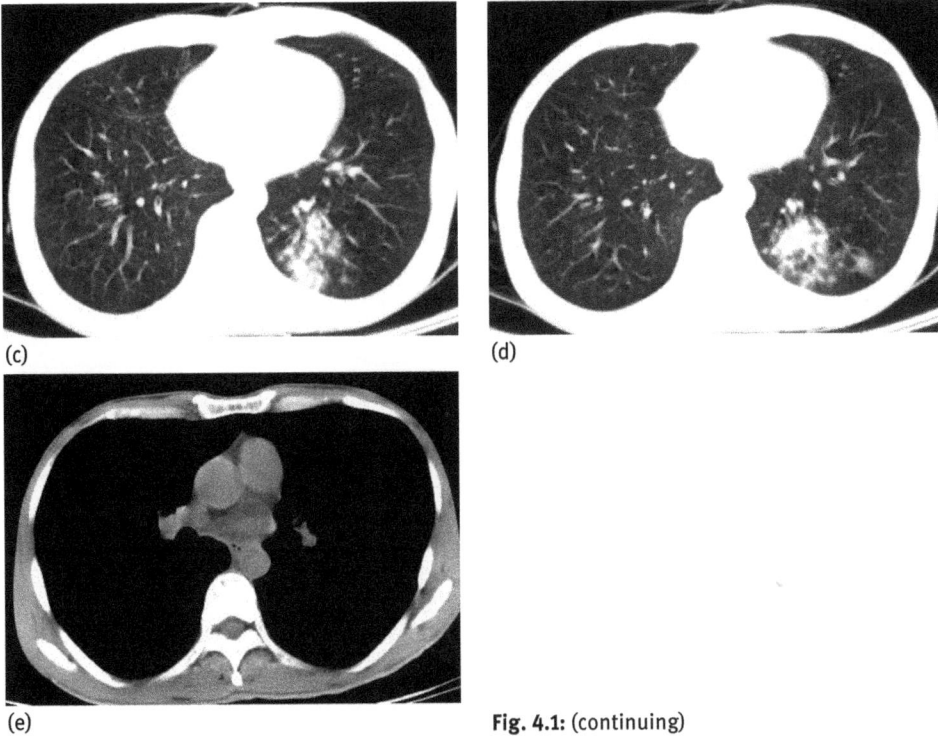

(c)

(d)

(e)

Fig. 4.1: (continuing)

The chest radiograph shows a small patchy opacity on the left lower lung and the heart postzone, with small blurring nodular shadows around the lesion (a). Chest CT scan with lung window showed multiple small nodules with blurring edges in the left posterior basal segment of lower lobe, some were fusing into patches, presenting a "tree-in-bud" sign (b–d). CT scan with mediastinal window demonstrated no enlarged lymph nodes (e).

Case 4.2 (Fig. 4.2 a–f)

A 26-year-old female, presented with paroxysmal cough due to catch a cold 2 months ago before admission, occasionally cough up little white phlegm. Appeared fever one month ago, temperature up to 39.1 °C, especially in afternoon, with slightly chilly, no shivering. Short of breath after exercise showed up one week ago, accompanied with 5 kg weight loss. CD4+ cell counted: 33/μl, CD4+/CD8+: 0.07; sputum smear: fungus positive, BALF culture: Aspergillus. The diagnosis was pulmonary aspergillosis with AIDS(C3).

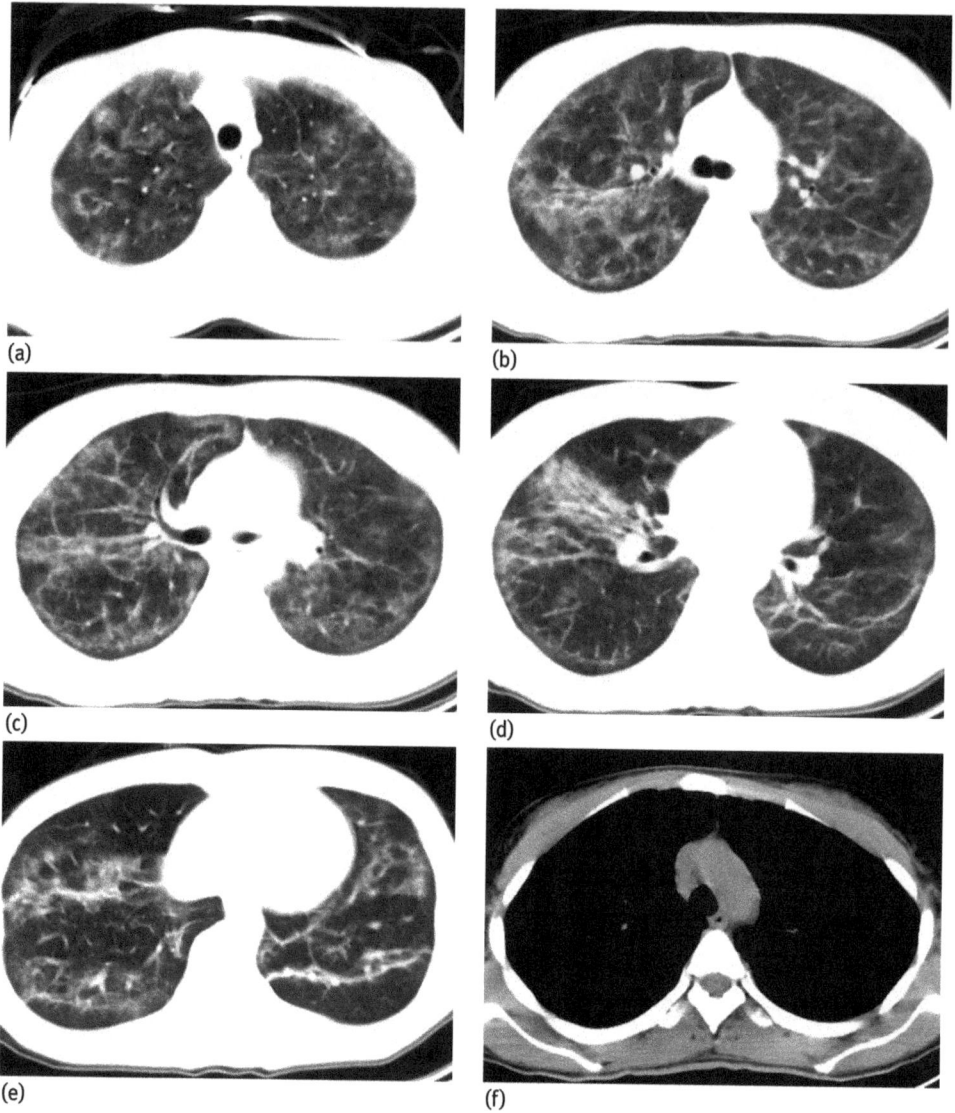

Fig. 4.2 a–f: Pulmonary aspergillosis.

Chest CT scan with lung window showed diffuse ground-glass appearance of the bilateral lungs, interlobular septal thickening and widely reticular fibrosis (a–e). CT scan with mediastinal window showed no enlarged lymph nodes (f).

Case 4.3 (Fig. 4.3 a–e)

A 32-year-old female, presented with sore throat, retrostenal pain for 14 days, aggravating and followed by fever for 3 days. The highest temperature was 39.0 °C, accompanied with chill, cough up amount of yellow phlegm. Bilateral lung sound increased and moist rales were heard in left lung. CD4+ cell counted: 46/μl, CD4+/CD8+: 0.12,

BALF culture: Aspergillus. The diagnosis was pulmonary aspergillosis, esophageal fungal infection with AIDS (C3).

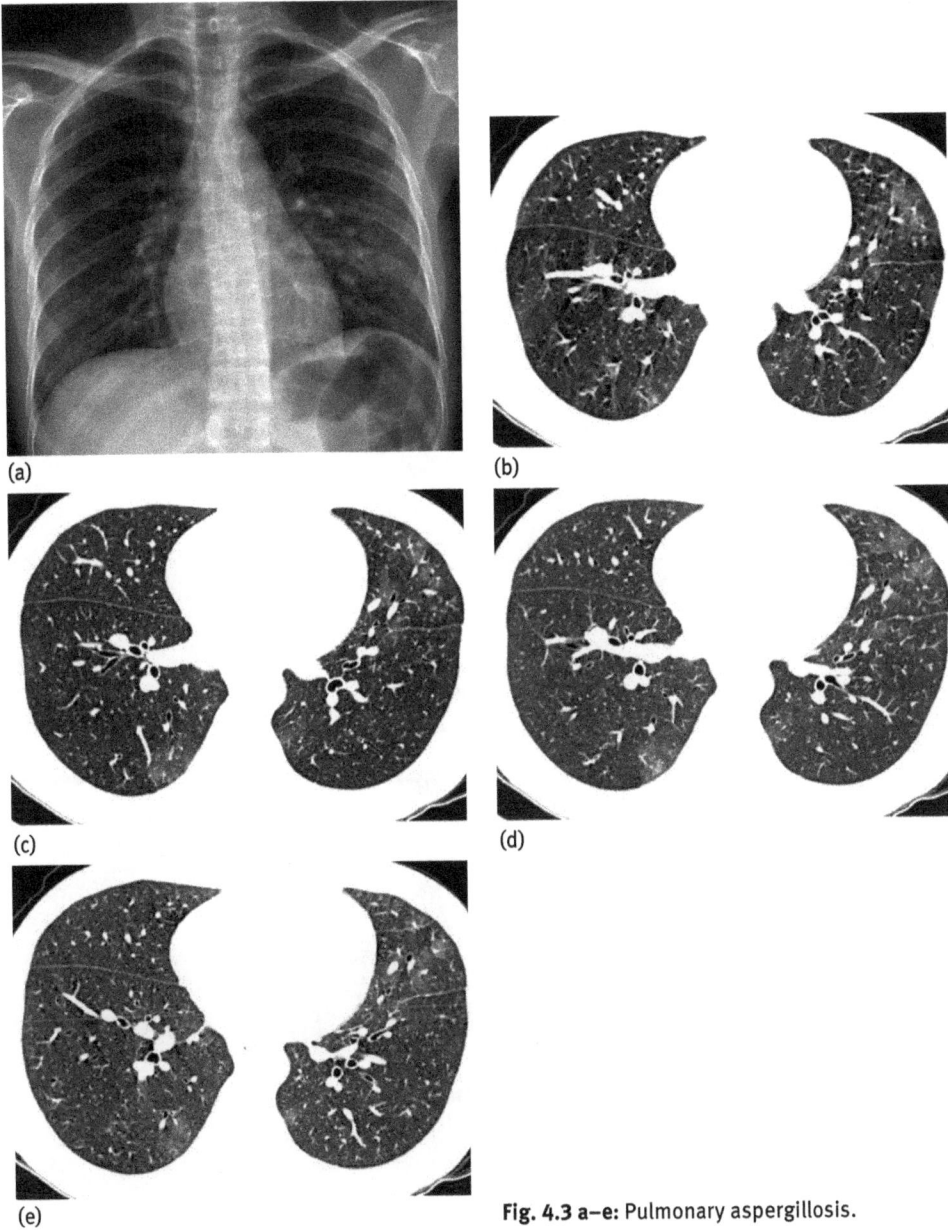

Fig. 4.3 a–e: Pulmonary aspergillosis.

The chest radiograph showed multiple small patchy opacities with blurring edge on bilateral lungs, mainly distributed in the left middle-lower field (a). The chest CT scans with lung window show multiple low-density small patchy opacities with blurring edge and ground-glass appearance, remarkably located in superior lingular segment of the left lung (b–e).

Case 4.4 (Fig. 4.4 a–f)

A 41-year-old man, presented with cough up with little white phlegm one month ago before admission, started to fever 10 days ago, obviously in afternoon, body temperature fluctuated at 38.39 °C, accompanied with 10kg weight loss recently. A 2 cm × 4 cm lymph node was touched in right side of neck. CD4+ cell counted: 46/µl, CD4+/CD8+, 0.17; BALF culture: Aspergillus. The diagnosis was pulmonary aspergillosis with AIDS (C3).

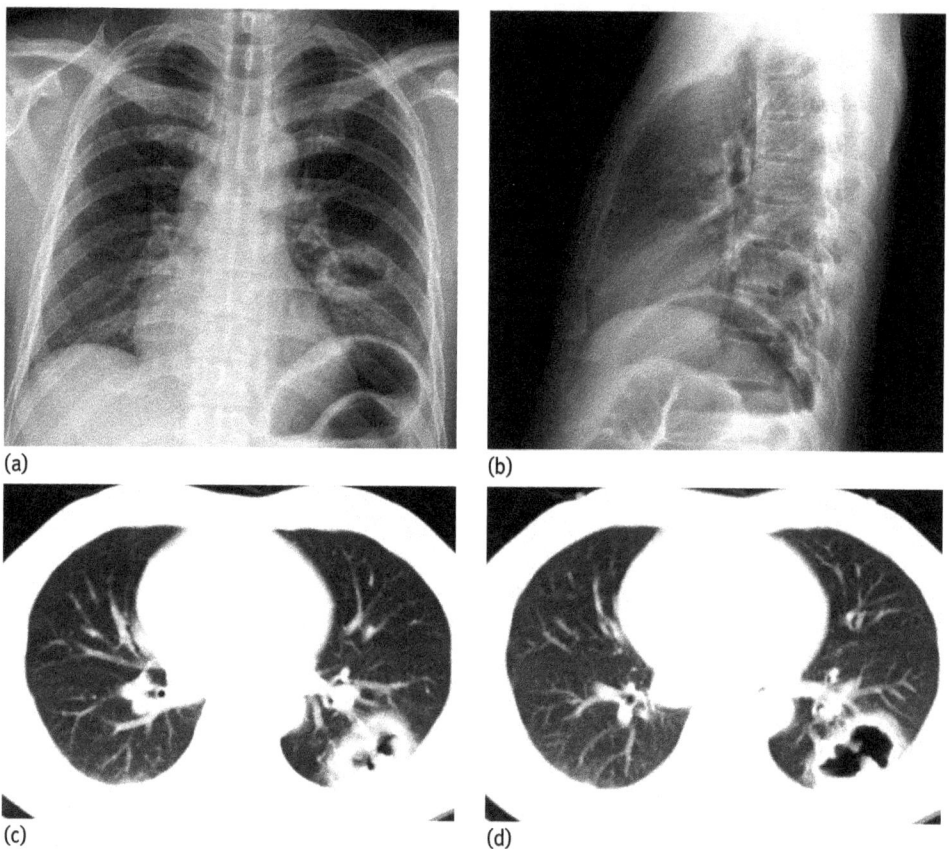

(a)

(b)

(c)

(d)

Fig. 4.4 a–f: Pulmonary aspergillosis.

The chest radiographs demonstrated a large nodule with blurring-edge located in the posterior basal segment of left lower lobe, accompanied with irregular thick-walled cavity in it (a–b). Chest CT scan with lung window demonstrated a large cavitary mass in posterior basal segment of left lower lobe, the inner wall of cavity was irregular,

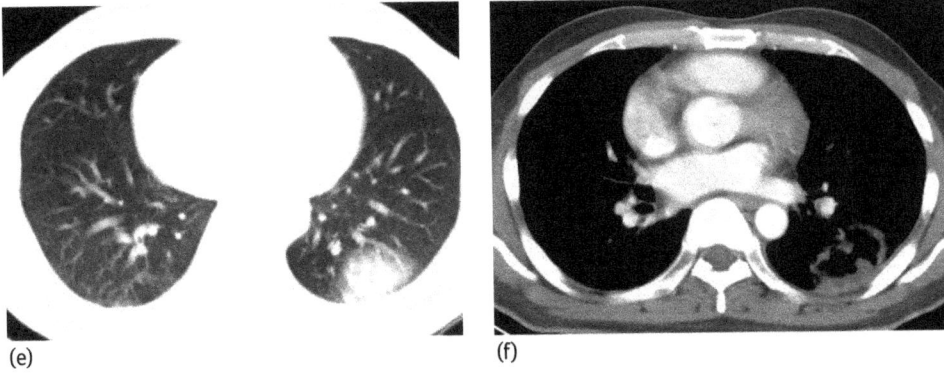

(e)   (f)

Fig. 4.4: (continuing)

with wall-attached small nodule(c–e). Enhanced CT scan with mediastinal window demonstrated non-enhanced multiple nodular protuberances located in the inner wall of the cavity, small air-fluid interface in it and adjacent pleural thickening (f).

Case 4.5 (Fig. 4.5 a–l)

A 58-year-old female, presented with history of recurrent fever and cough for one year, short of breath for one more month. Peaked temperature was 38.5 °C, accompanied with slight chilly, rigor and cough up white phlegm, cough symptom got worse while position change. Both lung sounds increased, tiny wet rales can be heard in lower lobes, no pleural friction sound. CD4+ cell counted: 196/μl, CD4+/CD8+: 0.08, BALF culture: Aspergillus. The diagnosis was pulmonary aspergillosis with AIDS (C3).

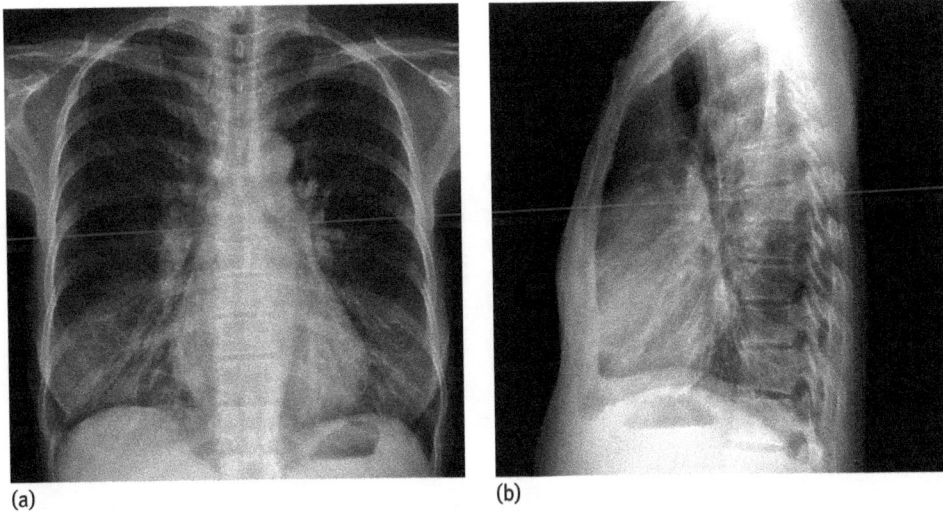

(a)   (b)

Fig. 4.5 a–l: Pulmonary aspergillosis.

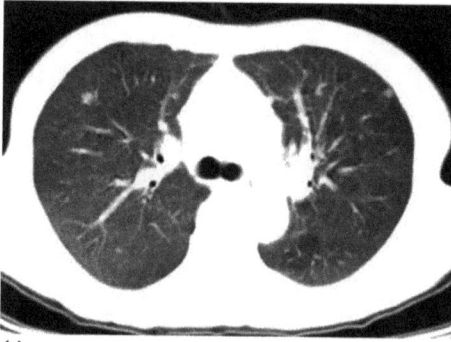

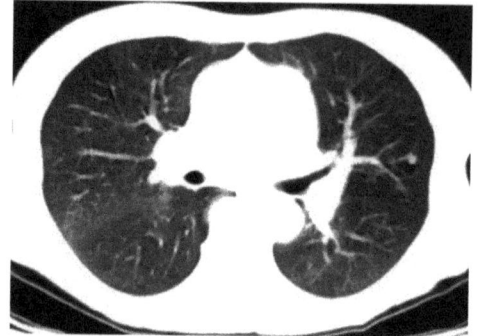

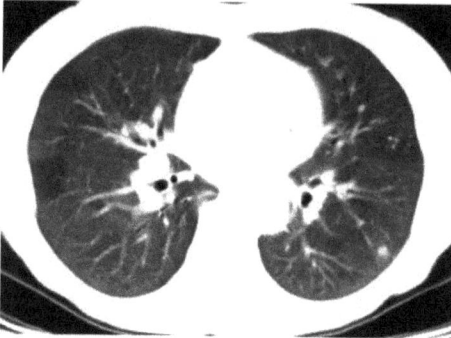

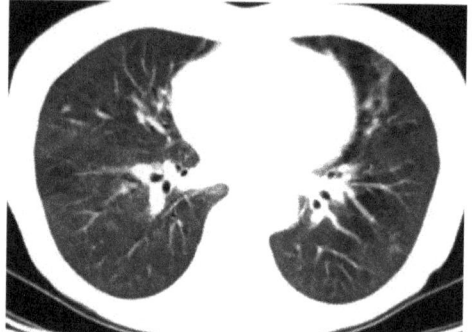

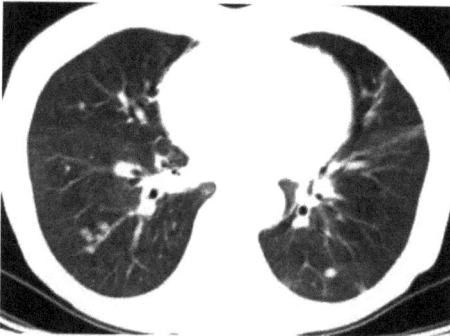

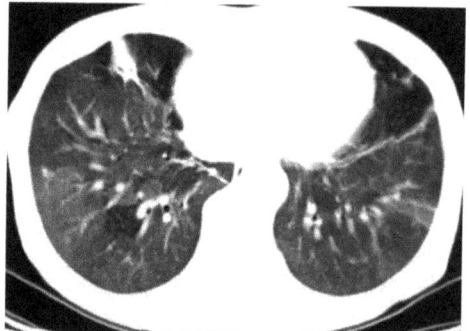

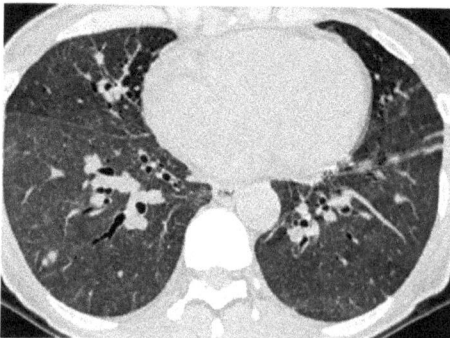

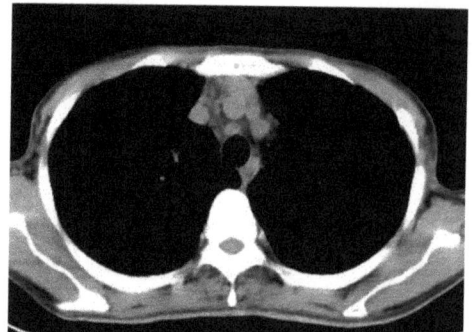

Fig. 4.5: (continuing)

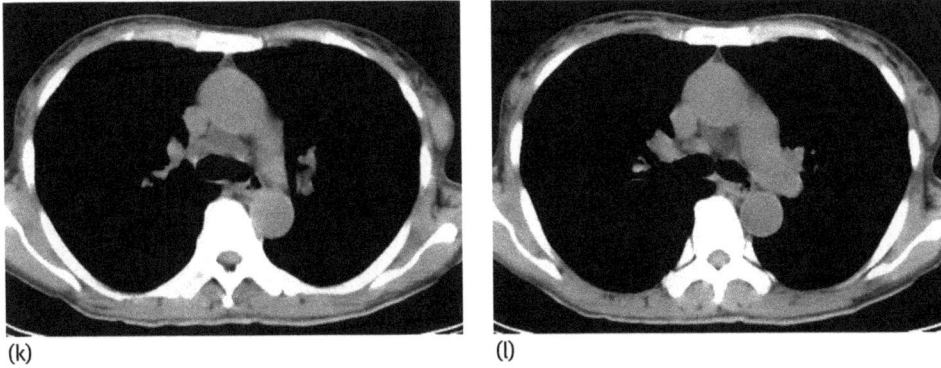

(k)   (l)

Fig. 4.5: (continuing)

The chest radiographs demonstrated multiple coarsened markings, obscure hilum in the bilateral lung, and a high density patchy opacity with blurring edge on right middle lobe (a, b). Chest CT scan with lung window demonstrated multiple nodular shadows of different sizes in the bilateral lung, with clear and smooth edges in some of them and a high-density patchy opacity with clear edge on the medialis segment of right middle lobe (c–h), presenting a typical tree-in-bud sign (g), demonstrating clearly in HRCT (i). CT scan with mediastinal window showed mediastinal slight lymph nodes enlargement (j–l).

Case 4.6 (Fig. 4.6 a–l)

A 37-year-old man, presented fever for 20 more days and cough for 3 days, peaked body temperature was 40 °C, accompanied with chilly and shivering, no obvious muscular soreness. Physical examination found no rash in whole body and no enlarged superficial lymph nodes. Both lung sounds coarsed, no dry or moist rales, no pleural-frictionsound. CD4+ cell counted: 12/µl, CD4+/CD8+, 0.05; BALF culture: Aspergillus. The diagnosis was pulmonary aspergillosis with AIDS (C3).

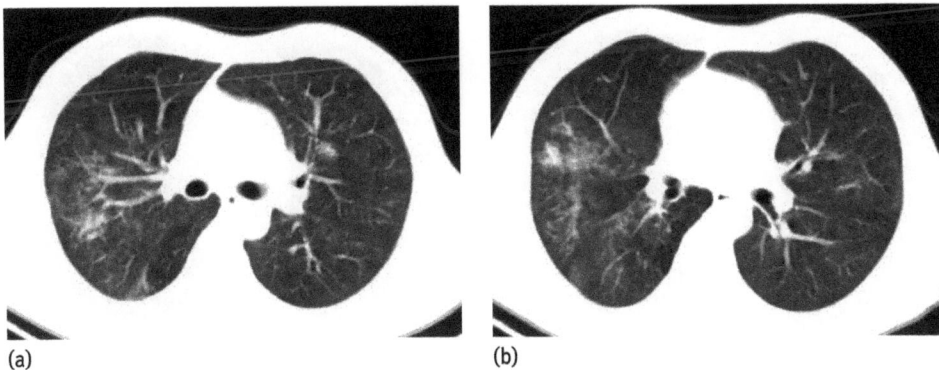

(a)   (b)

Fig. 4.6 a–l: Pulmonary aspergillosis.

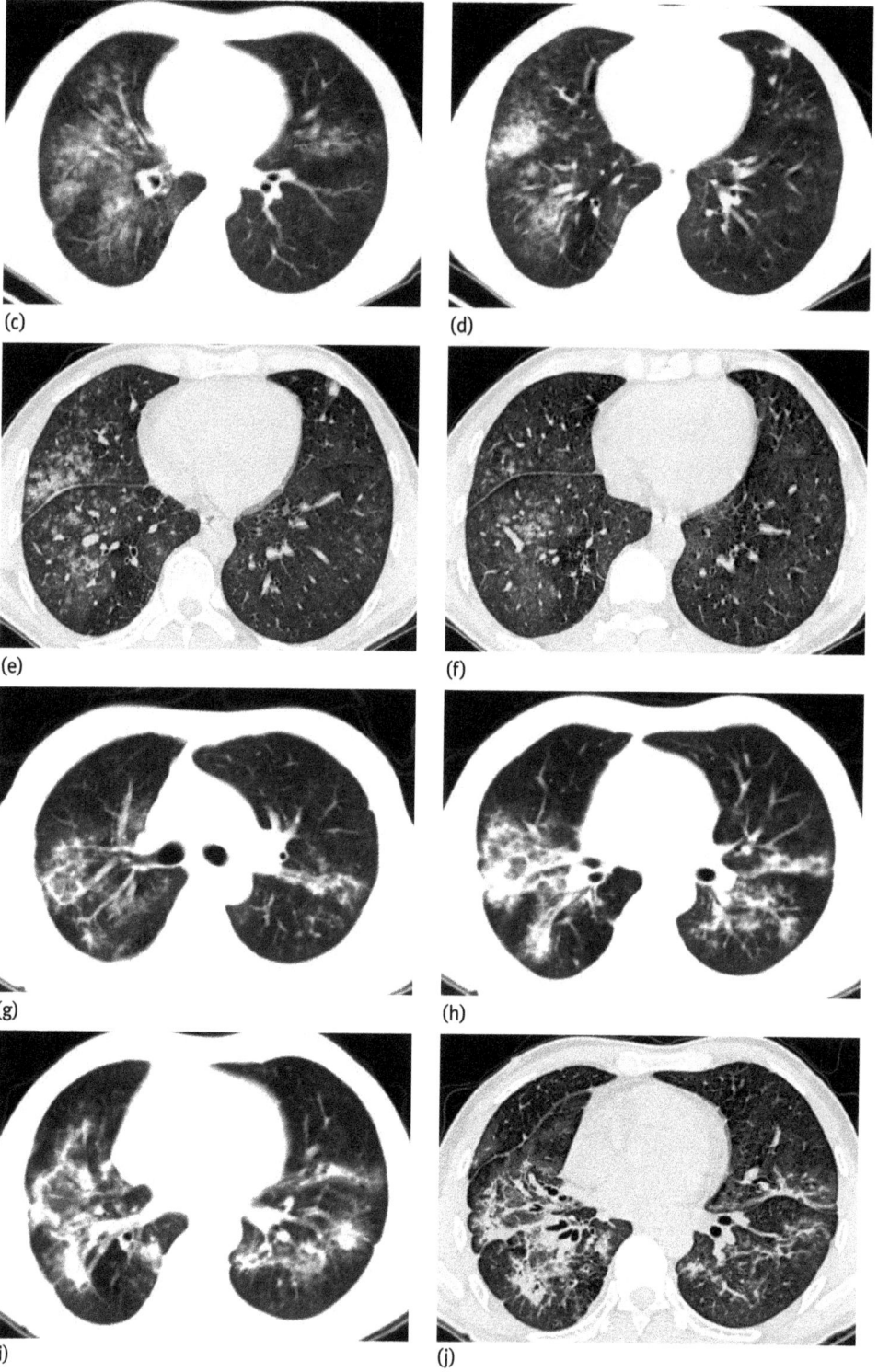

Fig. 4.6: (continuing)

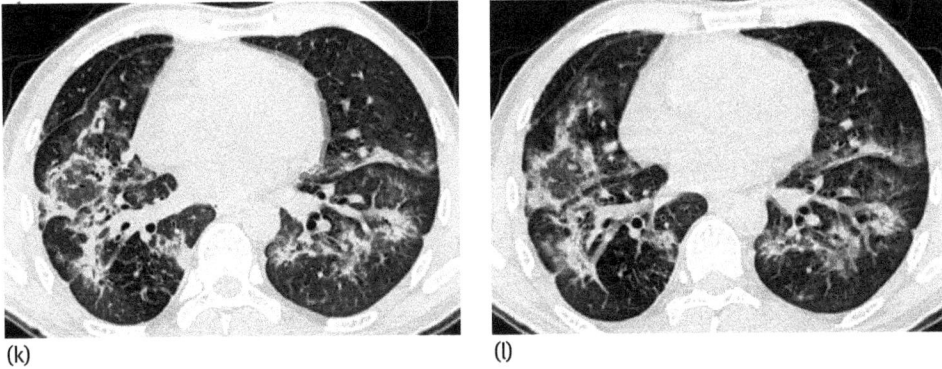

(k)   (l)

Fig. 4.6: (continuing)

Chest CT scan with lung window demonstrated ground-glass appearance of the bilateral lungs and multiple blurring-edged nodules of different sizes in the bilateral lungs, some nodules fusing into patches (a–f). After 5 weeks treatment, CT scan showed the lesions were obviously worsened, and multiple high-density patchy opacities with blurring edges on the bilateral lungs and honeycomb appearances in some lesions (g–i). HRCT scan demonstrated widely tractive bronchiectasis, interlobular septal thickening and reticular funicular fibrosis in the bilateral lungs (j–l).

4.3 Imaging features

The radiologic findings of IPA in AIDS patients are nonspecific. Multiple nodules with blurring edge in bilateral lungs can be seen in the early stage. They are located in the peripheral lung regions in most cases with a size of 1–2 cm in diameter. With the disease developing, the nodular shadows become sharper, showing a trend of fusing. Then in both middle-lower lobes appear scattered patchy round or crumby opacities, even with cavities in some lesions.

The chest CT findings of IPA in AIDS are characterized by multiple nodules surrounded by ground-glass-like rims, which is called halo sign typically in the early stage; and air-filled crescent sign typically in the late stage. Actually, for early diagnosis of invasive pulmonary aspergillosis (IPA), the halo sign and air-filled crescent sign are nonspecific on CT images. Besides, pleural effusion and mediastinal lymphadenectasis are less seen.

Editors: Xiaofeng Guo, Haolan He, Jinxin Liu, Yan Ding

5 Imaging findings of pulmonary mucormycosis in AIDS

5.1 Introduction

Mucormycosis, known as formerly zygomycosis or phycomycosis, is a rare opportunistic fungal infection caused by mucorales. Mucoraceae, belonging to zygomycetae under phycomyceteae, includes fungi commonly found in the natural world, such as rhizopus, lichtheimia and mucor. Mucor is not pathogenic in general but it may cause systemic infection on condition of the deteriorated immune function of a host by invading into the nose, affecting the ccessory nasal cavity and fossa orbitalis, and further causing meningitis and frontal abscess by invading the brain. Pulmonary mucormycosis is reported to be secondary to nasal and encephalic infections, followed by affections in skin, gastrointestinal tracks and other disseminated mucormycosis.

Pathologically, mucormycosis manifests itself with hemorrhagic gangrenous inflammations. A host affected by mucors, normally, reacts to kill the fungal spores by way of cytophagocytesis and oxidation mechanism.However, the host with depressed immune function may contract mucormysis only because of the impaired cytophagocytesis. Literature has reported few cases of mucormysis in AIDS patients. Its prevalence is dim so that it is rare and opportunistic. Recently, we admitted and treated only 13 AIDS patients with affirmatively-diagnosed pulmonary mucormysis in Guangzhou No. 8 hospital from January 2005 to September 2008.

It is reported that pulmonary mucormycosis is associated with high mortality (65%–96%) as the result of its speedy development. Clinically, it comes out with nonspecific pneumonia, with such common symptoms as fever, cough, hemoptysis, chest pain, tachypnea and hypoxia. The 13 AIDS patients mentioned above presented with almost the same symptoms except hemoptysis. Besides, we found bean curd-like thrushes on the tongues of 7 patients. However, the mortality among them was only 31%, lower than the figure internationally reported.

Of the 13 cases, 8 were confirmed to pulmonary mucors infection (2 patient ending up with death). 1 case was mucormysis combined with pneumocystis pneumonia (PCP), 1 case was mucormysis combined with *Penicillium marneffei (PM)*, *2 cases* were mucormysis combined with mycobacterial infections (1 died), and the last one died of mucormysis combined with *Penicillium marneffei* and mycobacterial infections.

The definite diagnosis of pulmonary mucormycosis (Color figure 5.0) is dependent on the detection of specific hyphae by microscopic examination of fungi as well as pathologic examination. The means of pathologic examination usually include fiber bronchoscopy, bronchial lavage fluid examination, exploratory thoracotomy and transthoracic needle aspiration biopsy of lung. Pitifully, the specimens of the pulmonary lesions are hard to get in AIDS patients so that the definite diagnosis of pulmonary muormysis becomes problematic.

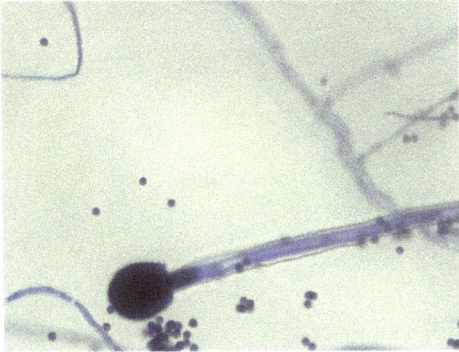

Fig. 5.0: Pulmonary mucomycosis, cotton blue stain, ×400. There were numerous nonseptate hyphae, suggestive of mucormycosis (medan staining, ×400).

5.2 Image findings

Case 5.1 (Fig. 5.1 a–j)

A 45-year-old male presented with a 4-mouth history of fever (up to 40 °C), accompanied with slight chills, cough with white phlegm. The progressive enlargement right cervical lymphadenopathy found 2 month ago was about the size of 1 cm × 2 cm. CD4+ cell counted: 11/μl, CD4+/CD8+: 0.04. Bronchoalveolar lavage fluid (BALF) culture: mucormycosis. Diagnosis: AIDS (C3) with pulmonary mucormycosis.

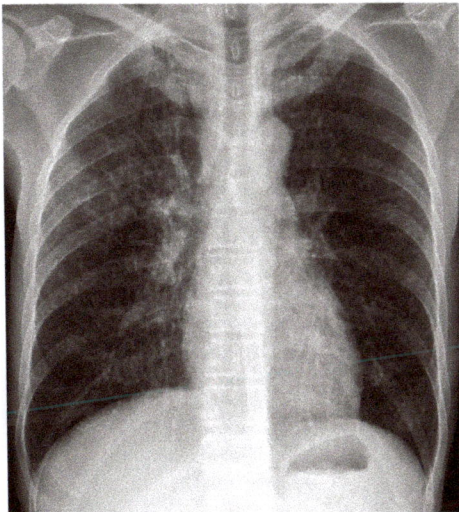

(a)

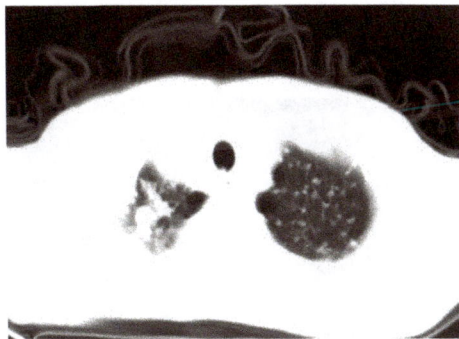

(b)

Fig. 5.1 a–j: Pulmonary mucormycosis.

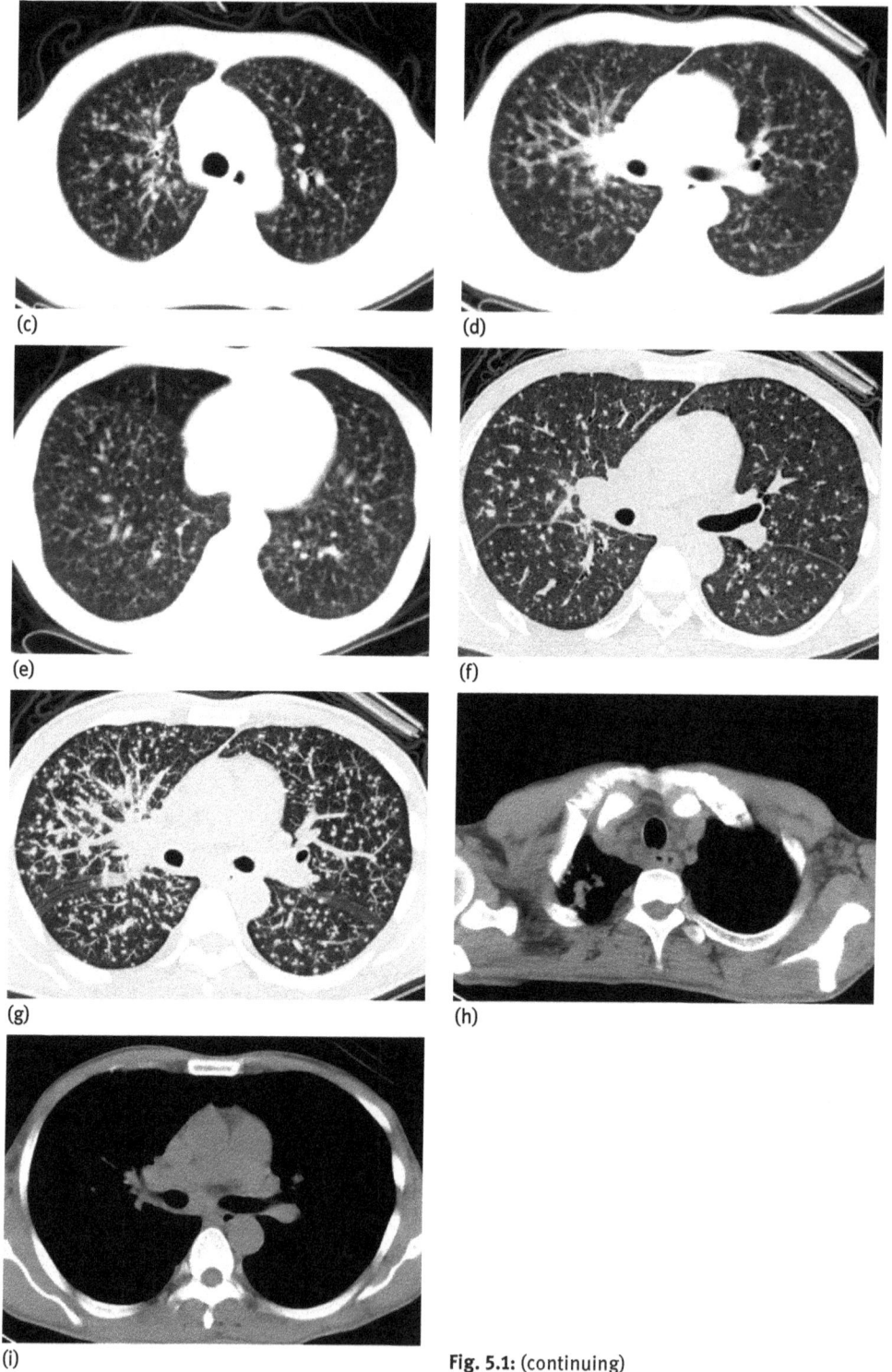

Fig. 5.1: (continuing)

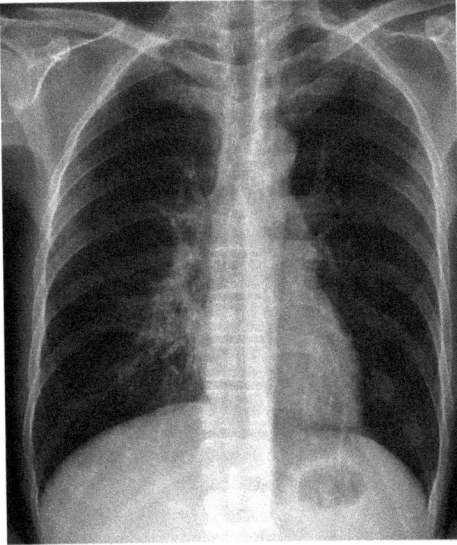

(j)   **Fig. 5.1:** (continuing)

The chest radiograph showed diffuse miliary nodules in the bilateral lungs (a). Chest CT scan with lung window showed diffuse miliary nodules in the bilateral lungs (b–e), small patchy and small funicular opacities on the right upper lobe (a). HRCT and MIP scans showed randomly distributed nodules with "tree-in-bud" sign (f–g). CT scan with mediastinal window showed lesions of soft tissue-like density in the right upper apex pulmonis, no enlarged lymph nodes in the mediastinum and bilateral porta pulmonis (h, i). After 7 months treatment, the small patchy opacity on the middle lobe of right lung was evidently much higher in density, the diffuse miliary nodules were remarkably absorbed in the bilateral lungs (j).

Case 5.2 (Fig. 5.2 a–l)

A 34-year-old male presented with a 4-week history of cough with white phlegm, and occasionally blood stained sputum. The confluence, slightly hard and poor activity cervical lymphadenopathy was about the size of 3 cm × 3 cm. Lots of rhonchi and a few moist rales have been audible over bilateral middle and lower lungs. CD4+ cell counted: 22/μl, CD4+/CD8+: 0.35. Bronchoalveolar lavage fluid (BALF) culture: mucormycosis. Diagnosis: AIDS (C3) with pulmonary mucormycosis.

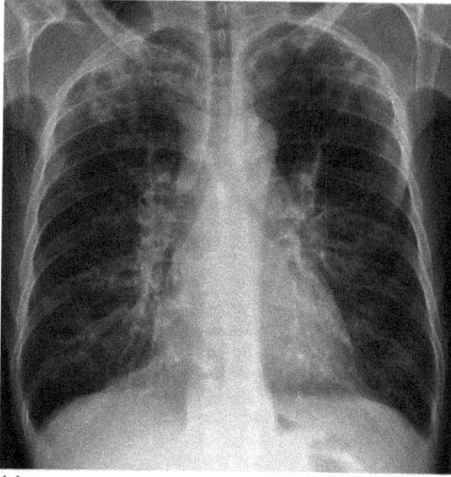
(a)

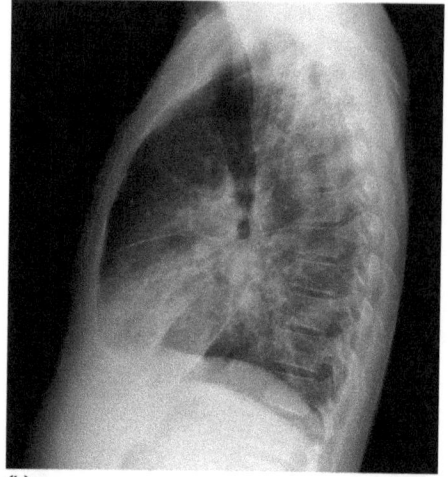
(b)

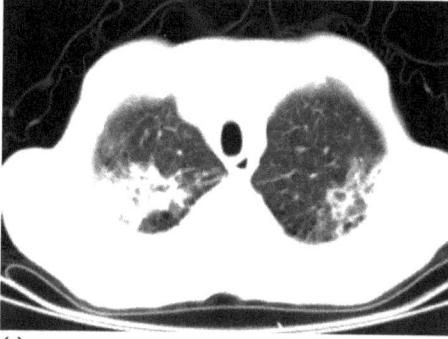
(c)

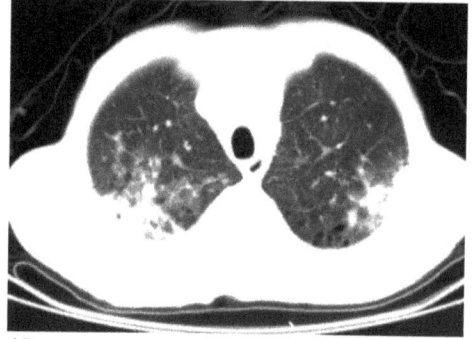
(d)

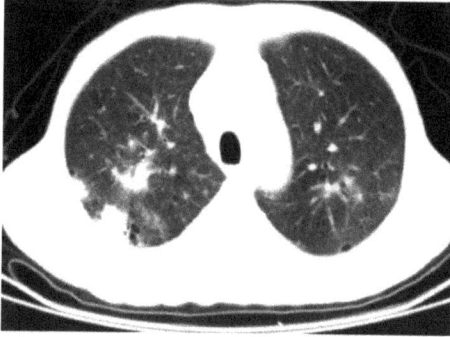
(e)

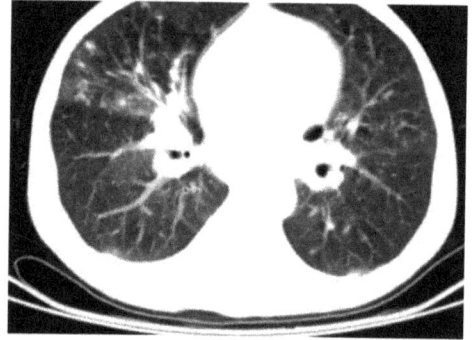
(f)

Fig. 5.2 a–l: Pulmonary mucormycosis.

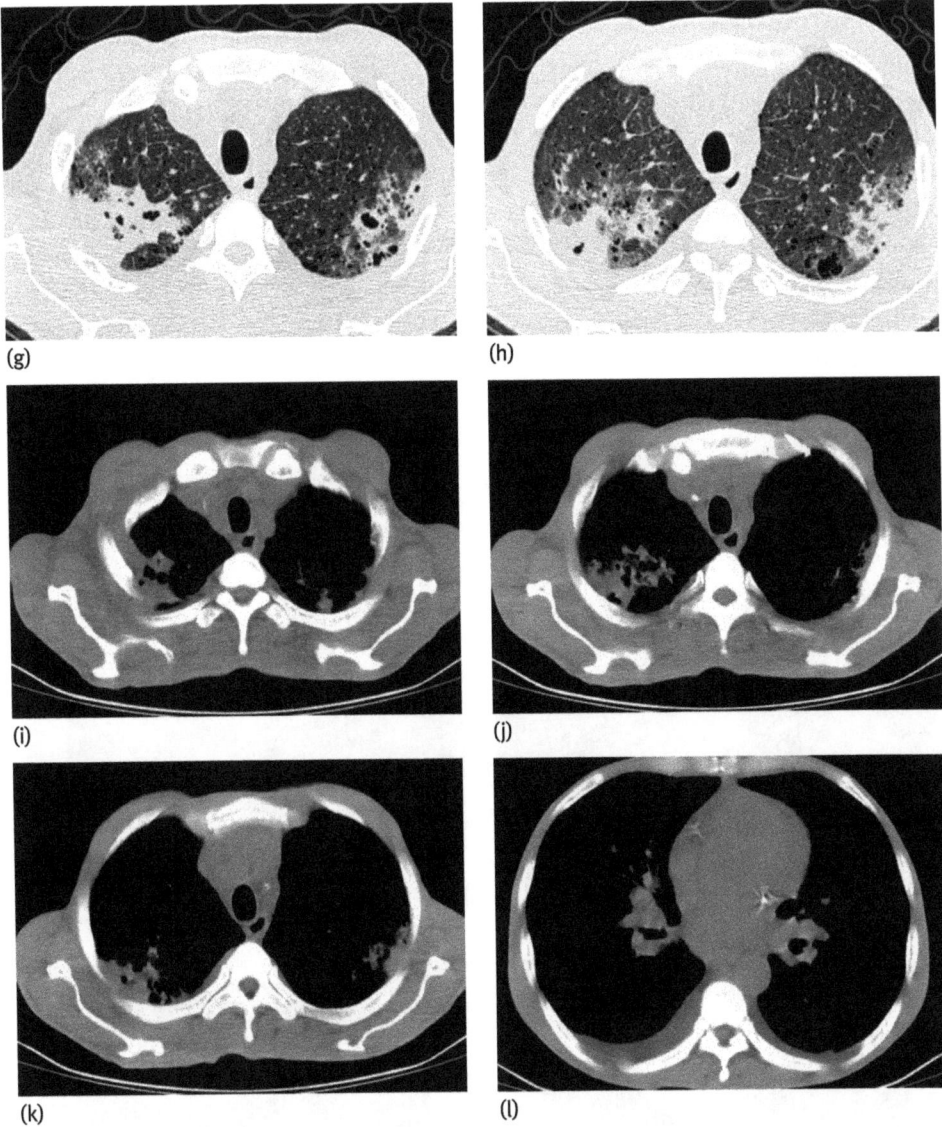

(g)   (h)

(i)   (j)

(k)   (l)

Fig. 5.2: (continuing)

The chest radiographs showed multiple patchy opacities with blurring edges on the bilateral lungs, mainly located in the apicoposterior segment of upper bilateral lung as well as the middle lobe of right lung (a, b). CT scan with lung window showed high-density patchy and nodular opacities with blurring edges on the apicoposterior segment of upper bilateral lungs as well as the middle lobe of right lung (c–f). HRCT scans presented multiple small cavities and bronchiectasis in the lesion with light ground-glass-like appearance around it and multiple small ballonets in adjacent lung tissue (g, h). CT scans with mediastinal window showed the opacities of soft tissue-like density on the bilateral lungs as well as cavities in the lesions, enlarged lymph nodes in the mediastinum and bilateral porta pulmonis and a little bilateral pleural effusions (i–l).

Case 5.3 (Fig. 5.3 a–l)

A 25-year-old male presented with a 3-month history of recurrent fever and cough before admission. The hard, activity and poor tenderness cervical lymphadenopathy with size around 0.5 cm × 0.5 cm was found on physical. CD4+ cell counted: 20/μl, CD4+/CD8+: 0.04. Bronchoalveolar lavage fluid (BALF) culture: mucormycosis. Diagnosis: AIDS (C3) with pulmonary mucormycosis.

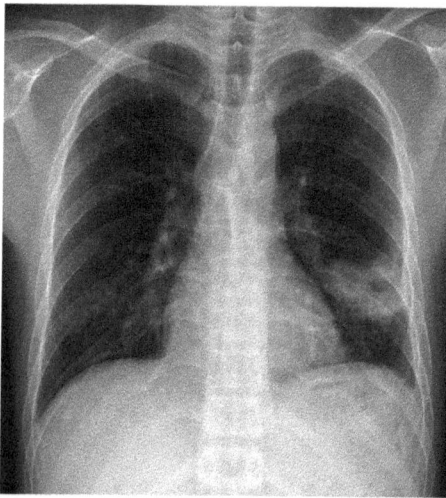
(a)

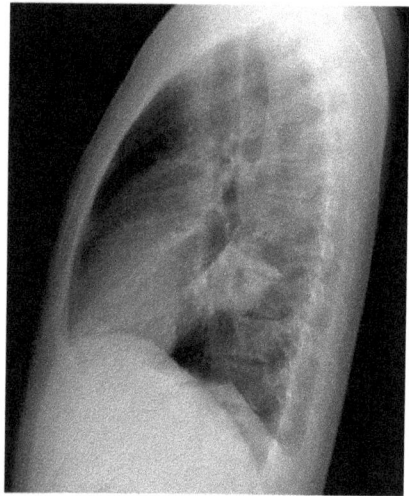
(b)

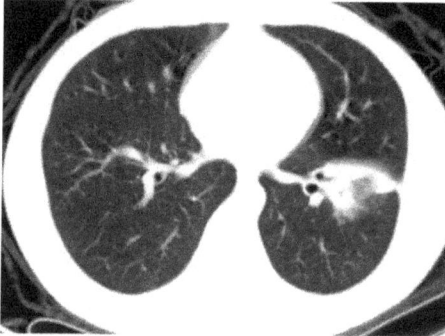
(c)

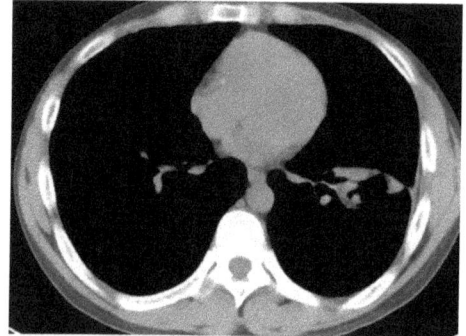
(d)

Fig. 5.3 a–l: Pulmonary mucormycosis.

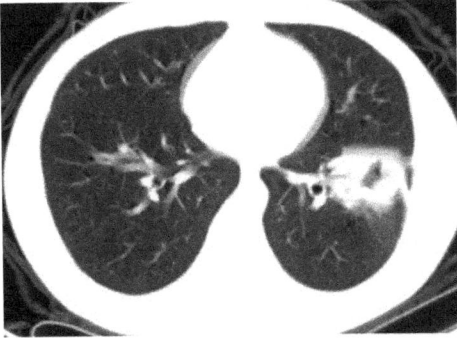
(e)

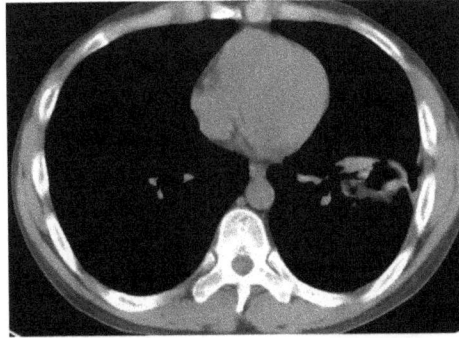
(f)

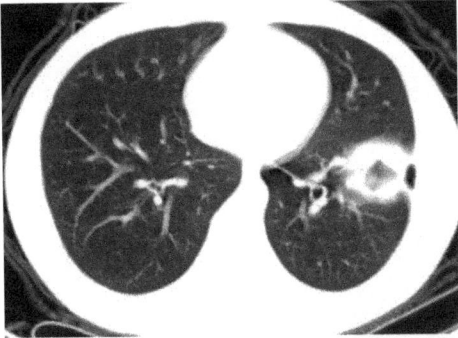
(g)

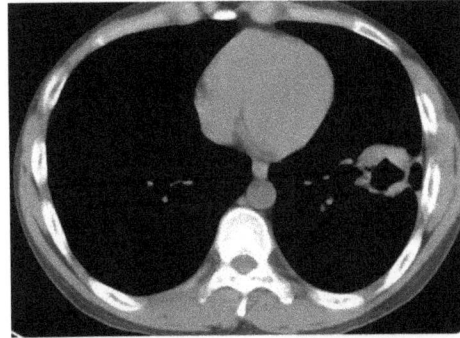
(h)

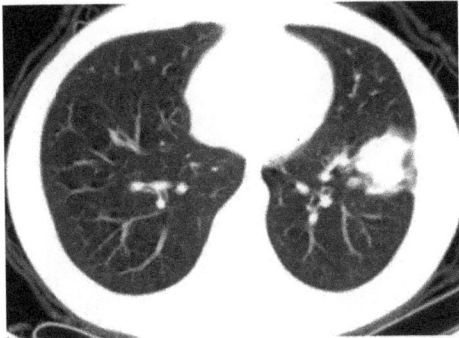
(i)

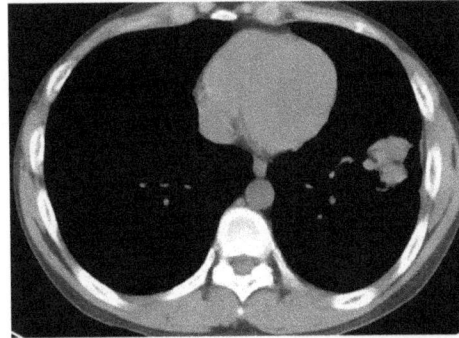
(j)

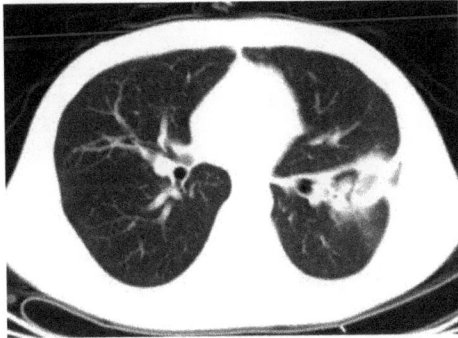
(k)

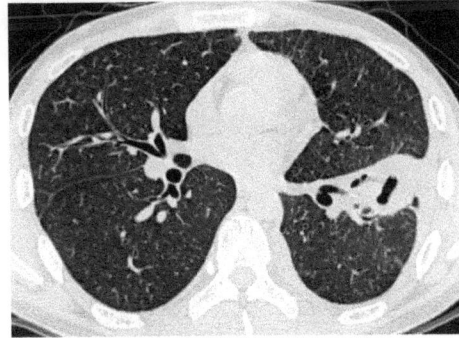
(l)

Fig. 5.3: (continuing)

The chest radiographs showed a lumpy opacity in the anterior medial segment and outer basal segment of left lower lung, with irregular cavity in it (a, b). CT scan with mediastinal window demonstrated an irregular leaflet-like nodule of soft tissue density in the anterior inner segment and outer basal segment of left lower lung, with an irregular cavity in it, and adhesive lateral corniform pleura (c–j). After 6 weeks treatment, the nodule of left anterior medial segment and outer basal segment of left lower lobe was smaller than before treatment and so was the cavity in it, with an obscure small nodule and irregular small bronchiectasis in the lesion, as showed in the CT scans with lung windows and HRCT scans (k). CT scans with mediastinal window show lateral pleural thickening and adhesion (l).

Case 5.4 (Fig. 5.4 a–k)

A 27-year-old male presented with fever, cough and tachypnea for a month, diarrhea for ten days which getting worse for 3 days, occurred blurring of vision for 3

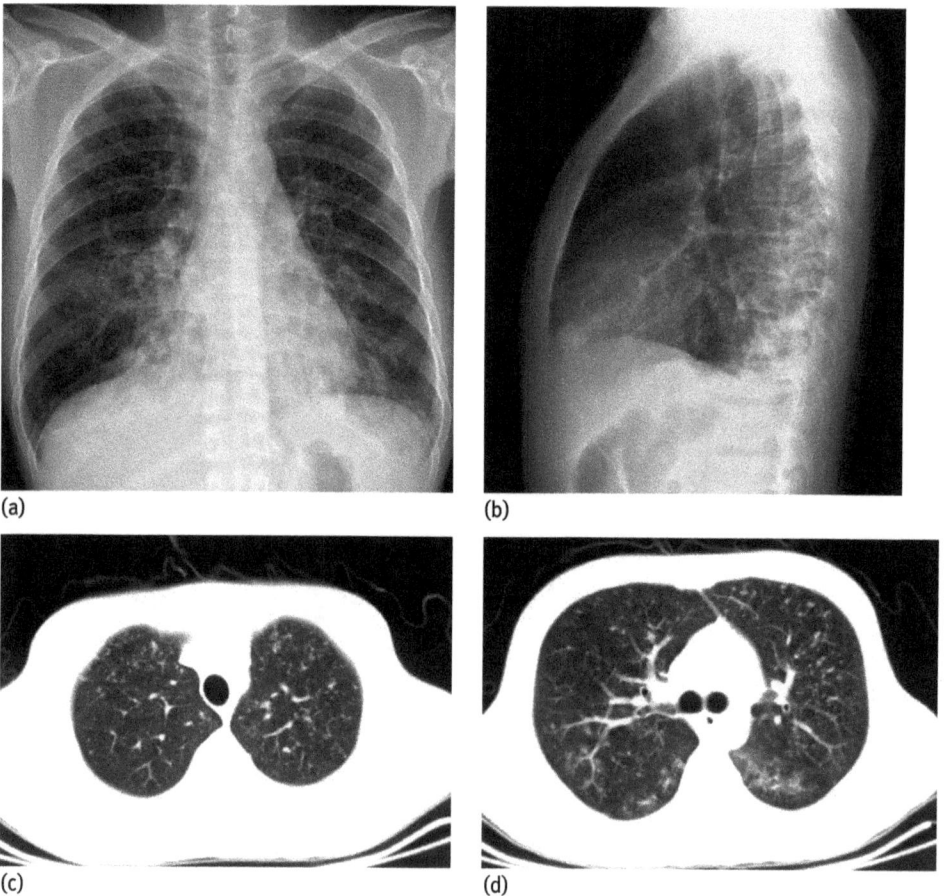

(a)

(b)

(c)

(d)

Fig. 5.4 a–k: Pulmonary mucormycosis.

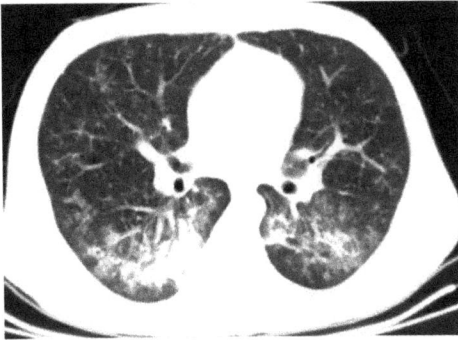
(e)

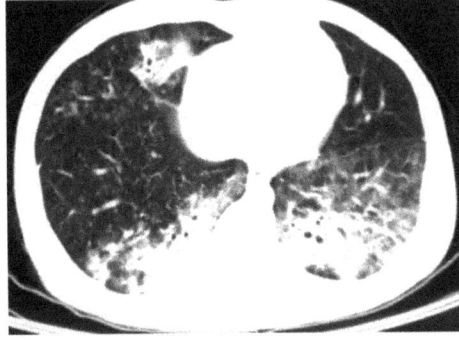
(f)

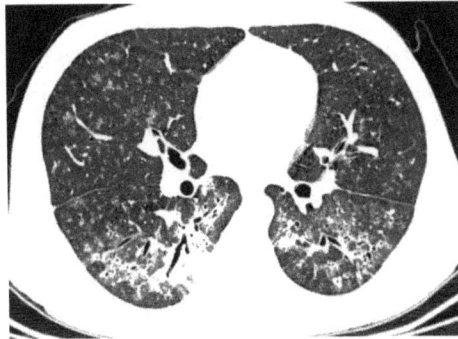
(g)

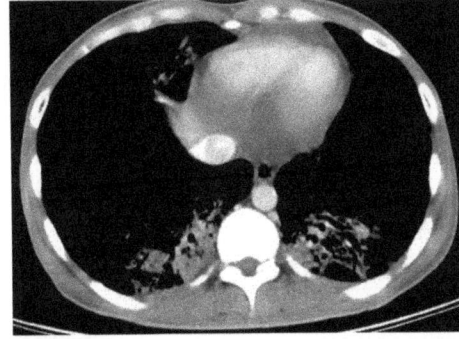
(h)

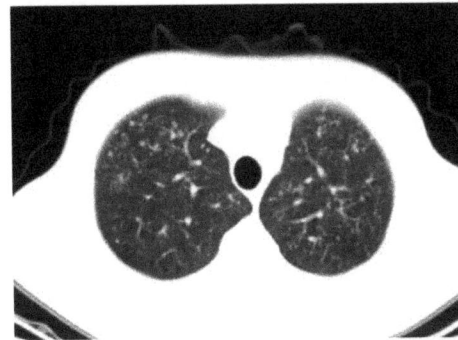
(i)

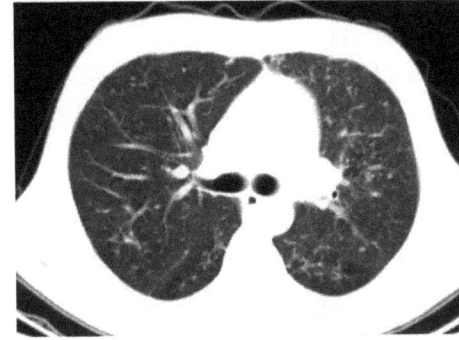
(j)

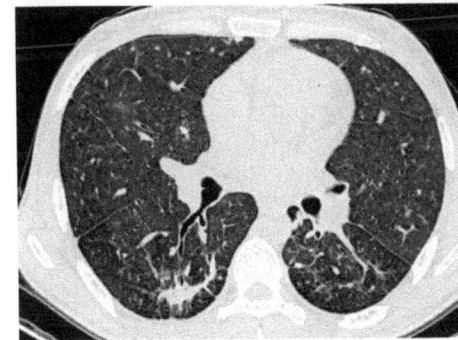
(k)

Fig. 5.4: (continuing)

days. CD4+ cell counted: 5/μl, CD4+/CD8+: 0.09. Bronchoalveolar lavage fluid (BALF) culture: mucormycosis. Diagnosis: AIDS (C3) with pulmonary mucormycosis.

The chest radiographs showed multiple patchy opacities distributed along the lung markings in the lower bilateral lung and diffuse miliary nodules in the bilateral lung (a, b). The CT scans with lung window present diffuse miliary nodules in the bilateral lung and multiple high-density patchy opacities with blurring edge in the bilateral lower lobes and middle lobe of right lung, mainly located in the lower lobe (c–f). HRCT demonstrated randomly distributed nodules and low-density central lobular nodules in the bilateral lung, with ground-grass-like appearance around it, patchy opacities with uneven density on the lower bilateral lung, mild bronchiectasis and interlobular septal thickening in the lesions (g). Enhanced CT scan with lung window showed opacities with soft tissue-like density in the bilateral lower lobes (h). After 3 weeks treatment, the diffuse military small nodules in bilateral lower lobes and middle lobe of right lungwere evidently absorbed and the shadows of the bilateral lungs were clearer than before treatment as showed in the CT scans with lung window as well as the HRCT scan (i–k).

Case 5.5 (Fig. 5.5 a–l)

A 34-year-old male presented with fever (up to 40 °C), accompanied with cough, white phlegm, chest distress and tachypnea (especially on exertion) for 20 days. He had weight loss of 5 kg. CD4+ cell counted: 48/μl, CD4+/CD8+: 0.04. Bronchoalveolar lavage fluid (BALF) culture: mucor positive, and the bronchoscopy biopsy suggested Pneumocystis pneumonia (PCP). Diagnosis: AIDS (C3) with pulmonary mucormycosis and PCP.

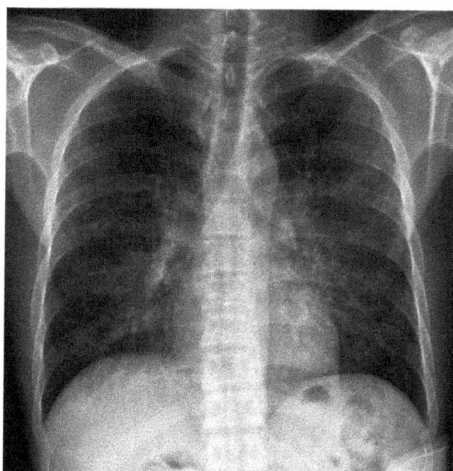

(a)

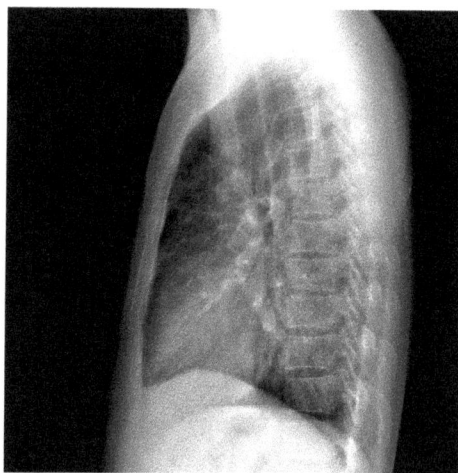

(b)

Fig. 5.5 a–l: Pulmonary mucormycosis and PCP.

(c)

(d)

(e)

(f)

(g)

(h)

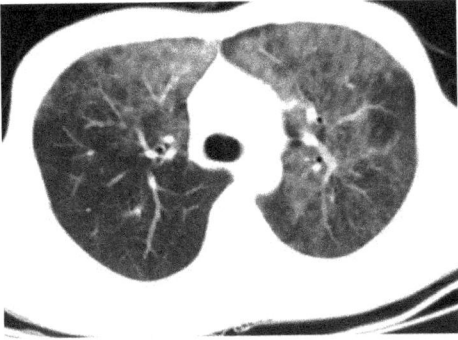

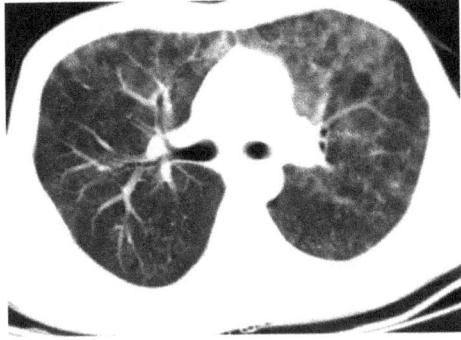

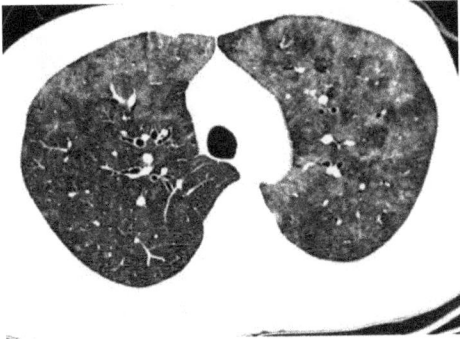

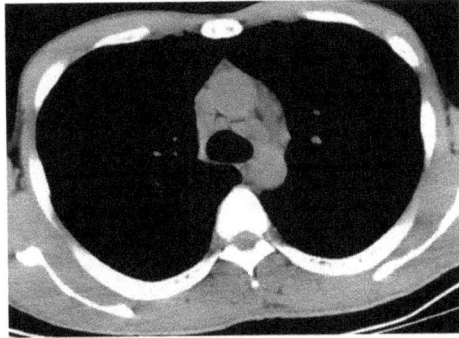

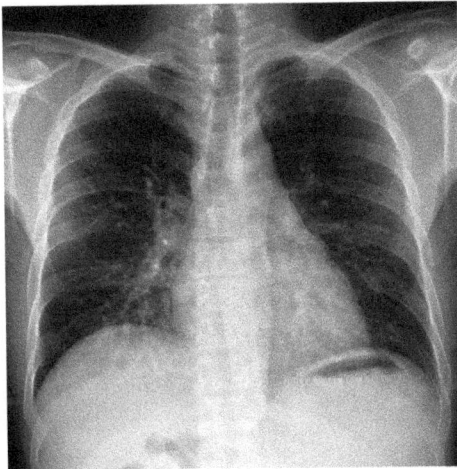

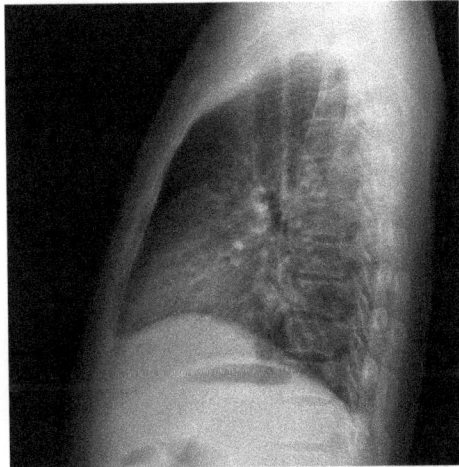

Fig. 5.5: (continuing)

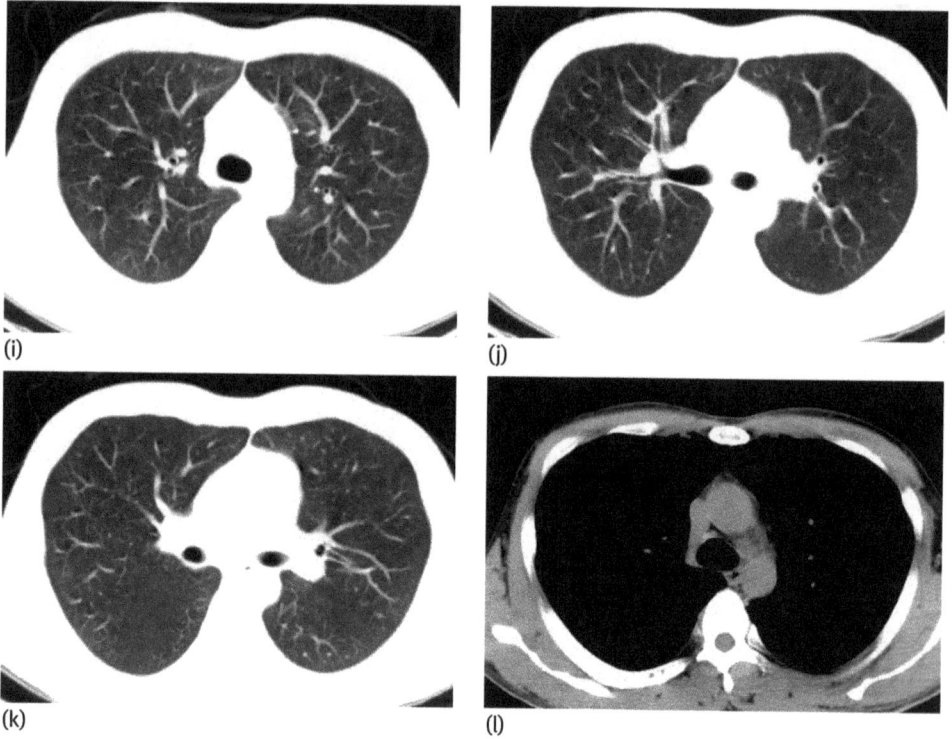

Fig. 5.5: (continuing)

The chest radiographs demonstrated decreased transparency and irregular ground-glass appearance of the bilateral lungs, with blurring lung-markings (a, b). The CT scans with lung window present diffuse irregular ground-glass-like lesions in the bilateral lung (c, d). HRCT scan demonstrated some small nodular and ground-glass-like opacities (e). CT scan with mediastinal window demonstrated enlarged lymph nodes of aortopulmonary (f). After 4 weeks treatment, the ground-glass-like lesions in the bilateral lungs were radically absorbed and dissipated as showed in the chest radiographs (g, h). The ground-glass-like lesions in the bilateral lung were absorbed as showed in the CT scans with lung windows (i–k) and the enlarged lymph nodes shrankas showed in the CT scan with lung window (l).

5.3 Imaging features

It is reported that the chest radiograghs of pulmonary mucormycosis (PM) in non-AIDS patients usually show progressive infiltrative consolidations, nodules, cavities or pleural effusions. Comparatively, our findings of pulmonary mucormycosis in the 13 AIDS patients identified in the Guangzhou No. 8 Hospital are concluded as follows:

1. Ediastinal lymphadenopathy
2. Interlobular septal thickening
3. Infiltration lesions within lung field
4. Diffused miliary nodules
5. Pleural effusions
6. Nodular opacity

Different from the imaging findings of non-AIDS PM patients, those in the AIDS PM patients typically present diffused miliary nodules. In our research, 4 AIDS patients only contracting pulmonary mucormycosis were found to have scattered miliary nodules (about 1 mm in diameter)in the bilateral lungs, which disappeared after 1–3 weeks effective therapy. In one patient contracting the combined infections by muc-orales and mycobacteria, scattered central nodules (3–5 mm in diameter) were found in the lung and then were well absorbed after 11 days treatment, which is different from the manifestations of tuberculous mycobacteria and therefore important for the differential diagnosis of PM.

Editors: Xiaofeng Guo, Haolan He, Yan Ding, Jinxin Liu

6 Imaging findings of pulmonary cryptococcosis in AIDS

6.1 Introduction

Pulmonary cryptococcosis (PC), an invasive fungal infection (IFI), is caused by the infections of *Cryptococcus neoformans*. *Cryptococcus* includes 37 categories and 8 varieties, among which only the *Cryptococcus neoformans* are pathogenic by most probably invading into human skin and respiratory tract. The neoformans have more affinity to central system, followed by skin and lung. It is reported that they affect lung at the rate of 20%, which is closely relevant to the conditions of the host immune system. Clinically, the external manifestations of PC are more severe than the internal ones. The high risk population PC may affect includes: 1. AIDS patients, taking up 6% to 10%; 2. long-term use of adrenal cortical hormone; 3. organ/cell recipients; 4. malignant cancer patients; 5. diabetic patients; 6. sarcoidosis patients and 7. those with chronic pulmonary diseases. They present nonspecific manifestations and symptoms of various severities clinically. AIDS patients with PC, however, may have high fever, tachypnea, hypoxemia but no thick foul sputum at coughing.

Diagnosis of PC is based on detection and isolation of cryptococcus from a pulmonary specimen (Color Figure 6.0), coupled with appropriate clinical and radiological findings.

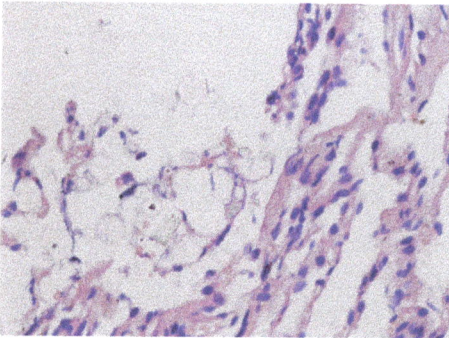

Fig. 6.0: Pulmonary cryptococcosis, HE stain, ×400.

6.2 Image findings

Case 6.1 (Fig. 6.1 a–n)

A 31-year-old male presented with productive cough for 20 days, occasionally accompanied with hemoptysisa, fever for 2 days (up to 39 °C). He responded well to the anti-bacteria drugs and the antitussive treatment before admission. CD4+ cell counted: 261/μl, CD4+/CD8+: 0.21. Bronchoalveolar lavage fluid (BALF) culture: cryptococcus, Diagnosis: AIDS (C3) with pulmonary cryptococcosis.

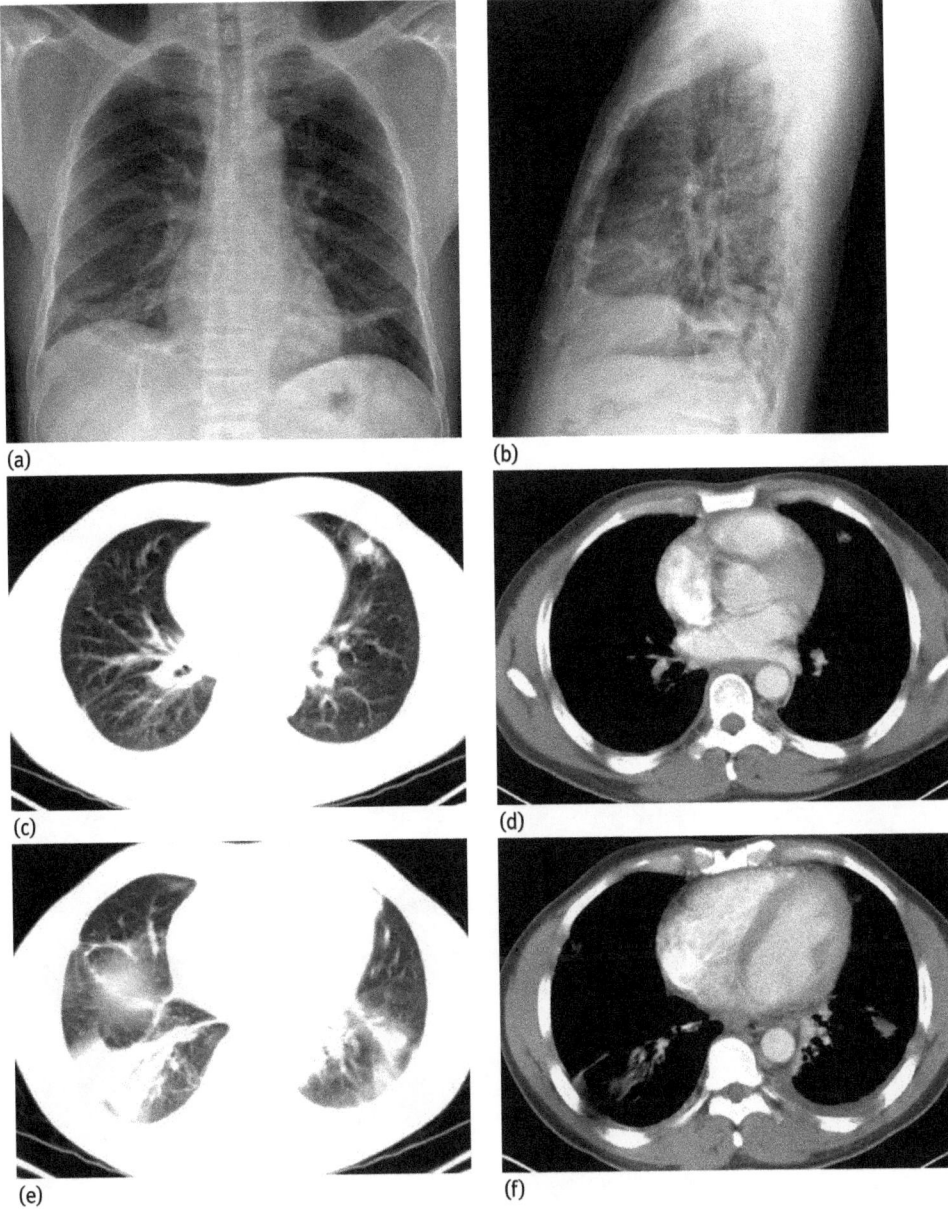

Fig. 6.1 a–n: Pulmonary cryptococcosis.

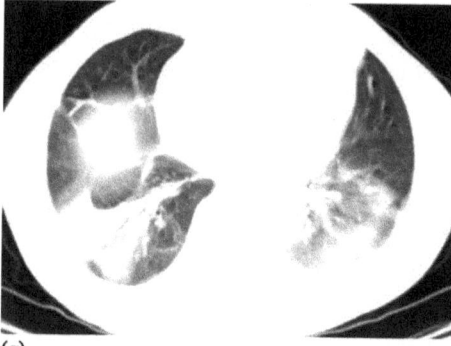

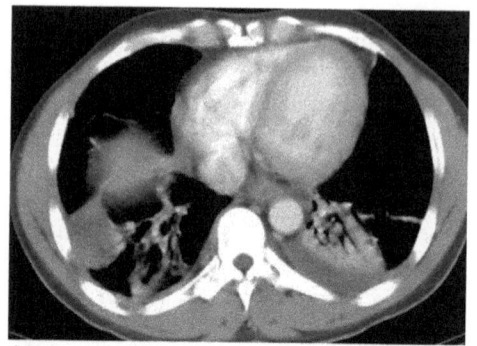

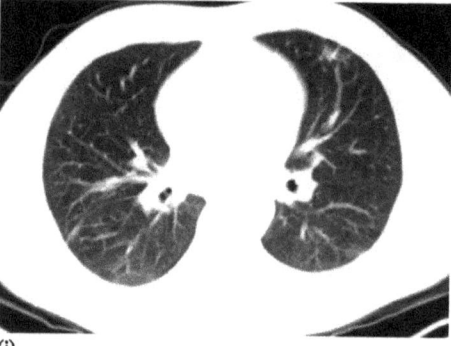

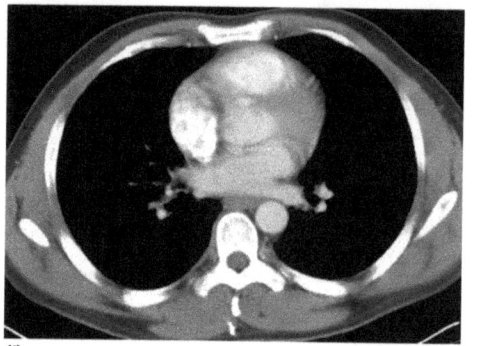

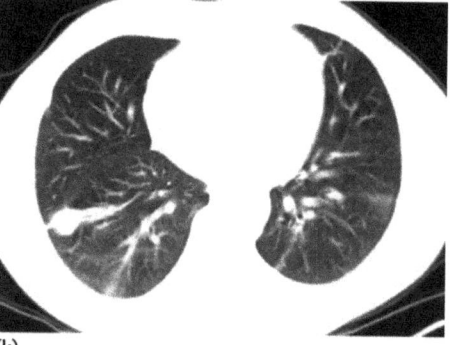

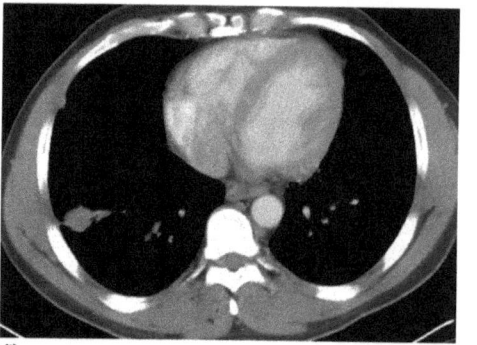

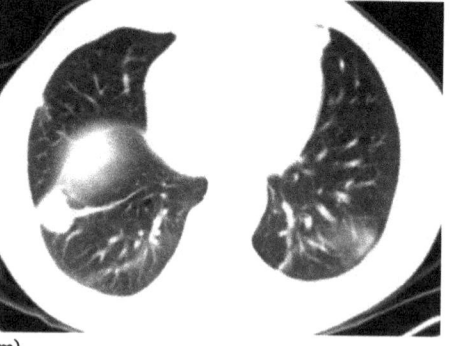

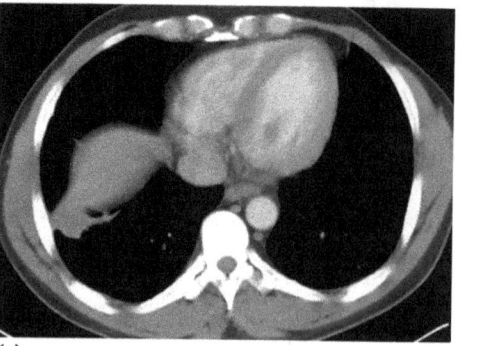

Fig. 6.1: (continuing)

The chest radiogragh demonstrated multiple high-density patchy opacities in the lower lobes of bilateral lungs (a). The radiograph of lateral projection demonstrated transversal stripy high-density shadows in the left lower lung as well as blunted posterior costophrenic angle in the bilateral lungs (b). The CT scans with lung and mediastinal window demonstrated high-density patchy shadows on lingual segment of upper lobe of left lungand the bilateral lower lobes, presenting pulmonary segmental consolidation (c–h). After treatment for 6 weeks, the lesions of bilateral lungs were remarkably absorbed in spite of a few stripy fibrous opacities remained, the bilateral pleural effusions were completely absorbed (i–n).

Case 6.2 (Fig. 6.2 a–f)

A 45-year-old female presented with cough and skin rash for 4 months, headache and vomit for half a month. Signs of meningeal irritation were positive (neck rigidity). CD4+ cell counted: 4/µl, CD4+/CD8+: 0.01. Cerebrospinal fluid (CSF) smear: *cryptococcus* positive (India ink stain). Culture of blood and bone marrow grew *Cryptococcus neoformans*. Diagnosis: AIDS (C3) with disseminated cryptococcosis.

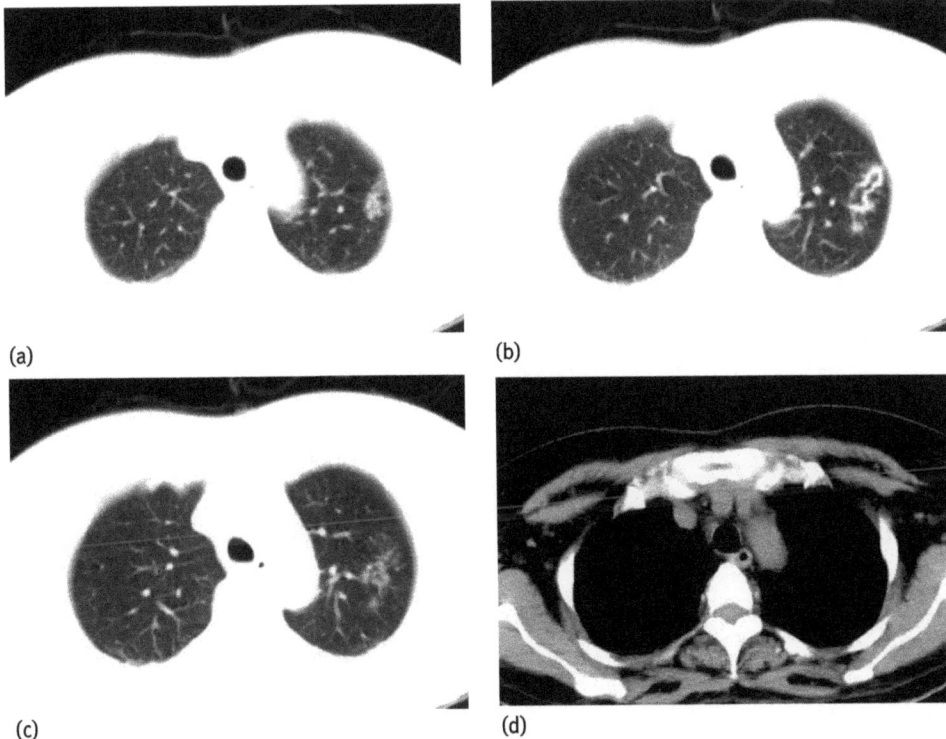

(a)

(b)

(c)

(d)

Fig. 6.2 a–f: Disseminated cryptococcosis.

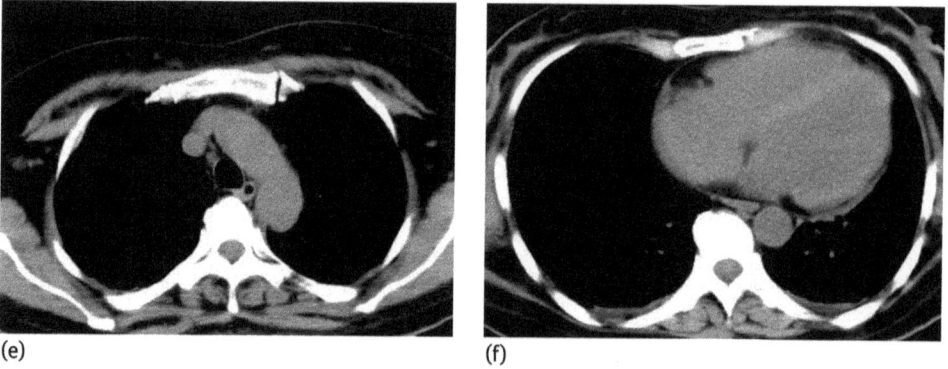

(e)   (f)

Fig. 6.2: (continuing)

Chest CT scan with lung window demonstrated the irregular nodules in the apicoposterior segment of the left upper lobe, the thin-walled irregular cavities and small stripy shadows and small burry nodules around them (a–c). The CT scans with mediastinal window demonstrated no enlarged mediastinal lymph nodes (d–e) and a few pericardial effusion and pleural effusion in both sides (f).

Case 6.3 (Fig. 6.3 a–j)

A 39-year-old female presented with irregular fever (up to 38.6 °C) with chilly and paroxysmal headache (more conspicuous of forehead) without any reason for half a month. She did not experience improvement of symptoms at hospital discharge at local hospital. 6 days ago before hospitalized, she presented with non-projectile and non-coffee ground vomiting without hematemesis for 3–8 times a day. CD4+ cell counted: 7/μl, CD4+/CD8+: 0.03. Smear and culture of cerebrospinal fluid (CSF): *Cryptococcus neoformans*. Cultures of blood and bone marrow also grew *Cryptococcus neoformans*. Diagnosis: AIDS (C3) with disseminated cryptococcosis.

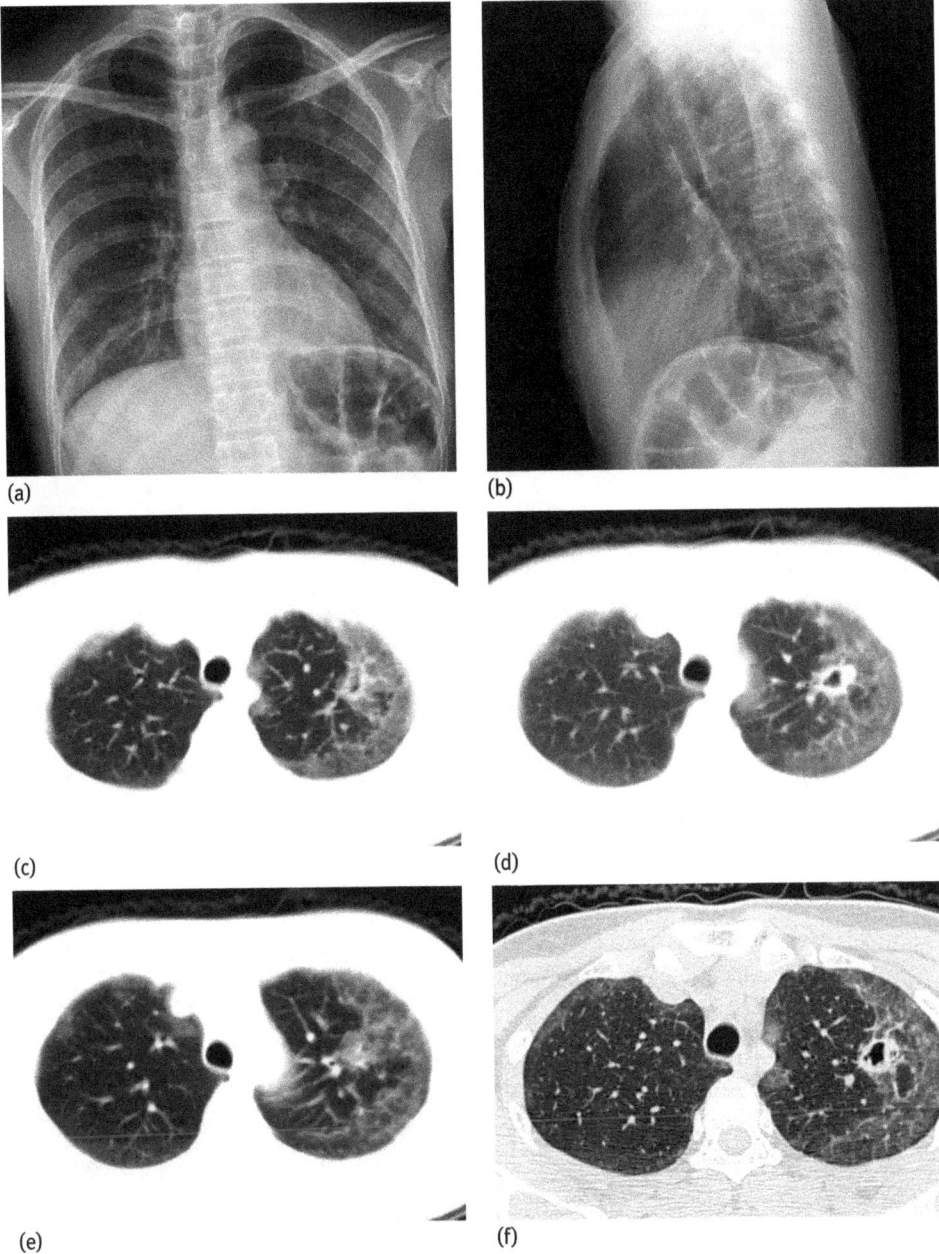

Fig. 6.3 a–j: Disseminated cryptococcosis. The chest radiograghs demonstrated the reduced translucence of pulmonary field, especially on the upper lung, and an ill-defined nodule on the first anterior intercostals space of the left upper lung (a, b). CT scan with lung window and HRCT demonstrated the irregular cavity and high-density ground-glass-like patchy opacity in the left upper lung, mild ground-glass-like opacity in the right upper lung (c–g). CT scan with mediastinal window revealed the enlarged paratracheal and subaortic lymph nodes (h–j).

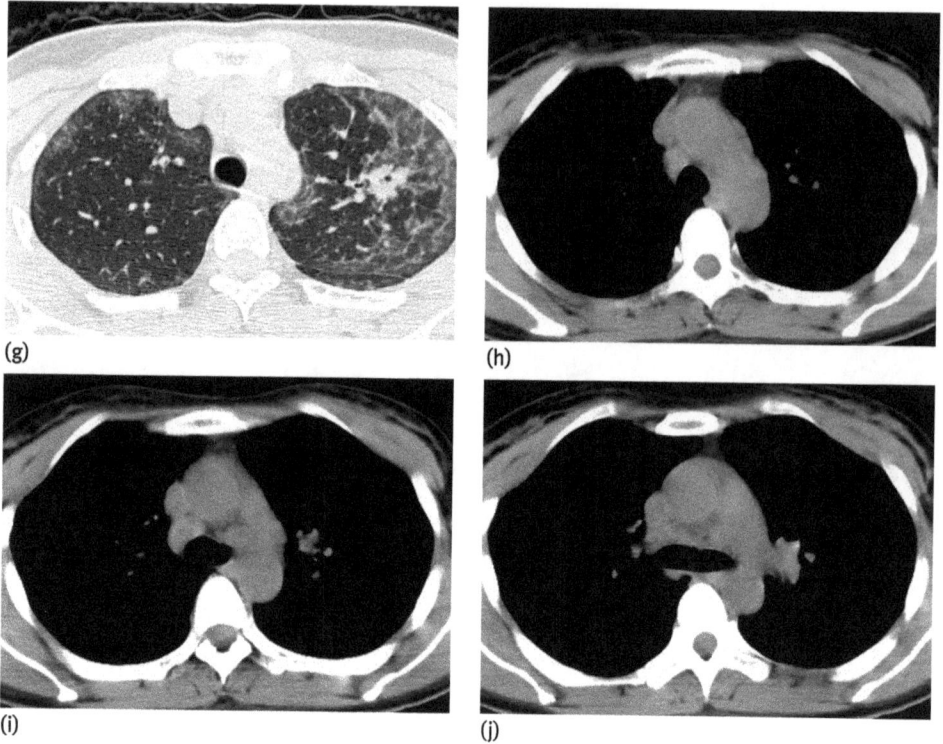

(g)

(h)

(i)

(j)

Fig. 6.3: (continuing)

6.3 Imaging features

The image findings of pulmonary cryptococcosis in AIDS patients are characterized by the variety. In radiography, the findings generally include:

1. Lung interstitial changes involved predominantly, usually widespread and proceeding rapidly, presenting as ground-glass attenuation and small nodules.
2. multiple infiltration of lung parenchyma.
3. Cavities: the inner wall of the cavity is always smooth, and high incidence of cavity is likely to be a characteristic performance of pulmonary cryptococcosis in AIDS.
4. pleural effusions usually associated with subpleural nodules.
5. enlargement of hilar lymph nodes similar with hilar tuberlulous lymphadenitis, but without calcification.
6. nodular masses that usually located subpleural, with a variety of size, well-defined or ill-defined or with short burrs.

Editors: Wanshan Chen, Bihua Chen, Yan Ding, Fuchun Zhang

7 Imaging features of penicilliosis marneffei in AIDS

7.1 Introduction

Penicilliosis marneffei (PSM) is an opportunistic infection caused by *Penicillium marneffei* (PM) in immunocompromised individuals, especially the AIDS patients, in Southeast Asia and Southern China.

The first case of effuse PSM in lymphoma patients was reported in 1973. Since then, more and more PSM cases have been reported across the world. Right now, AIDS patients contract PSM by 85% so that it is identified as a specific indicator of AIDS clinically. In recent years, the identified PSM cases increase in Guangdong province, China, at a very fast speed, only because PM is a major pathogen for opportunistic infections due to the humid and warm weather in Guangdong.

In mycology, PM is the only dimorphic fungus in the genus of penicillium. It exists in mycelial form at 25°–30 °C but yeast form at 35°–37 °C and produce red diffusible pigment which stains the PM culture in typical color of red wind. Microscopically, fruiting structures are found at 25°–30 °C. The definite identification of PSM in AIDS patients requires mycological testing on cultures of the organism from skin aspirates, blood, sputum, or fine needle aspirate/biopsy materials (Color figure 7.0 a–c).

Pathologically, PM usually invades into the mononuclear phagocytic system and presents the manifestations in three histological forms, e. g., granuloma, abscesses like skin pustules and multiple lung abscesses, and weak reaction or even necrotic reaction.

Clinically, the AIDS patients with PSM may have fever, weight loss, cough, sputum aspiration, shortness of breath, anemia, and diarrhea. In most cases, the fever is remittent or irregular, often combined with chills but no shivering as well as weight loss.

For PSM patients, skin lesions are specific. 50%–75% of the patients have skin lesions such as subcutaneous abscesses and papule-like ulcers distributed mainly at face, trunk of a body and limbs (Color figure 7.0 d). The skin between the lesions is normal with mild itching. 40% of the patients have hepatosplenomegaly and lymphadenopathy.

In AIDS patients with PSM, the CD4+ lymph cell count is extremely low, less than 50/μl in most of them.

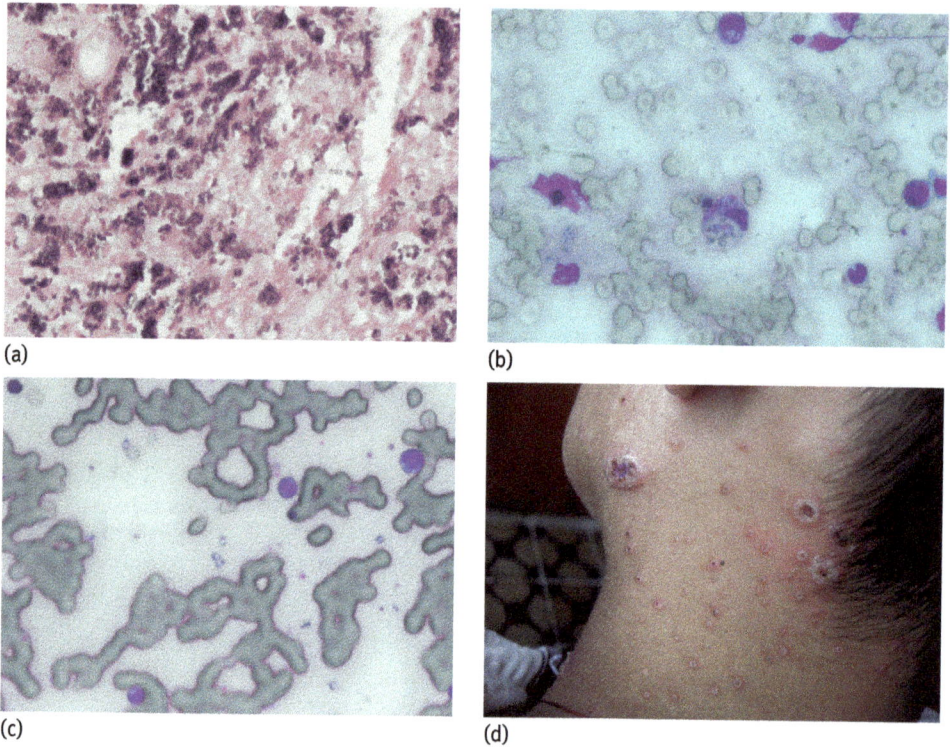

Fig. 7.0: Lung biopsy P. marneffei, hexamine silver staining, ×400 (aA). Bone marrow P. marneffei, Wright-Giemsa's staining, ×400 (b). Blood smear P. marneffei, Wright-Giemsa's staining, ×400 (c) Umbilical concave necrotic papulae (d).

7.2 Image findings

Case 7.1 (Fig. 7.1 a–e)

A 38-year-old female presented with hypodynamia and skin rash for 9 days.The patient was a 38-year-old female. She had hypodynamia and skin rashes for 9 days. Body temperature at admission was 36.5 °C. On examination, there were herpes zosters on the right side of the chest and on the back but without ulceration. There were no enlargements of the systemic superficial lymph nodes. The breath sounds of the bilateral lungs were slightly rough but without dry or moist rales. The CD4+ cell count was 63/μL. Blood culture was PM positive. Diagnosis: AIDS (C3) complicated with PSM.

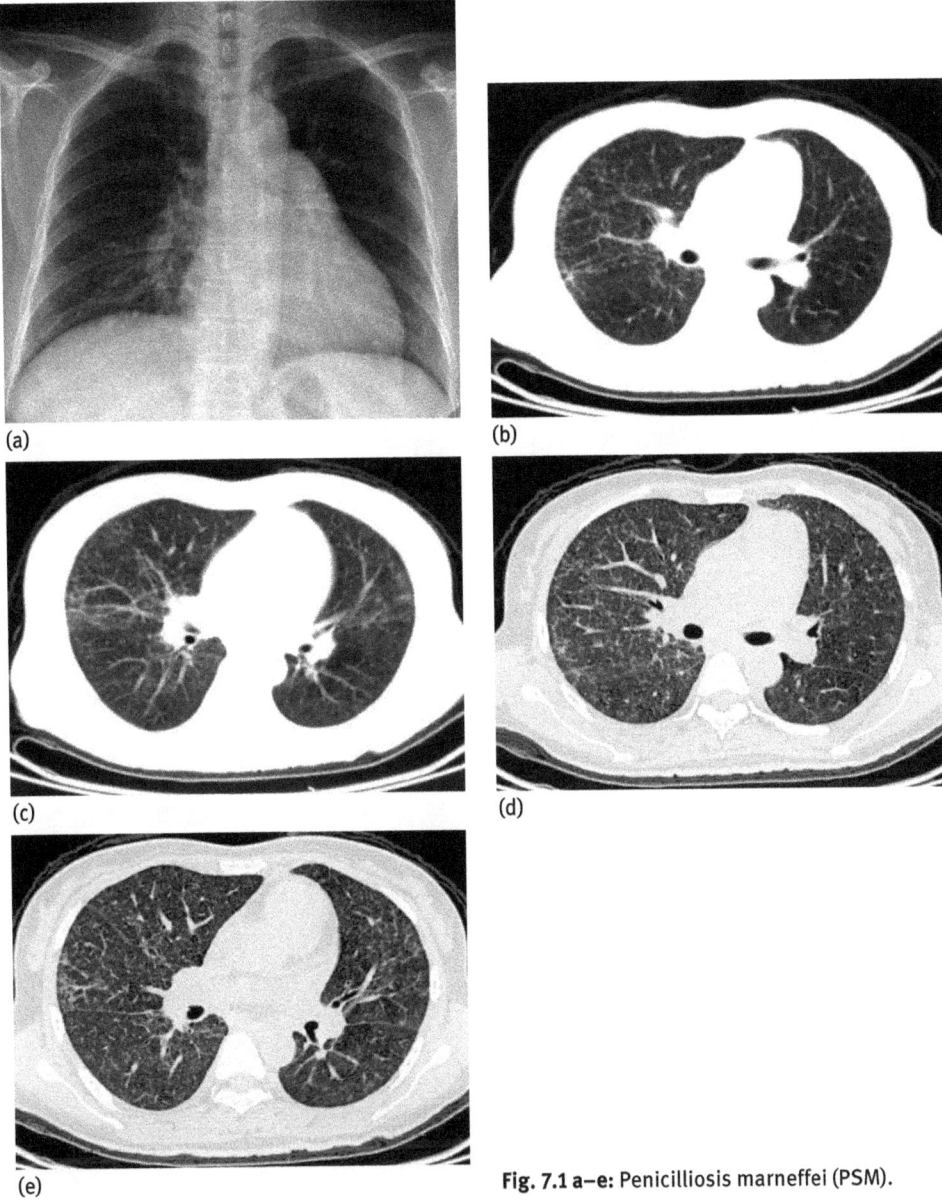

Fig. 7.1 a–e: Penicilliosis marneffei (PSM).

The chest radiograph revealed increasing, thickened and disordered markings in the lung (a). CT scan demonstrated reticular markings in the lung (b, c). HRCT demonstrated the thickened interlobular septa (d, e).

Case 7.2 (Fig. 7.2 a–e)

A 30-year-old female presented with fever, cough and dyspnea for 2weeks. Her body temperature at admission was 39.5 °C. On examination, there were no bean-curd-like materials on the surface of the tongue and no hairy leukoplakia on either side of the tongue. The enlarged lymph nodes were palpable in the bilateral inguinal fold. The bilateral lung sounds were rough but with no dry or moist rales. The CD4+ cell count was 4/μL. Blood culture was PM positive. Diagnosis: AIDS (C3) complicated with PSM.

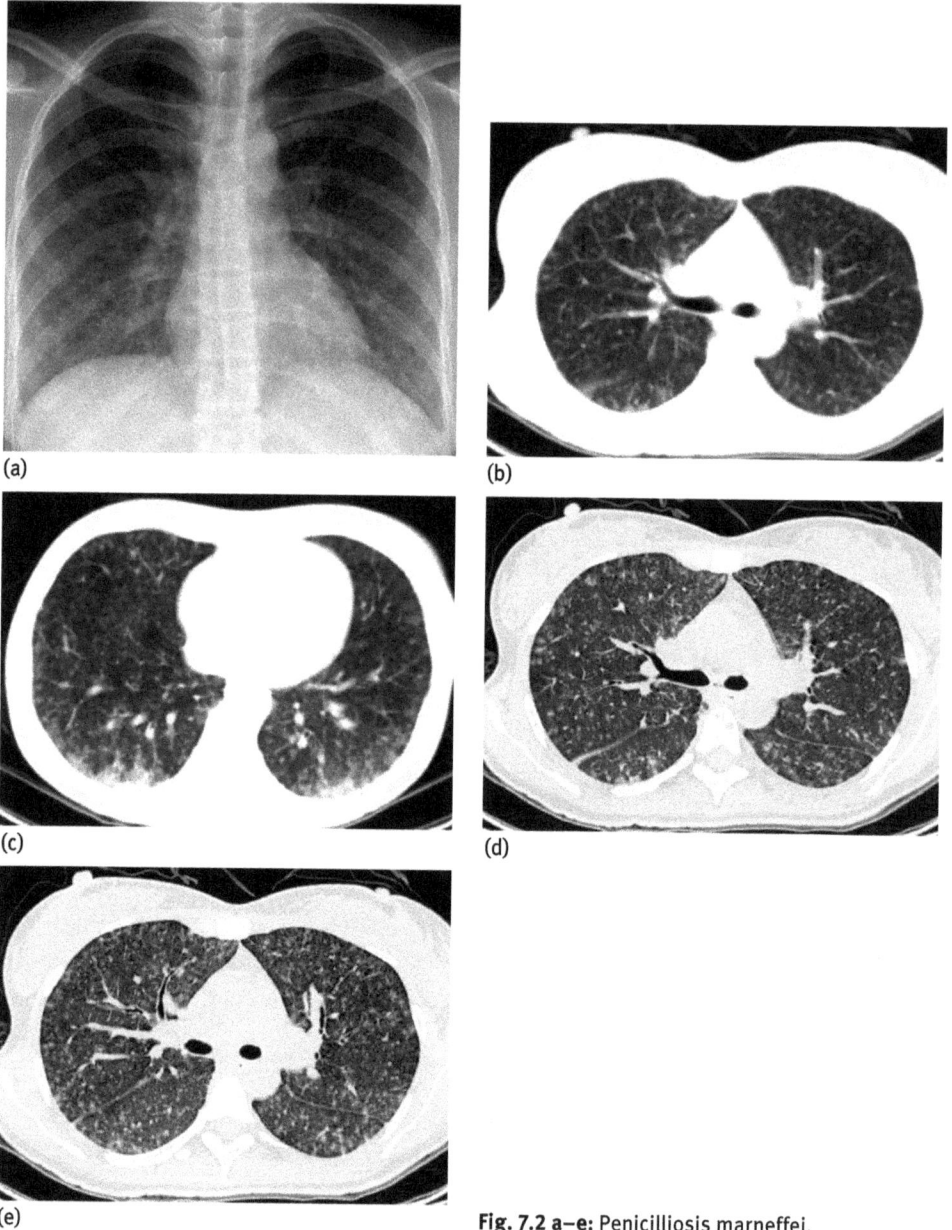

(a)

(b)

(c)

(d)

(e)

Fig. 7.2 a–e: Penicilliosis marneffei.

The chest radiograph demonstrated the reticular markings and miliary lesions in both lungs and multiple lesions in the lower lungs (a). CT scan (b, c) and HRCT scan (d, e) both showed miliary lesions in the lung, and ill-defined high-density small patchy shadows in the posterior basal segment of the lung.

Case 7.3 (Fig. 7.3 a–l)

A 42-year-old male presented with fever (between 38 °C–40 °C) with no apparent cause and cough for 2 months. His cervical tumors were found one month ago. Body temperature at admission was 39.5 °C. There were bean-curd-like materials on the surface and hairy leukoplakia on both sides of the tongue. The lymph nodes in the bilateral neck, armpit, supraclavicular fossa and groin were enlarged and palpable. The bilateral lung sounds were rough but without dry or moist rales. The CD4+ cell count was 13/μL. Culture of bone marrow was PM positive. Diagnosis: AIDS (C3) complicated with PSM.

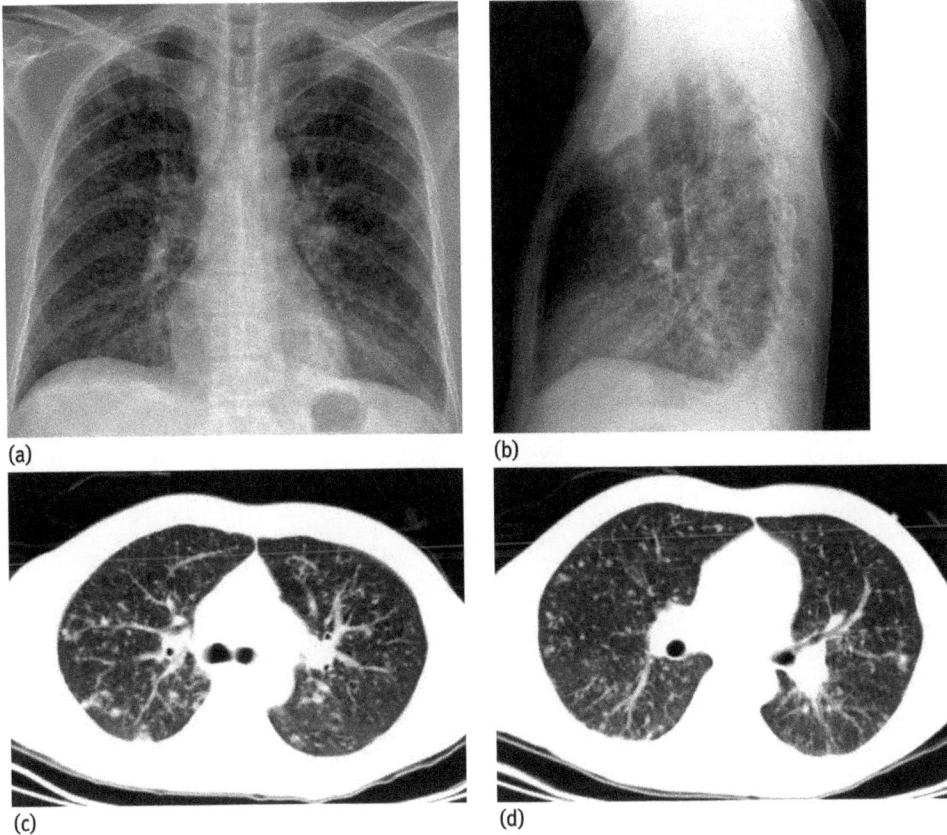

(a)

(b)

(c)

(d)

Fig. 7.3 a–l: Penicilliosis marneffei.

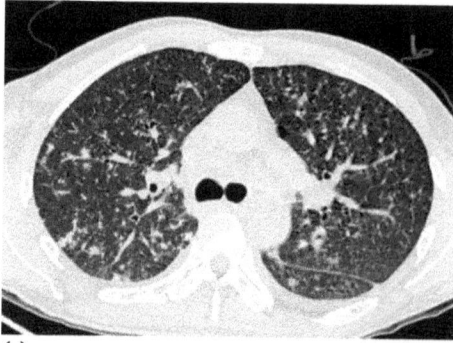
(e)

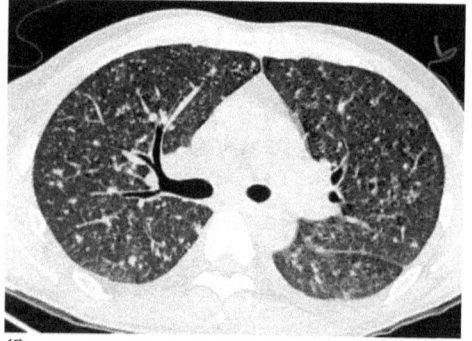
(f)

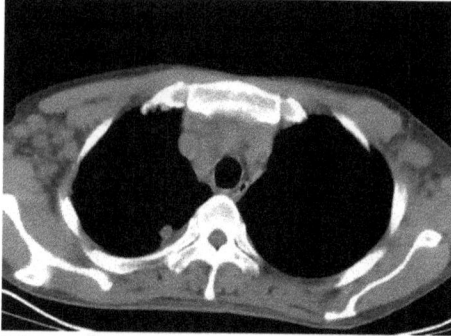
(g)

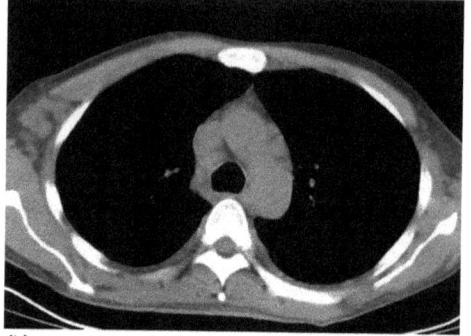
(h)

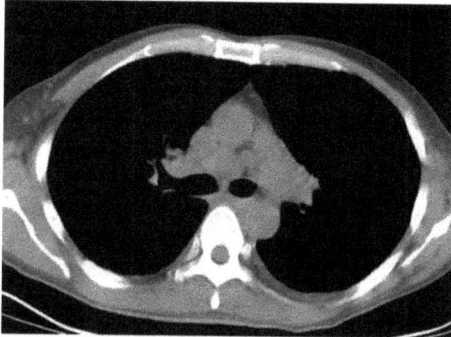
(i)

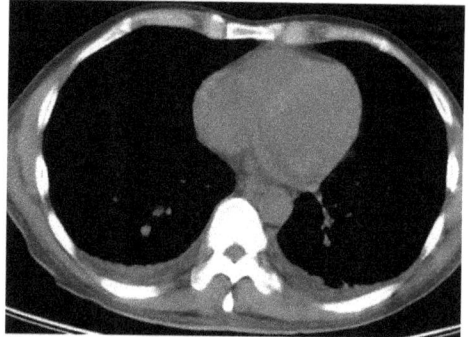
(j)

Fig. 7.3: (continuing)

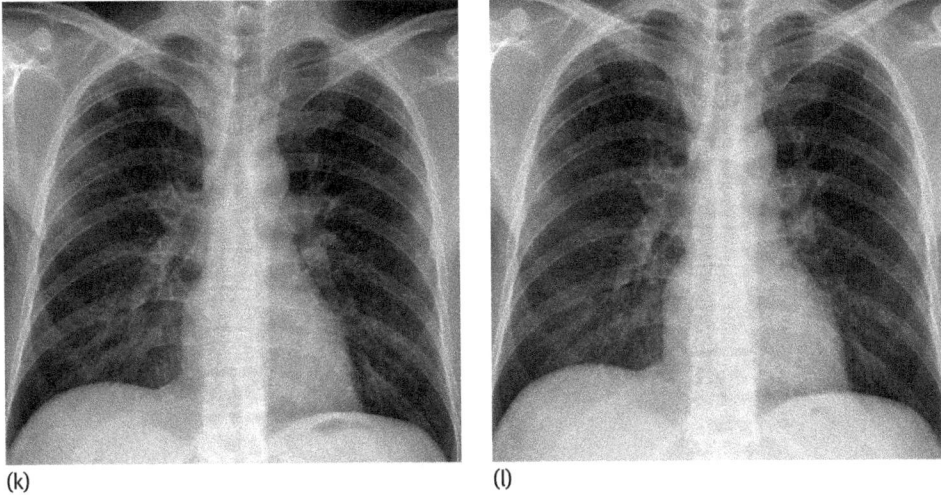

(k)   (l)

Fig. 7.3: (continuing)

The chest radiograph demonstrated the reticular markings, widely-but-unevenly distributed miliary lesions of different sizes and a few effusions in the bilateral lungs (a, b). CT scan showed the same findings as in the chest radiographs (c, d). HRCT scan demonstrated the thickened interlobular septa (e, f). CT scan with mediastinal window (g, j) demonstrated widespread lymphadenectasis (g–i) and a few pleural effusions in the bilateral thoracic cavity (i–j). After 3 weeks therapy, the lesions of lung were significantly absorbed in the bilateral lungs as showed in the chest radiograph (k) and after 11 weeks therapy, they were fundamentally absorbed as showed in the chest radiograph (l) .

Case 7.4 (Fig. 7.4 a–g)

A 31-year-old male presented with recurrent fever for six months and headache for one week. Body temperature at admission was 38.2 °C. There were bean-curd-like materials on the surface and hairy leukoplakia on the side of the tongue. There was no systemic enlargement of the lymph nodes. The bilateral lung sounds were rough but without moist or dry rales. The CD4+ cell count was 13/μL. Culture of bone marrow was PM positive. Diagnosis: AIDS (C3) complicated with PSM.

The chest radiograph revealed reticular markings in the lung and the effuse miliary lesions gradually increasing from superior to inferior in the lung (a), which are confirmed on CT scans (b–c). HRCT scan demonstrated pneumathodes in the superior lingular segment of left lung (d). After 11 days therapy, the markings became limpid and the miliary lesions were significantly reduced in the lung as showed in the chest radiograph (f). After 23 days therapy the lesions in the lung were completely absorbed as showed in the chest radiograph (g).

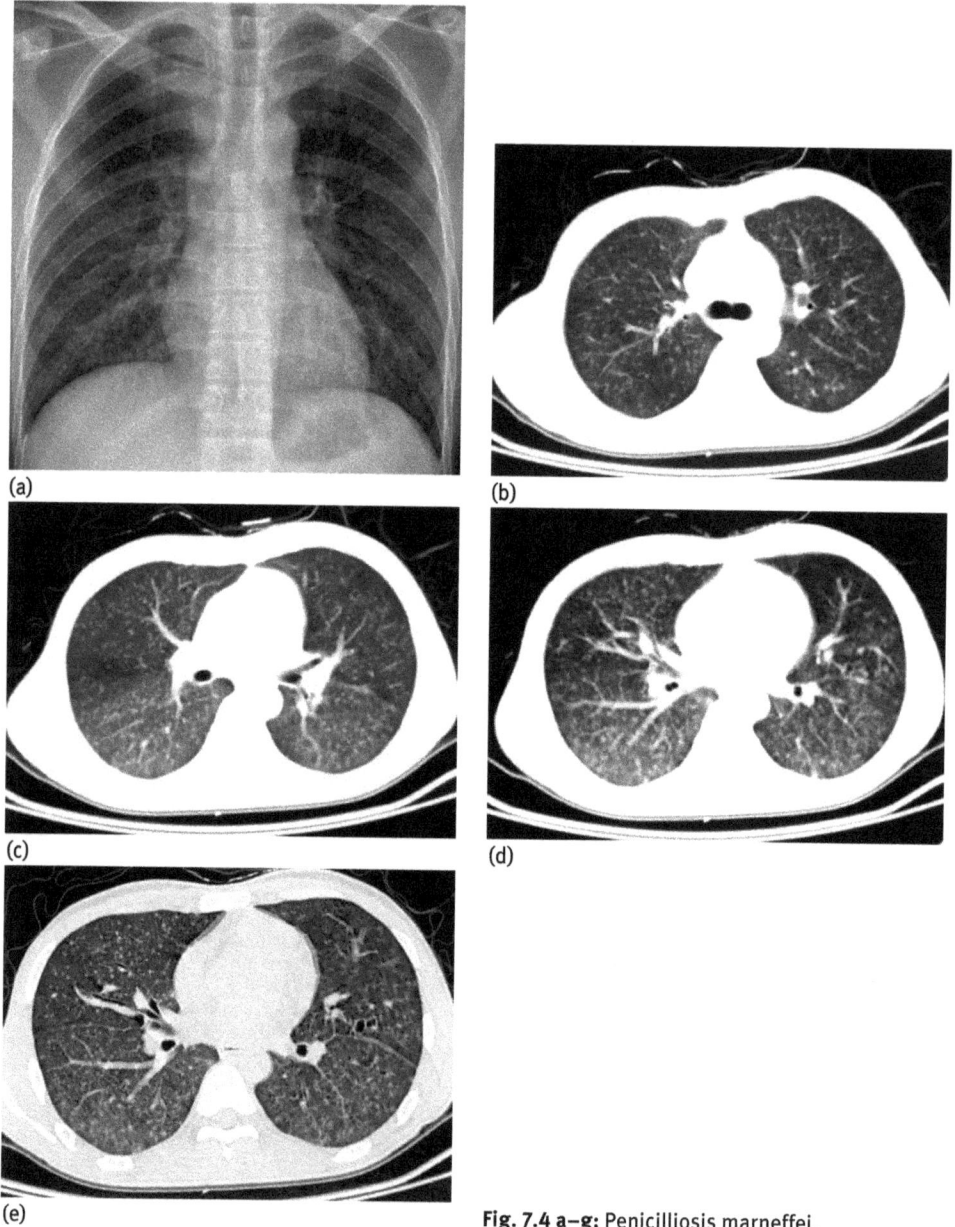

(a)

(b)

(c)

(d)

(e)

Fig. 7.4 a–g: Penicilliosis marneffei.

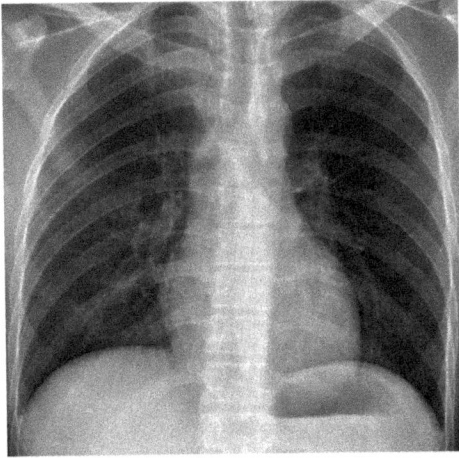

(f)

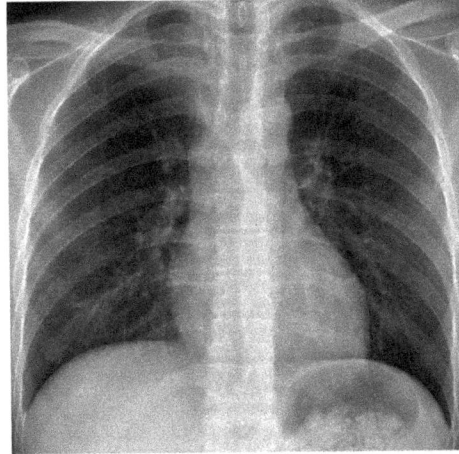

(g)

Fig. 7.4: (continuing)

Case 7.5 (Fig. 7.5 a–k)

A 30-year-old male presented with irregular fever (up to 39.7 °C) with chilly but no rigor for 3 months, accompanied with productive cough. Body temperature at admission was 38.2 °C. There were bean-curd-like materials on the surface and hairy leukoplakia on the sides of the tongue. There was no systemic enlargement of the lymph nodes. The bilateral lung sounds were clear on percussion with slight moist rales in the lower part and the breath sounds were rough. The CD4+ cell count was 7/μL. The fibrobronchoscopy test of specimen from lung biopsy was PM positive. Diagnosis: AIDS (C3) complicated with PSM.

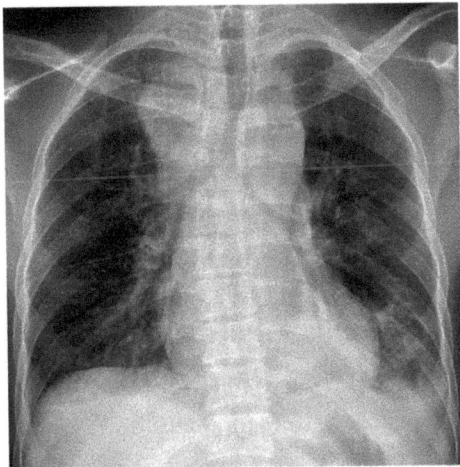

(a)

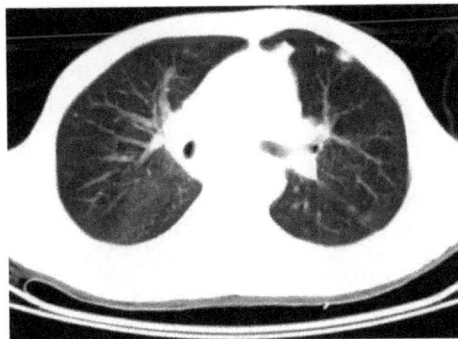

(b)

Fig. 7.5 a–k: Penicilliosis marneffei.

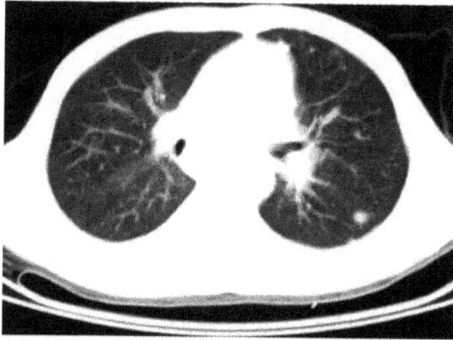
(c)

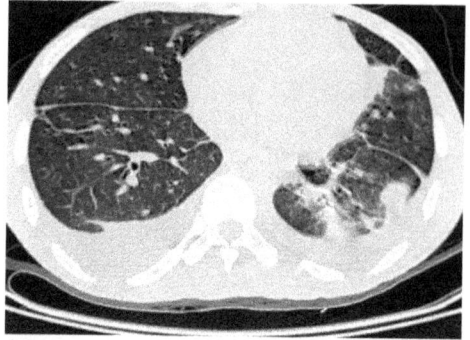
(d)

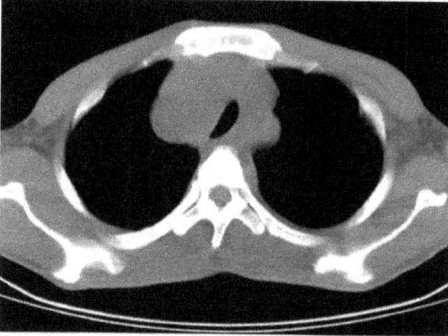
(e)

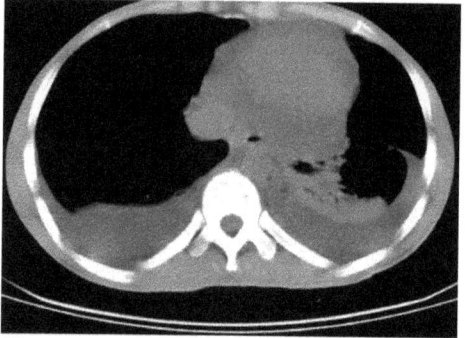
(f)

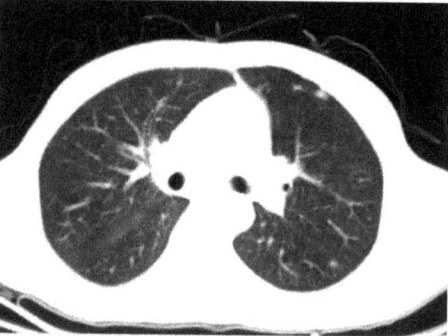
(g)

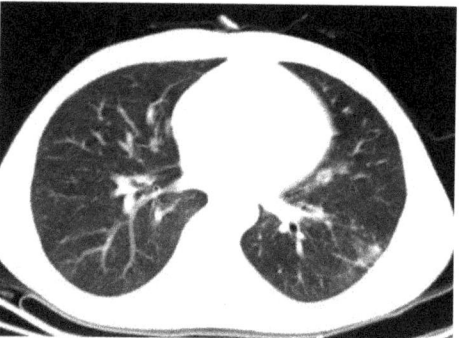
(h)

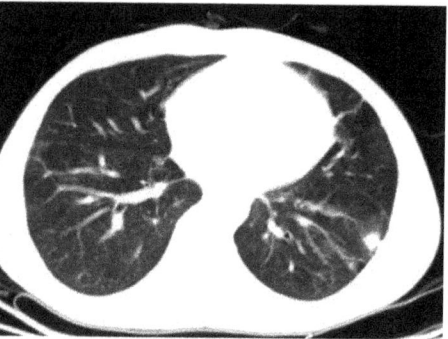
(i)

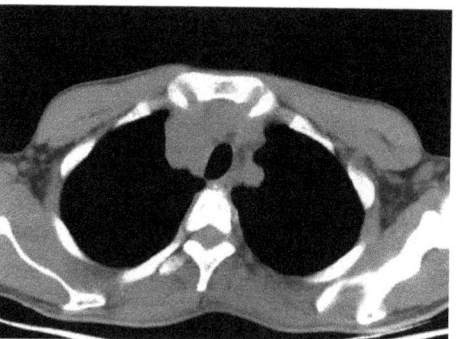
(j)

Fig. 7.5: (continuing)

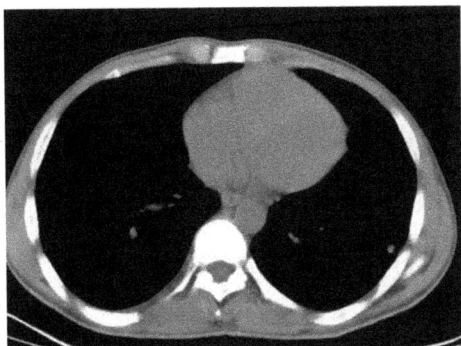

(k)   **Fig. 7.5:** (continuing)

The chest radiograph showed reticular markings in the lung, ill-defined patchy dense shadows with blurring edges in the left lower lung, slight hydrothorax in the left and widened mediastinum in the right (a). CT scan demonstrated small nodules in various sizes in the lung and increased patchy dense shadows in the left lower lung (b–d). CT with mediastinal window demonstrated the enlarged paratracheal lymph nodes especially in the right side, narrowed trachea by pressure (e), a few pleural effusions in the bilateral pleural cavity and compressive atelectasis in the left lower lung (f). After 2 weeks therapy, the lesions of lungs significantly shrank as showed in the CT scans (g, i), so did the enlarged paratracheal lymph nodes as showed in the scan (i) and the pleural effusions were absorbed in the bilateral cavitas thoracis as showed in the scans (j–k).

Case 7.6 (Fig. 7.6 a–k)
A 22-year-old male presented with fever (up to 39.7 °C) with slightly chilly and occasionally cough for 2 weeks. The symptoms were getting worse and accompanied with tachypnea for 4 days. Body temperature at admission was 38.5 °C. On examination, there were several green bean-sized erythematous maculopapular rashes scattered on cephal-facial and pectoral skin. The rashes were sunken in the middle and those in the cephal-facial shin had scabbed. There were bean-curd-like materials on the surface of the tongue. There was no systemic enlargement of lymph nodes. The throat was congestive, the breath was slightly fast, and the breath sounds of the bilateral lungs were rough but without dry or moist rales. The CD4+ cell count was 49/μL. Cultures of blood and bone marrow were PM positive. Diagnosis: AIDS (C3) complicated with PSM.

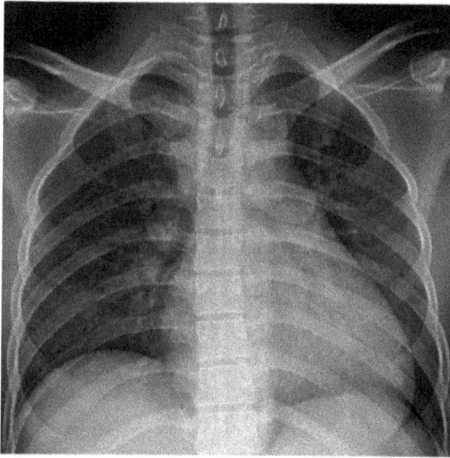
(a)

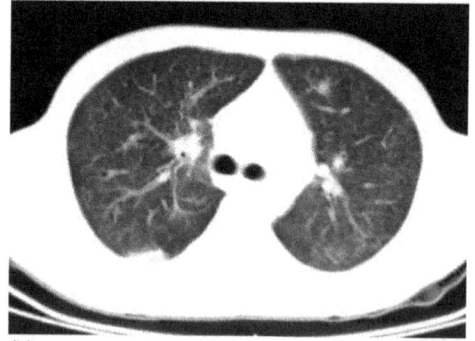
(b)

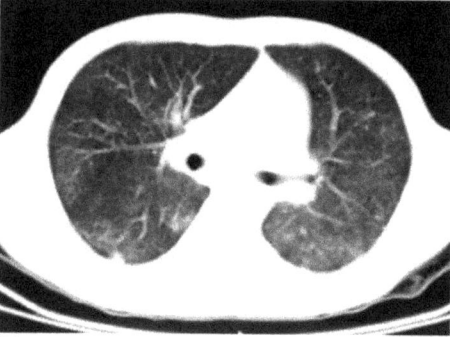
(c)

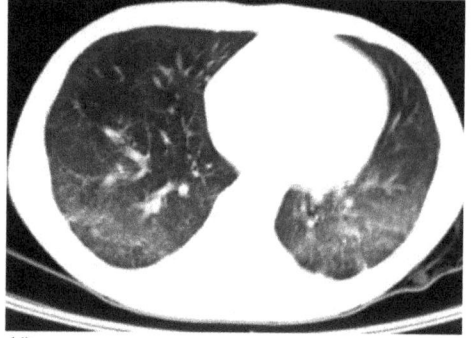
(d)

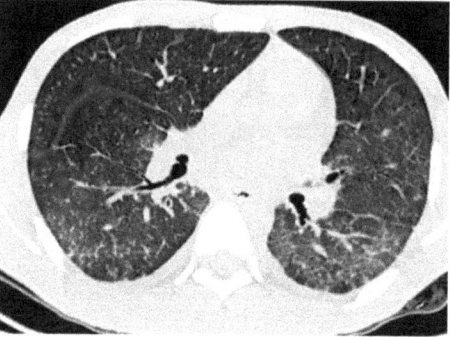
(e)

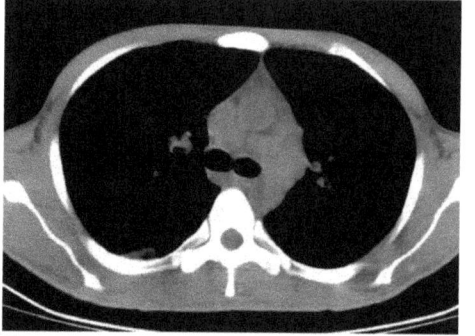
(f)

Fig. 7.6 a–k: Penicilliosis marneffei.

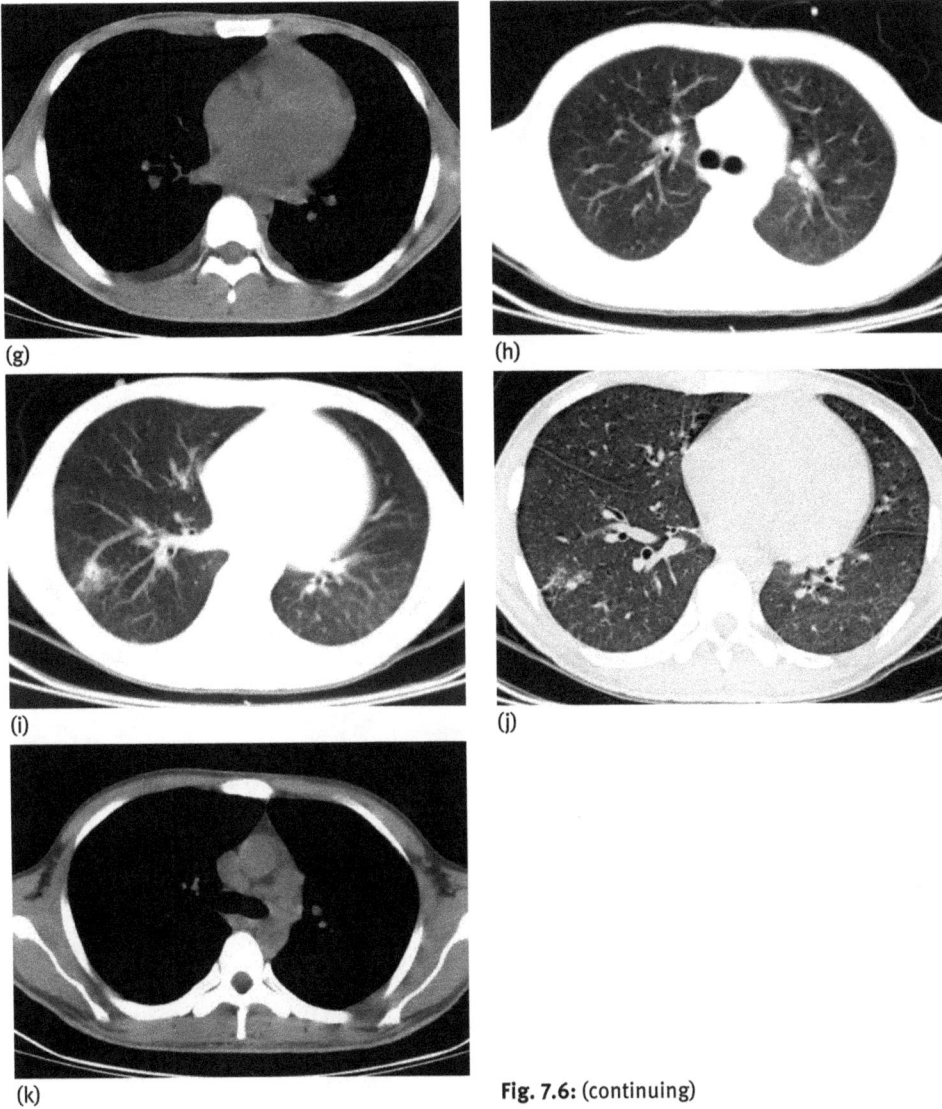

(g)

(h)

(i)

(j)

(k)

Fig. 7.6: (continuing)

The chest radiograph revealed reticular markings in the lung, high-dense patchy shadows in the bilateral lower lung and mild ground-glass-like shadow in lungs (a). This is confirmed on CT scan (b–d). HRCT scan demonstrated the thickened interlobular septa (e). CT scans with mediastinal window showed the enlarged tracheobronchial lymph nodes and slight pleural effusion (f, g). After 5 weeks therapy, the lesions in the lung were significantly decreased in number in the axial CT scans (h–i) and shrank in size as showed in the HRCT scan (j) and the enlarged tracheobronchial lymph nodes were significantly shrunken as showed in CT scan (k).

Case 7.7 (Fig. 7.7 a–e)

A 46-year-old male had a 5-month history of recurrent fever, cough and tachypnea. Body temperature at admission was 38 °C. There were enlarged lymph nodes in the bilateral upper clavicles. The bilateral breath sounds were rough but with no dry or moist rales. The CD4+ cell count was 2/µL. Cultures of blood, bone marrow and bronchoalveolar lavage fluid (BALF) were PM positive. Diagnosis: AIDS (C3) complicated with PSM.

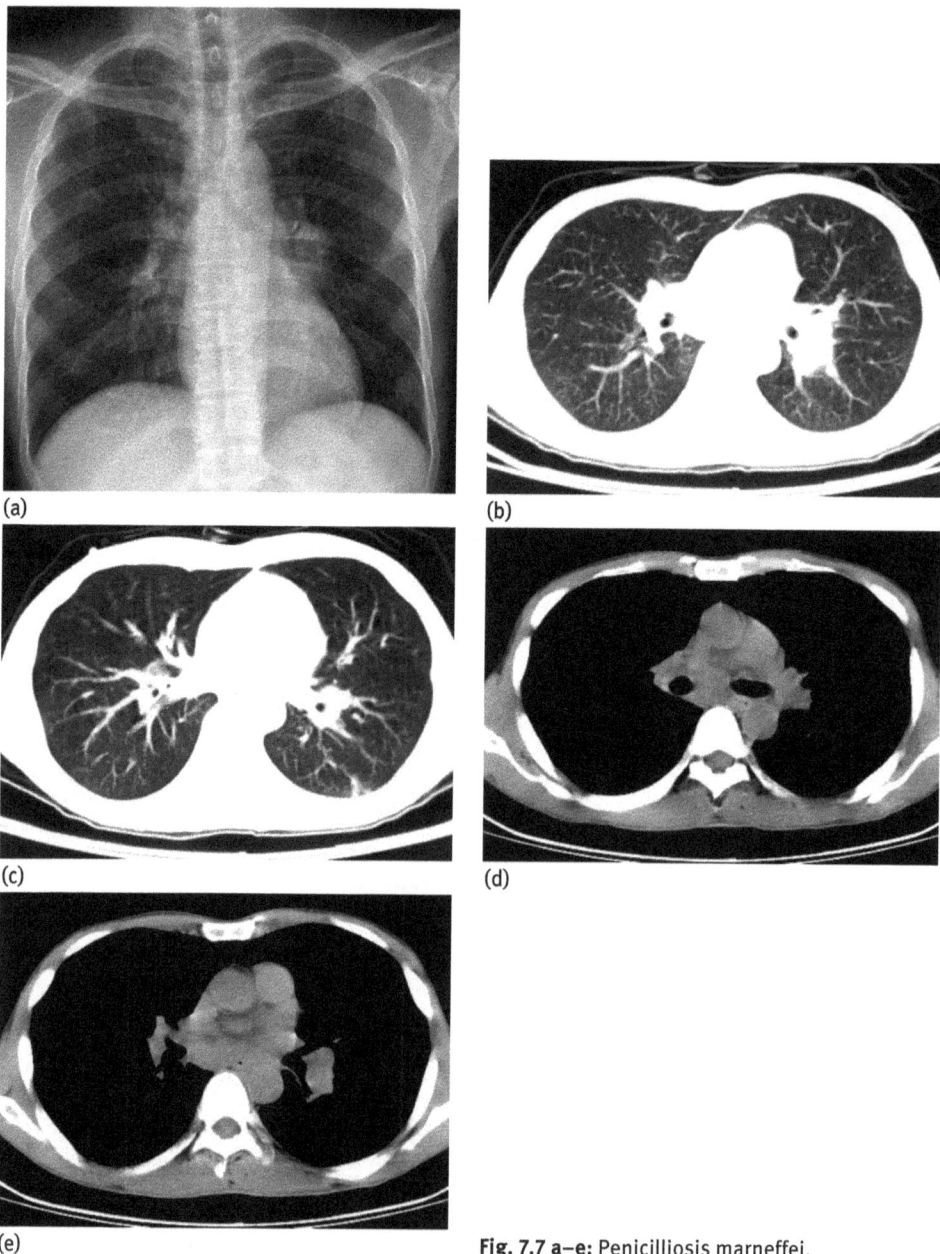

(a)

(b)

(c)

(d)

(e)

Fig. 7.7 a–e: Penicilliosis marneffei.

The chest radiograph revealed the enlarged left hilar shadow (a). Chest CT confirmed the hilar enlargement of left lung (b) and showed small nodular foci in the left posterior basal segment of the lung (c). CT scan with mediastinal window demonstrated lymphadenectasis in the mediastina and hilum of left lung (d, e).

Case 7.8 (Fig. 7.8a–e)

A 48-year-old male had a 1-month history of recurrent fever and bellyache. Body temperature at admission was 38.6 °C. On examination, the enlarged cervical lymph nodes were palpable. The sounds of bilateral lungs were clear on percussion and the breath sounds were diminished but without no dry or moist rales. The CD4+ cell count was 4/μL. Cultures of bone marrow and BALF were PM positive. Diagnosis: AIDS (C3) complicated by PSM.

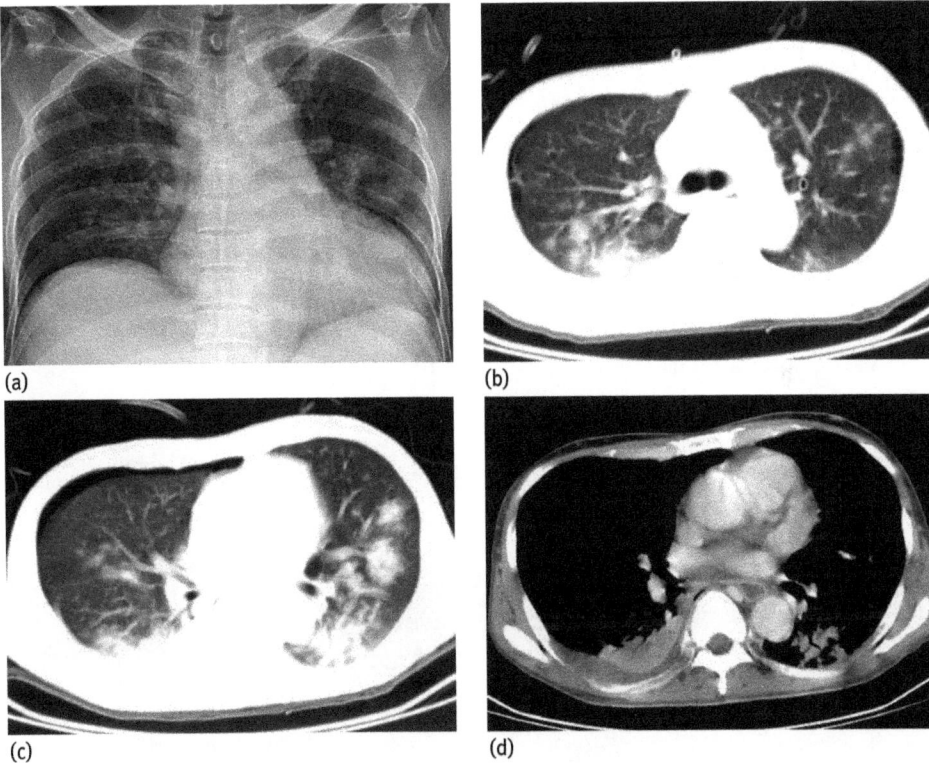

(a) (b) (c) (d)

Fig. 7.8 a–e: Penicilliosis marneffei.

The chest radiograph revealed patchy dense shadows in the bilateral lungs, slight pneumothorax in the right lung and the enlarged cardiac shadow (a). CT scan showed multiple high-density patchy opacities of different sizes with blurring edge, paraseptal emphysema of left upper lung and pneumothorax in the right lung (b, c). CT scan

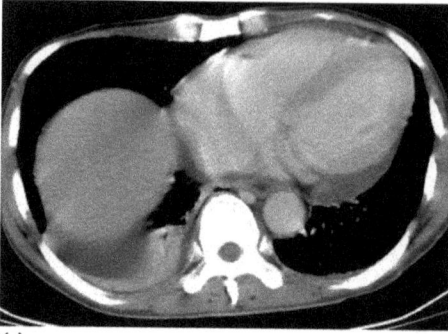

(e)   **Fig. 7.8:** (continuing)

with mediastinal window demonstrated the right-sided pleural effusion, a few peri-cardial effusions and compressed atelectasis in the posterior basal segment of right lung (d, e).

Case 7.9 (Fig. 7.9 a–j)

A 38-year-old male who had weight loss for four months, occurred fever four days ago with temperature up to 40 °C, complicated with slight chills and shivering.Body temperature at admission was 40 °C. On examination, there was white membranoid substance on the mucous membrante of mouth. The lymph nodes behind the ears, in the submaxillary, cervical and left supraclavicular fossa were enlarged. The breath sounds of the bilateral lungs were clear with no dry or moist rales. The CD4+ cell count was 56/μL. Cultures of bone marrow and sputum were PM positive. Diagnosis: AIDS (C3) complicated by PSM.

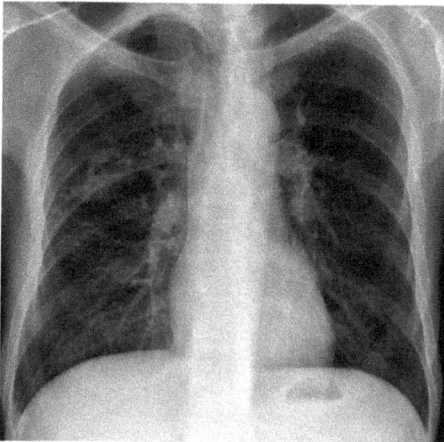
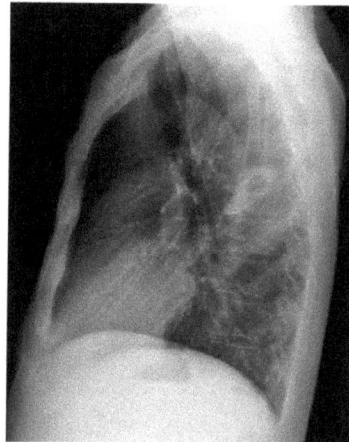

(a)   (b)

Fig. 7.9 a–j: Penicilliosis marneffei.

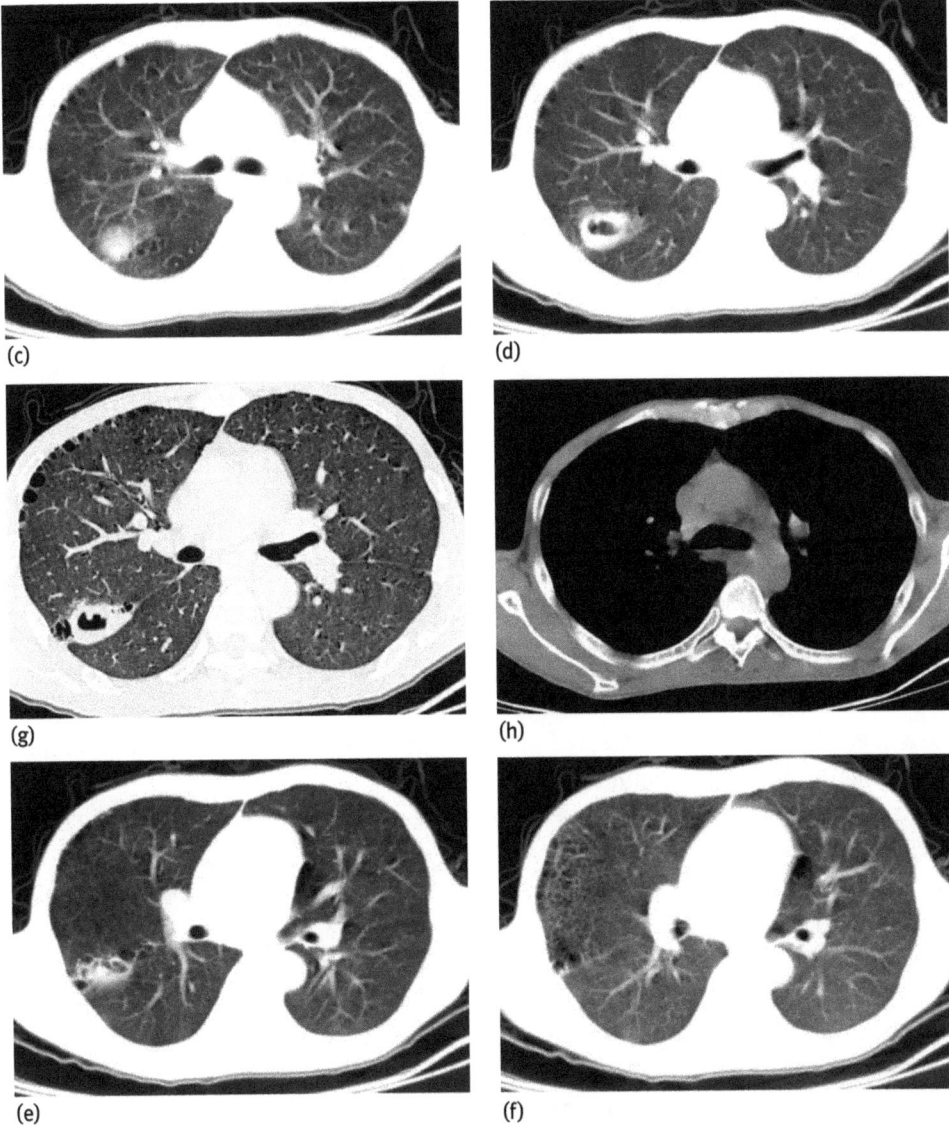

Fig. 7.9: (continuing)

The chest radiographs revealed nodular foci in the posterior segment of right superior lobe lung and irregularly-walled cavities (a, b). CT scan with lung window (c–f) together with HRCT scan (g) demonstrated the nodular foci surrounded by multiple thin-walled cavities, cavities in the lesions and liquid-air interfaces in the cavities in the posterior segment of the right superior lobe, a few small nodular foci in the bilateral lungs, and subpleural paraseptal emphysema in the right upper lung. CT scan with mediastinal window showed mediastinal lymphadenectasis (h). After 4 weeks treatment, the foci in the right upper lung were evidently absorbed and the cavities disappeared as showed in the chest radiograph (i). After 8 weeks therapy, the foci in the right upper lung were further absorbed as showed in the chest radiograph (j).

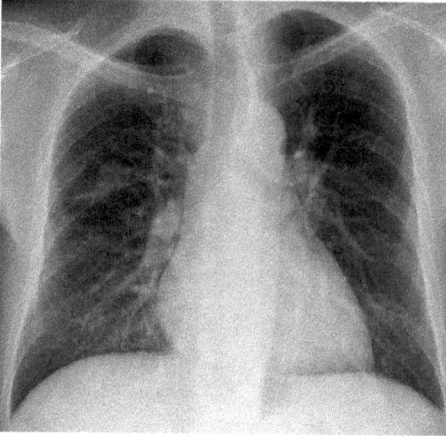 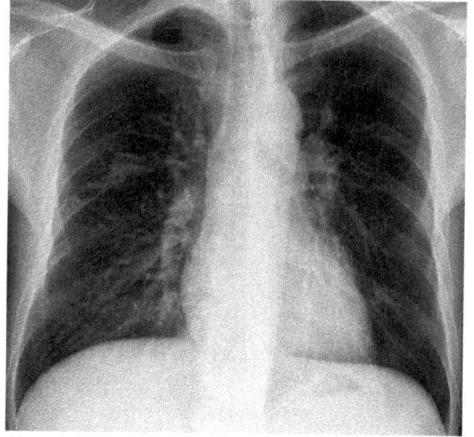

(i) (j)

Fig. 7.9: (continuing)

7.3 Imaging features

Between January 2007 and December 2011, 765 HIV-infected adult patients seeking for medical care in the Guangzhou No. 8 People's Hospital were diagnosed with PSM by pathological examination and 281 of them took thoracic scans as clinical evaluation. Their imaging features are summarized as follows:
1. Interstitial lung fibrosis: pulmonary markings increase in number, growing reticular and miliary;
2. Multiple intropulmonary invasive lesions or local pulmonary consolidation and ground-glass-like shadows;
3. Hilar lymphadenopathy and/or mediastinal lymphadenopathy;
4. Plural effusions;
5. Cavitary lesions.

Among them, hilar lymphadenopathy and/or mediastinal lymphadenopathy and miliary lung fibrosis are significant for the differential diagnosis because they are at a higher rate of incurrence among the AIDS patients.

In spite of non-specificity in PSM diagnosis of AIDS patients clinically and imageologically leading to possibility of confusing PSM with other opportunistic infections in AIDS patients, the above-mentioned imaging features side by side with extremely lower counts of CD4+ T lymph cell, are affirmatively attributive to the identification of PSM in AIDS patients. In this case, bacteria culture becomes a need for its definite diagnosis.

Editors: Songfeng Jiang, Haolan He, Xiaoping Tang, Yi Liang

8 Image findings of pneumocystis pneumonia (PCP) in AIDS

8.1 Introduction

Pneumocystis pneumonia (PCP) is an opportunistic infection that caused by *Pneumocystis jirovecii*, which was used to be mistaken as a protozoan and has recently been reclassified as a fungus because its genetic analysis are more similar to those of fungi. It is a ubiquitous organism that is found worldwide, causing an asymptomatic or mild infection in the normal host but fulminate pneumonia (PCP) in the immunocompromised host. About 65%–80% of AIDS patients may be infected by *Pneumocystis jirovecii* once or more. PCP is one of the most common opportunistic infections and one of the common causes of death among patients with AIDS.

Pneumocystis jirovecii has characteristics of both protozoa and fungi. On histopathologic examination, life cycle including cysts (Figure 8.0) and trophozoites are found. Microscopically, the cysts appear as small black organisms typical of *P. jiroveci* by Gomori methenamine silver stains, and violet blue organisms by toluidine blue O stains.

P. jiroveci lives almost exclusively in the pulmonary alveoli, which can lead to pulmonary interstitial edema and interstitial pneumonia, with typical change of full-filled foamy alveolar exudates and enlarged alveolar. Pulmonary interstitial edema along with interstitial pneumonia that caused by inflammatory cells (mainly lymphocytes, macrophages and eosinophils) may lead to epithelial hyperplasia, septal thickening, transparent coating (advanced stage), and finally pulmonary fibrosis, weakening alveolar-capillary exchange.

All these pathological reactions can lead to progressive hypoxemia and respiratory failure. The clinical features are nonspecific, including: fever, dry cough, oxygenation impairment, tachypnea, and so on. Pneumocystis is difficult to culture, and definitive diagnosis requires the visualuzation of *P. carinii* in pulmonary tissue or lower airway fluids (such as bronchoalveolar lavage and induced sputum).

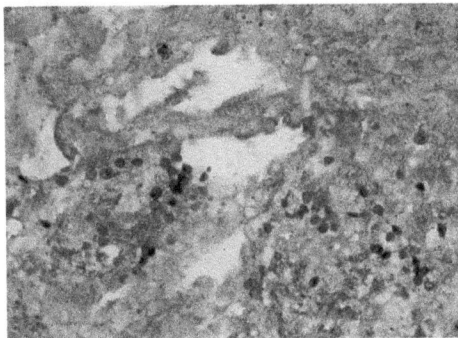

Fig. 8.0: Lung biopsy *P. jiroveci gomori* methenamine silver staining, ×400.

8.2 Image findings

Case 8.1 (Fig. 8.1 a-j)

A 42-year-old male presented with fever and cough for 10 days, tachypnea for 8 days. His body temperature at admission was 37.7 °C. The CD4+ cell count was 16/μL. The

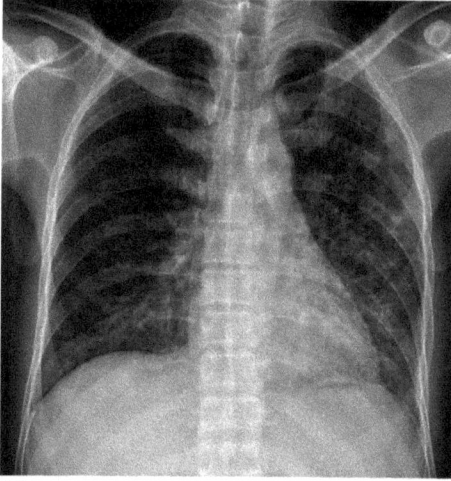

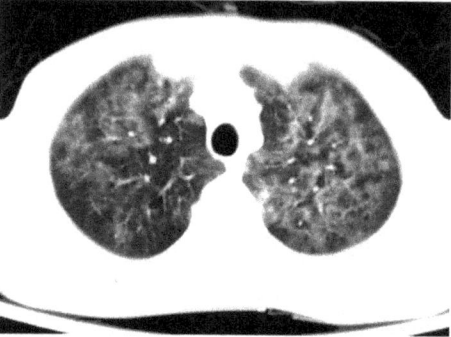

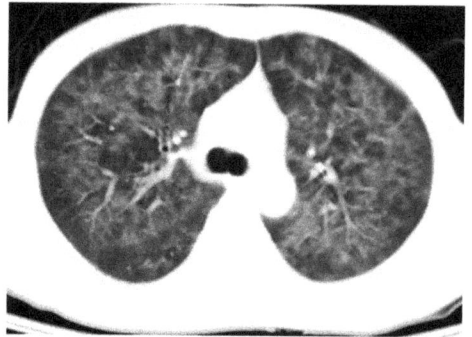

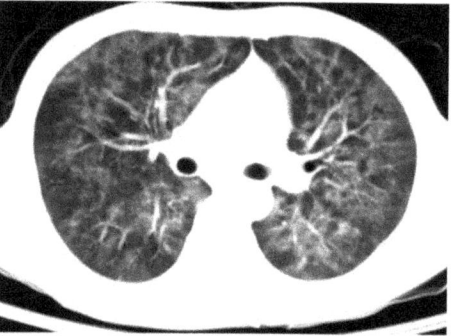

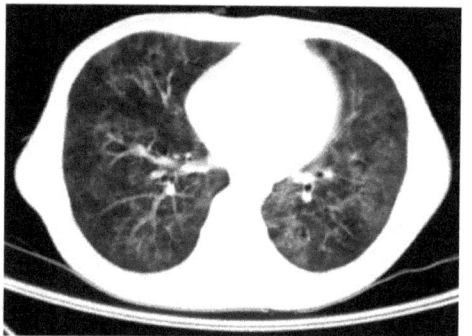

Fig. 8.1 a–j: Pneumocystis pneumonia (PCP).

histopathological findings based on branchofiberoscopy of lung tissue indicated pneumocystis pneumonia. The patient was diagnosed with AIDS (C3) complicated with PCP.

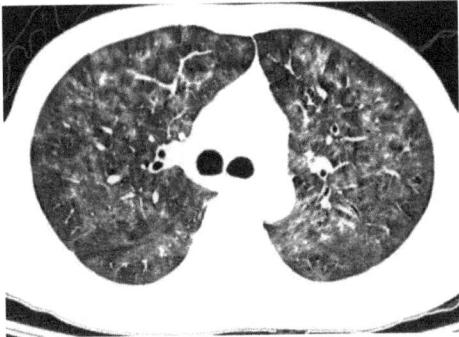
(f)

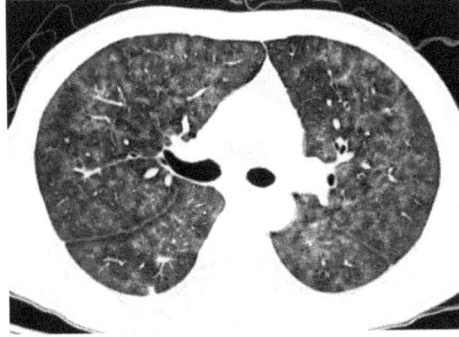
(g)

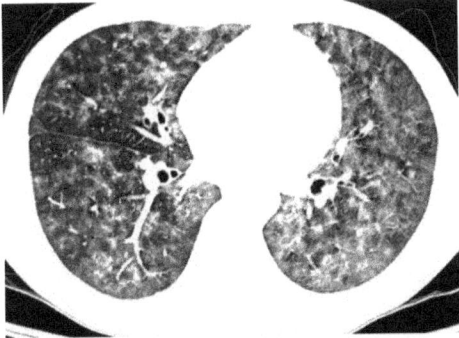
(h)

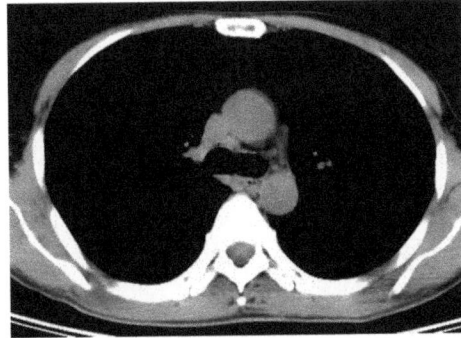
(i)

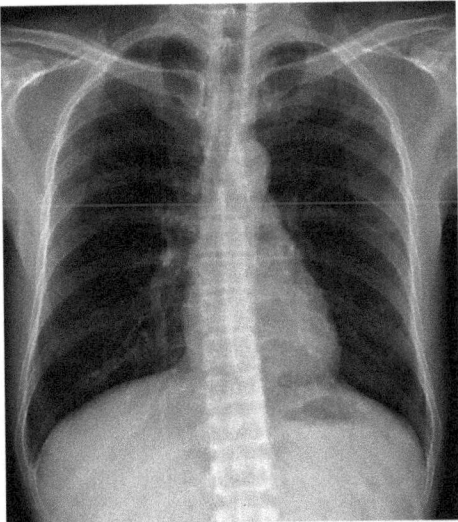
(j)

Fig. 8.1: (continuing)

Chest radiograghs revealed reduced diaphaneity in the bilateral pulmonary field, presenting ground-glass-like change, with increased and blur markings of both lungs (a). CT scans (b–e) and HRCT scans (f–h) demonstrated widespread ground-glass attenuation without mediastinal lymphadenopathy (i). The chest radiograghs obtained a 20-days treatment showed the fundamental absorption of bilateral lesions, the pulmonary field became limpid (j).

Case 8.2 (Fig. 8.2 a–k)

A 37-year-old male had a one month history of fever, cough and tachypnea. His body temperature at admission was 38.7 °C. The CD4+ cell count was 48/μL. The histopathological findings based on branchofiberoscopy of lung tissue indicated pneumocystis pneumonia. Diagnosis: AIDS (C3) complicated with PCP.

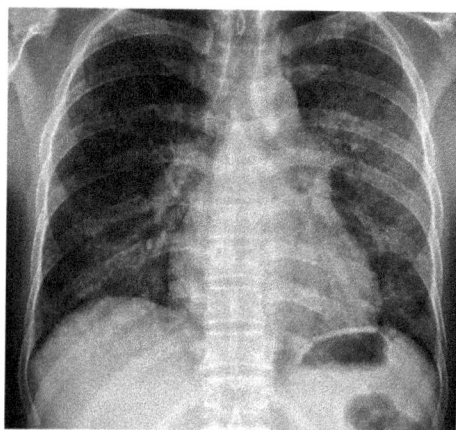

(a)

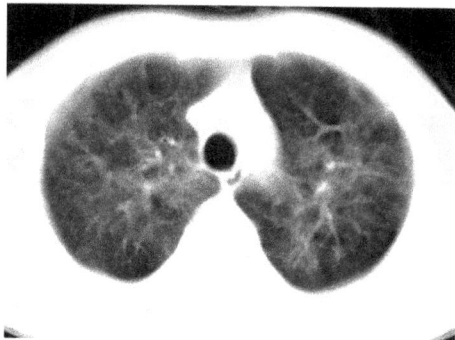

(b)

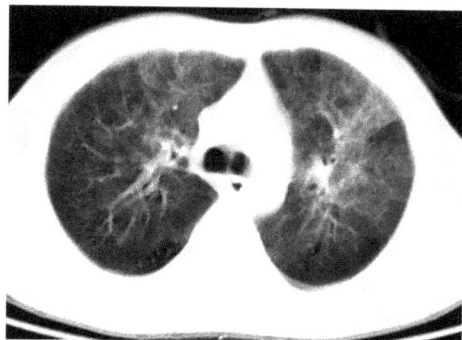

(c)

Fig. 8.2 a–k: Pneumocystis pneumonia (PCP).

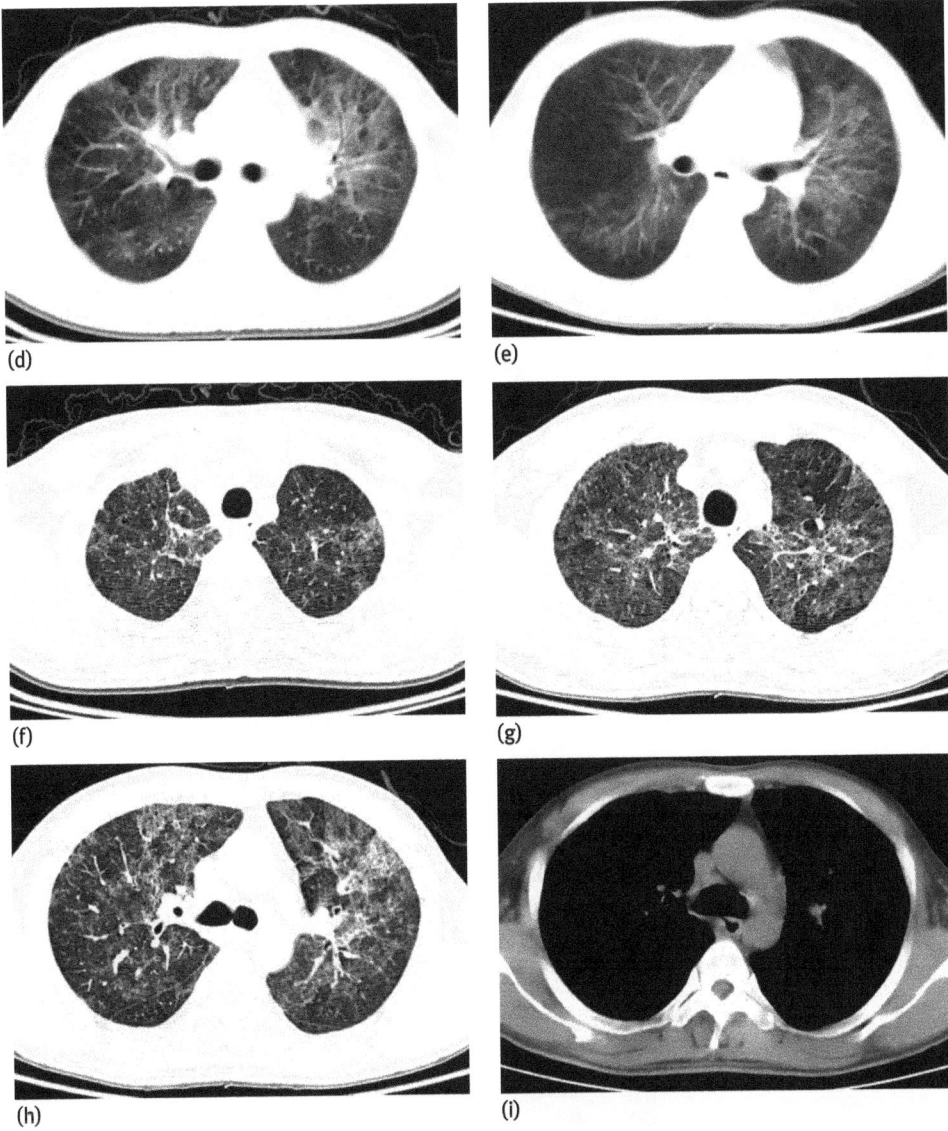

Fig. 8.2: (continuing)

The chest radiographs (a) revealed reduced diaphaneity and ground-glass-like shadow on the bilateral lungs, and thickened reticular markings of lung. CT scans (b–h) revealed the thickened asystematic reticular markings and a hyaline shadow on the bilateral lungs. HRCT scans (f–h) show. The scan with mediastinal window showed no lymphadenectasis (i). HRCT scans (f–h) showed "crazy paving" appearance. Chest radiographs (j, k) obtained after 20 days and 42 days therapy respectively revealed the gradually absorption of lesions in the lung and the limpid pulmonary field.

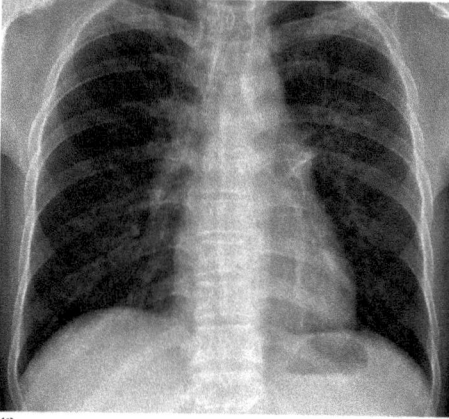

(j)

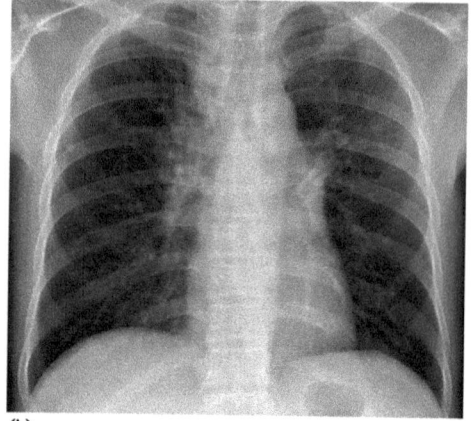

(k)

Fig. 8.2: (continuing)

Case 8.3 (Fig. 8.3 a–k)

A 35-year-old male presented with recurrent fever and cough for 3 months, symptom getting worse and accompanied with tachypnea for I month. Body temperature at admission was 38.4 °C. The CD4+ cell count was 65/μL. Histopathological diagnosis was based on the direct visualized of *P. carinii* in tissue obtained from branchofibero-scope. Diagnosis: AIDS (C3) complicated with PCP.

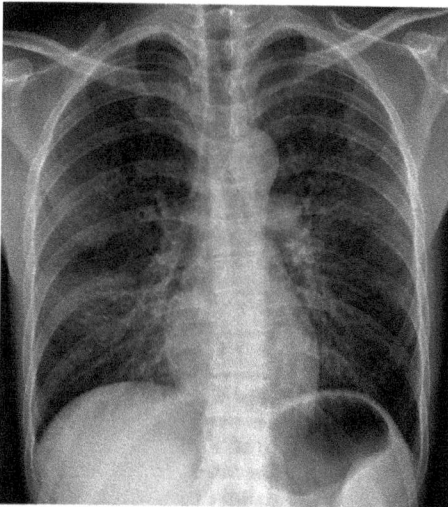

(a)

Fig. 8.3 a–k: Pneumocystis pneumonia (PCP).

(b)

(c)

(d)

(e)

(f)

(g)

(h)

(i)

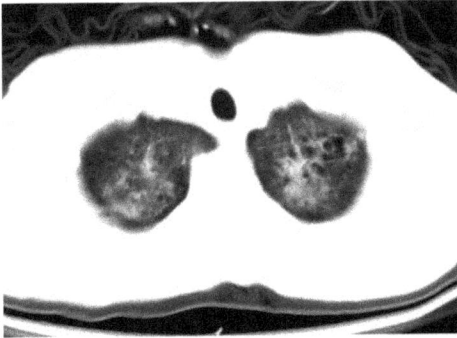

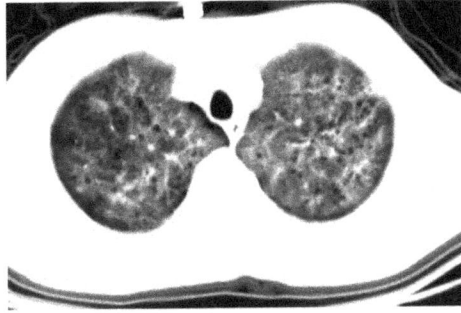

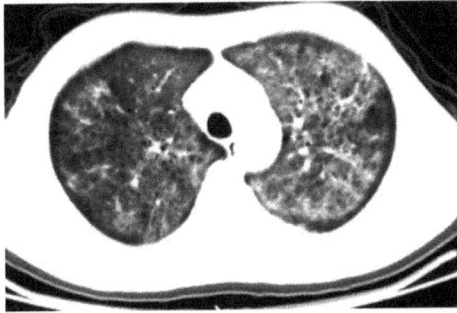

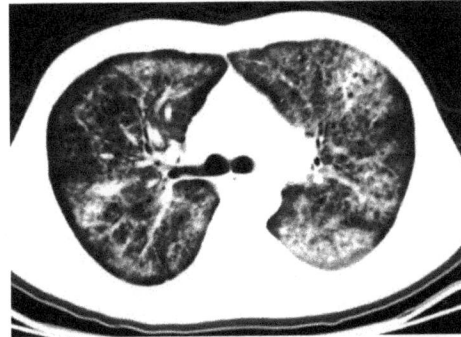

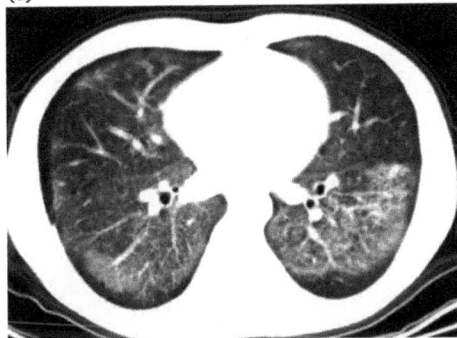

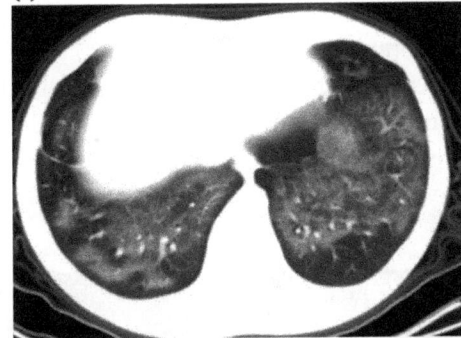

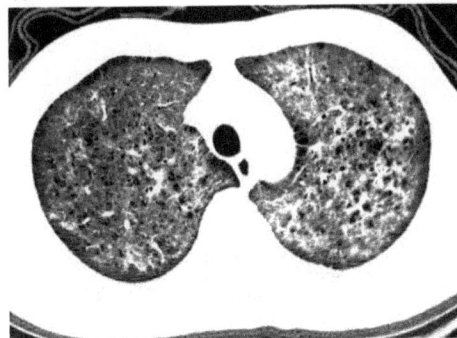

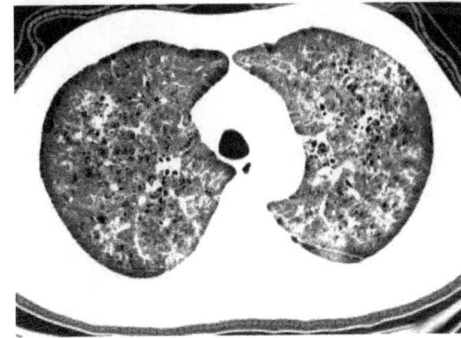

Fig. 8.3: (continuing)

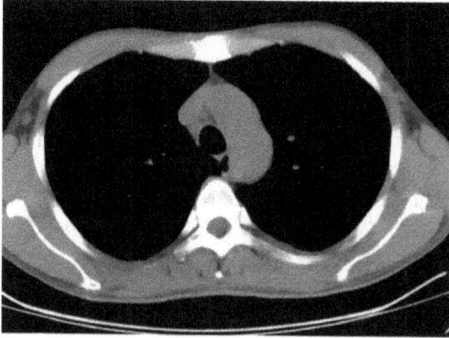
(j)

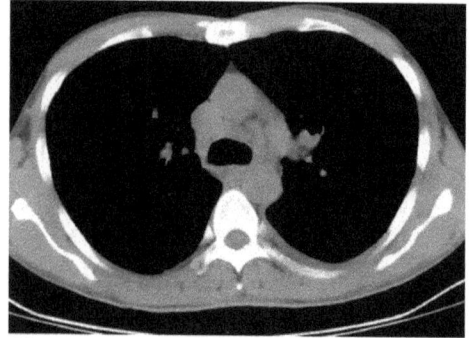
(k)

Fig. 8.3: (continuing)

Chest radiogragh (a) revealed the bilateral reduced pulmonary field translucent associated with gridding-like interstitial shadow. CT scans (b–g) revealed widespread ground-glass attenuation associated with the gridding-like thickening of interlobular septa. HRCT (h, i) demonstrated bilateral "gravel road" appearance. CT scans with mediastinal window showed multiple small lymph nodes in the mediastina (j, k).

Case 8.4 (Fig. 8.4 a–j)
A 45-year-old female presented with cough for 1 month and fever for 2 weeks. Body temperature at admission was 38.7 °C. The CD4+ cell count was 4/μL. Histopathological diagnosis was based on the direct visualized of *P. carinii* in tissue obtained from branchofiberoscope. The clinical diagnosis was AIDS (C3) complicated with PCP. Eventually, her condition deteriorated and died during hospitalization due to respiratory failure.

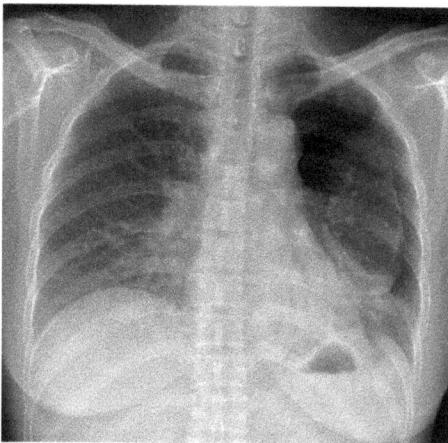
(a)

Fig. 8.4 a–j: Pneumocystis pneumonia (PCP).

(b)

(c)

(d)

(e)

(f)

(g)

(h)

(i)

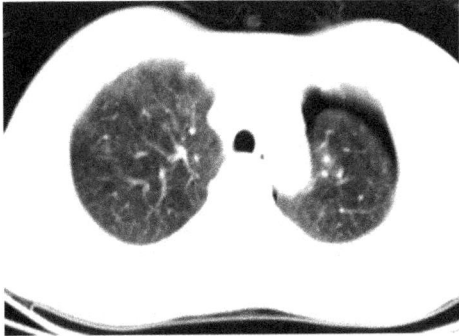

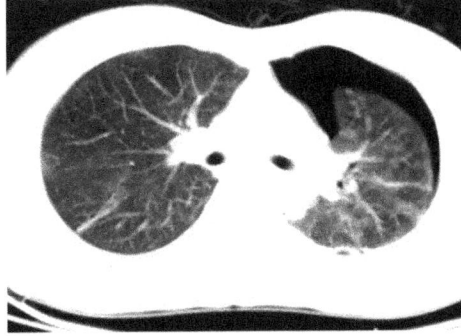

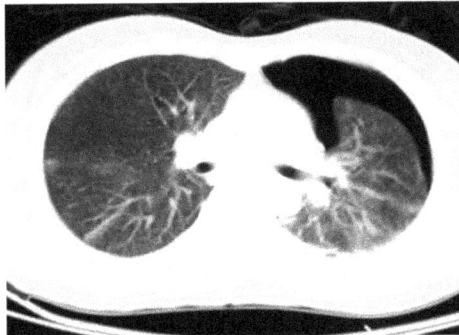

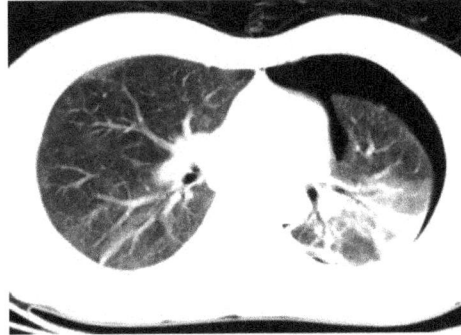

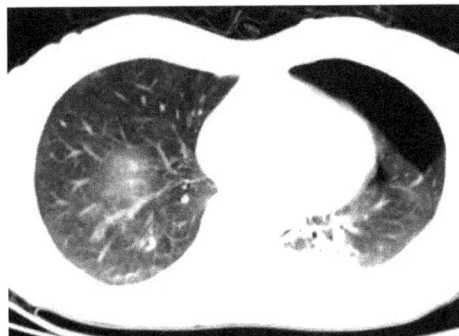

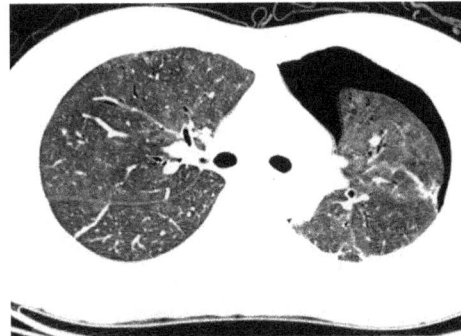

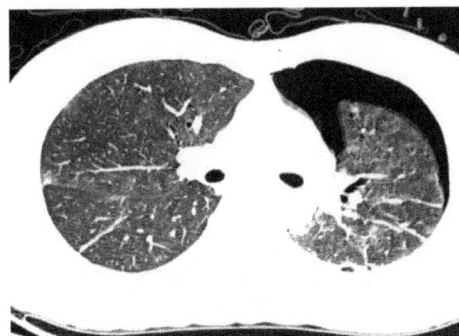

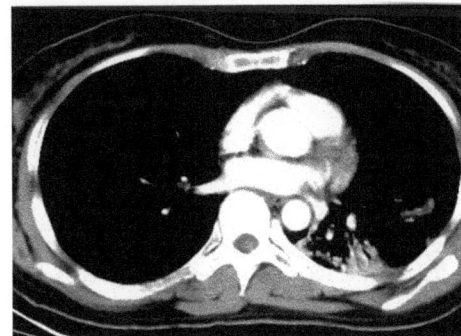

Fig. 8.4: (continuing)

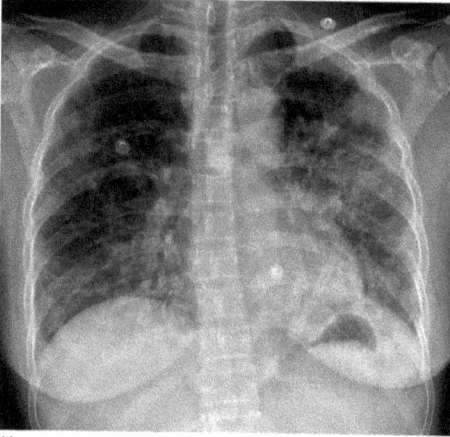

(j)

Fig. 8.4: (continuing)

Chest radiograghs (a) revealed bilateral reduced pulmonary field translucent associated with increased markings of lungs and left-side pneumthorax. CT scans (b–f, g and h stand of HRCT scans and i for enhanced mediastinal window scan) demonstrated widespread ground-glass-like attenuation associated with left-side penumthorax and atelectasis of left lower lobe. The bed-side X ray (j) obtained 14 days after treatment showed the absorption of pneumthorax but widespread of the bilateral interstitial shadow, indicating pulmonary multiplicity of infections which resulted in respiratory failure.

Case 8.5 (Fig. 8.5 a–l)
A 39-year-old male presented with productive cough for 3 months, fever for 2 weeks. Body temperature at admission was 38.3 °C. The CD4+ cell count was 88/μL. His-

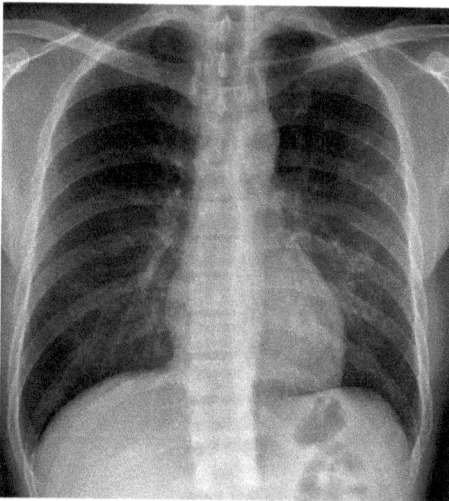

(a)

Fig. 8.5 a–l: Pneumocystis pneumonia (PCP).

topathological diagnosis was based on the direct visualized of *P. carinii* in tissue obtained from branchofiberoscope. Diagnosis: AIDS (C3) complicated with PCP.

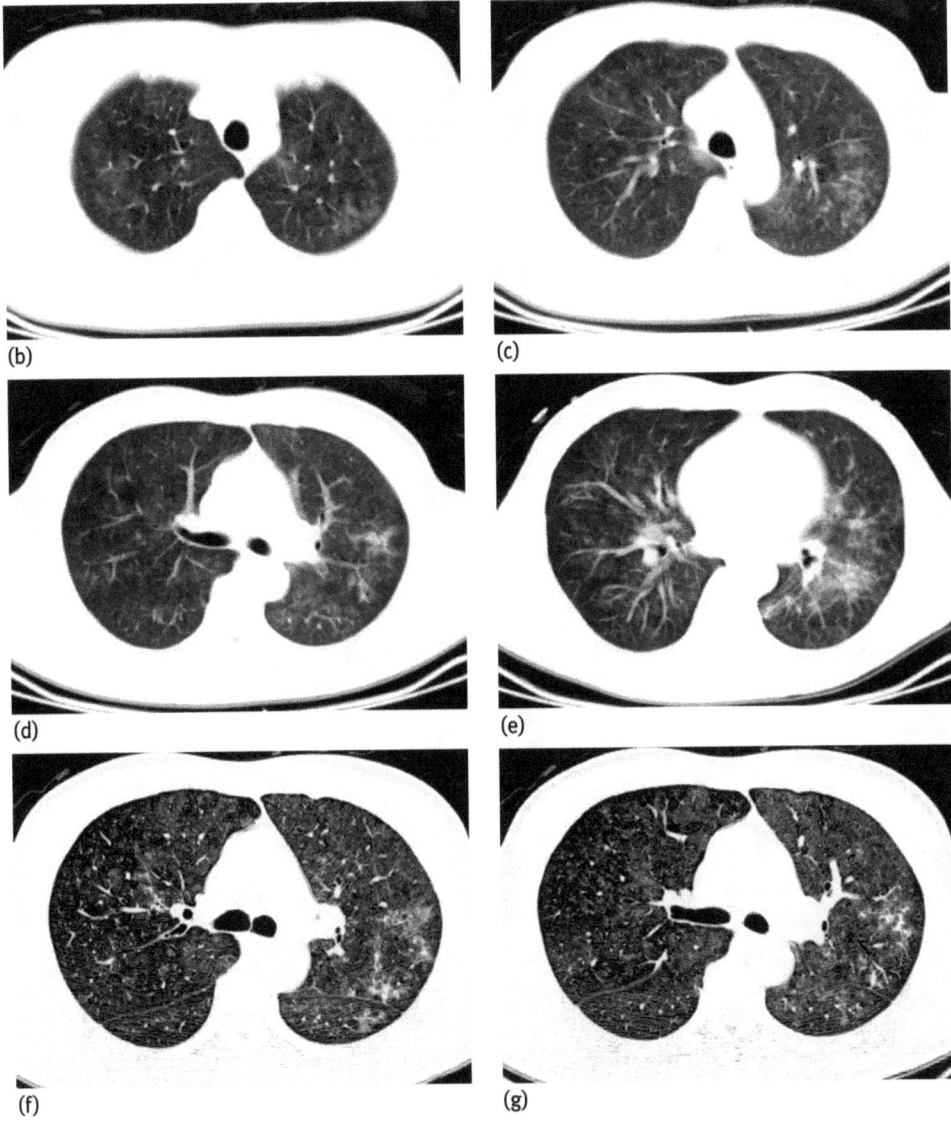

(b)

(c)

(d)

(e)

(f)

(g)

Fig. 8.5: (continuing)

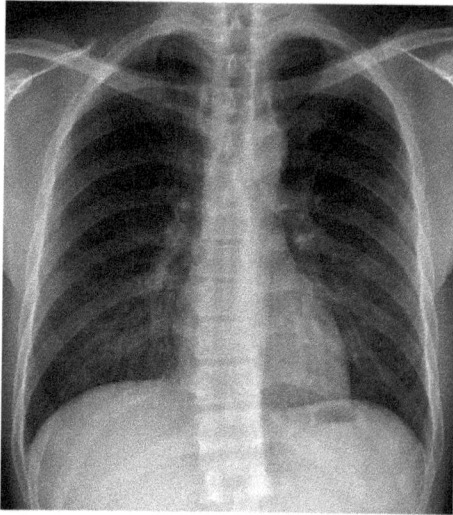
(h)

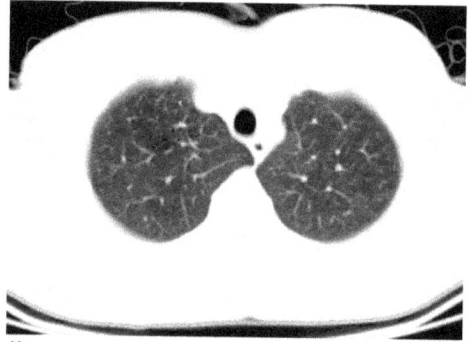
(i)

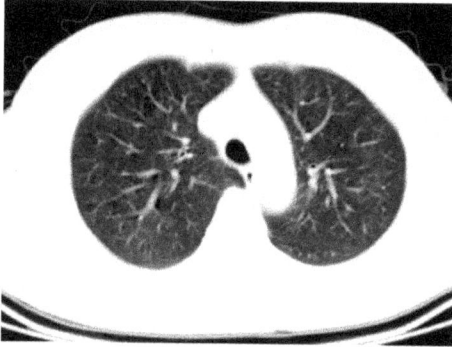
(j)

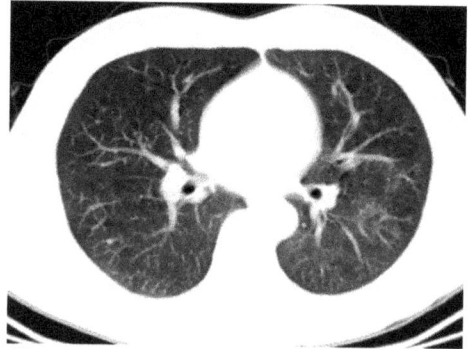
(k)

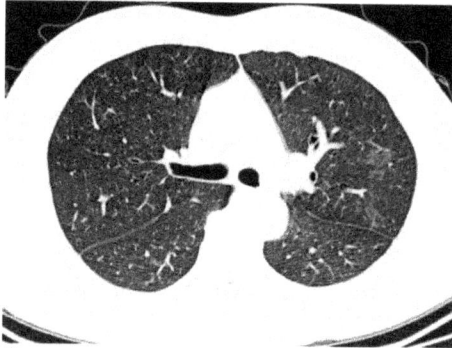
(l)

Fig. 8.5: (continuing)

Chest radiograghs (a) revealed bilateral reduced pulmonary field translucent associated with increased markings of lungs. CT scans (b–e) and HRCT (f, g) revealed bilateral ground-glass attenuation associated with the thickening of interlobular septa, more widespread on the left lobes. The obvious absorption of lung lesions was presented on the chest radoigragh (h) and CT scans (i–l) obtained 28 days after treatment.

Case 8.6 (Fig. 8.6 a–j)

A 50-year-old male presented with tachypnea for 20 days, fever and cough for 2 weeks. Body temperature at admissionxwas 37.4 °C. CD4+ cell count was 2/μL. Histopathological diagnosis was based on the direct visualized of *P. carinii* in tissue obtained from branchofiberoscope. Diagnosis: AIDS (C3) complicated with PCP.

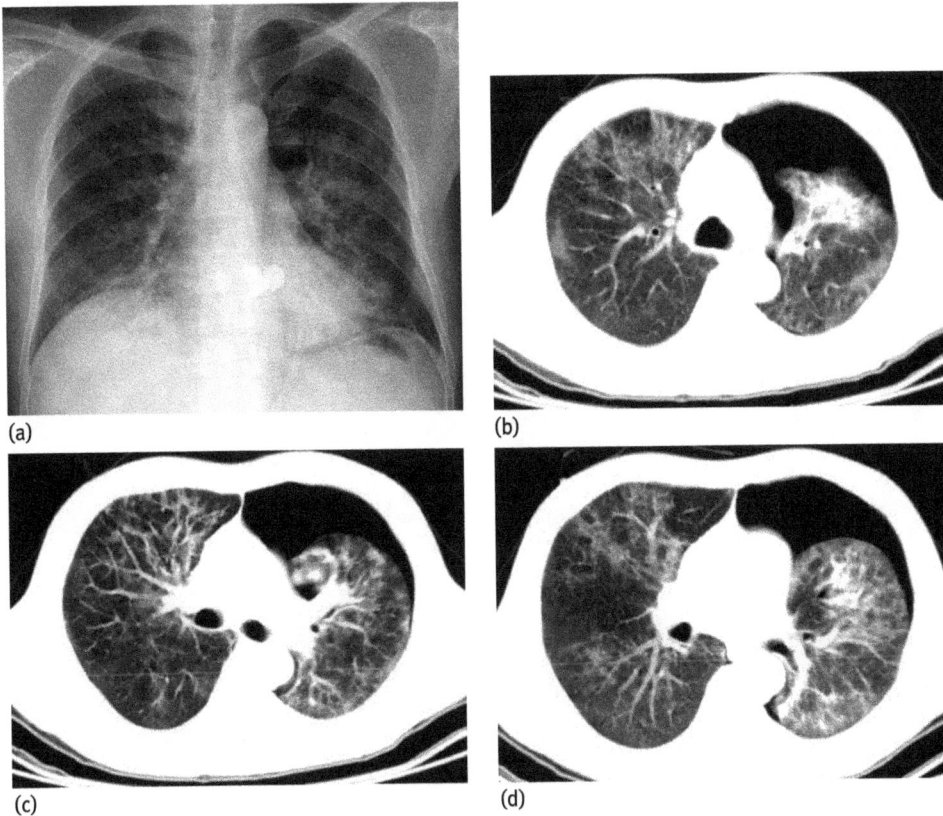

Fig. 8.6 a–j: Pneumocystis pneumonia (PCP).

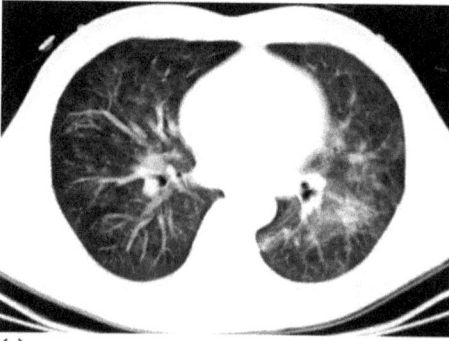

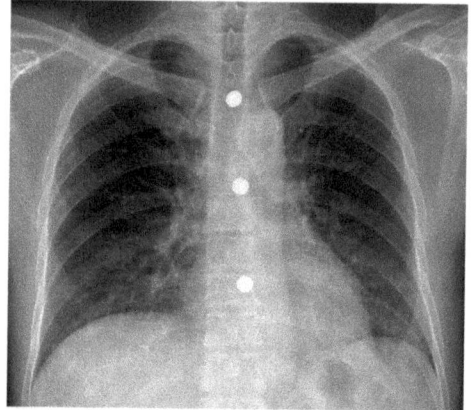

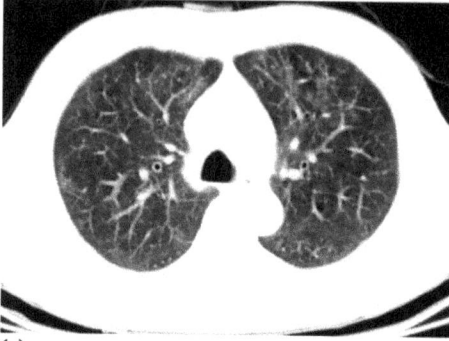

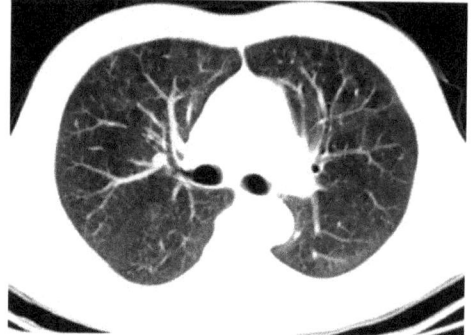

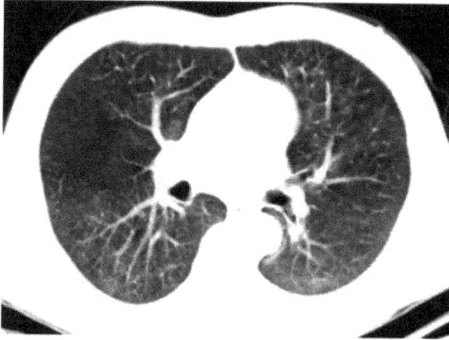

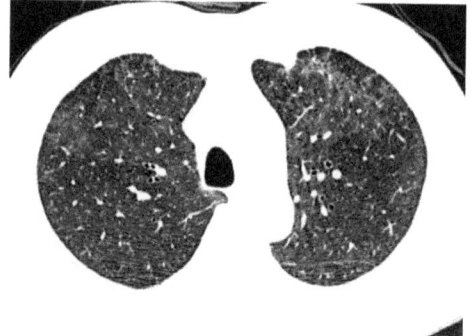

Fig. 8.6: (continuing)

Chest radiogragh (a) revealed thickened markings of lung, ground-glass-like shadow in the pulmonary field and pneumothorax in the left lung. CT scans (b–e) revealed widespread ground-glass attenuation associated with the gridding-like thickening of interlobular septa and numerous thin-walled pneumathodes on lower lobe of left lund and middle lobe of the right lung. Chest radiograghs (f) obtained 24 days and CT scans (g–j) obtained 2 months respectively after the treatment reveal the gradually absorption of the lesions including pneumthorax and pneumathodes, leaving scatter of ground-glass attenuation.

Case 8.7 (Fig. 8.7 a–d)

A 31-year-old male presented with recurrent fever and productive cough for 9 months, symptom got worse and accompanied with tachypnea for 1 month. Body temperature at admission was 38.5 °C. CD4+ cell count was 14/μL. Histopathological diagnosis was based on the direct visualized of *P. carinii* in tissue obtained from branchofiberoscope. Diagnosis: AIDS (C3) complicated with PCP.

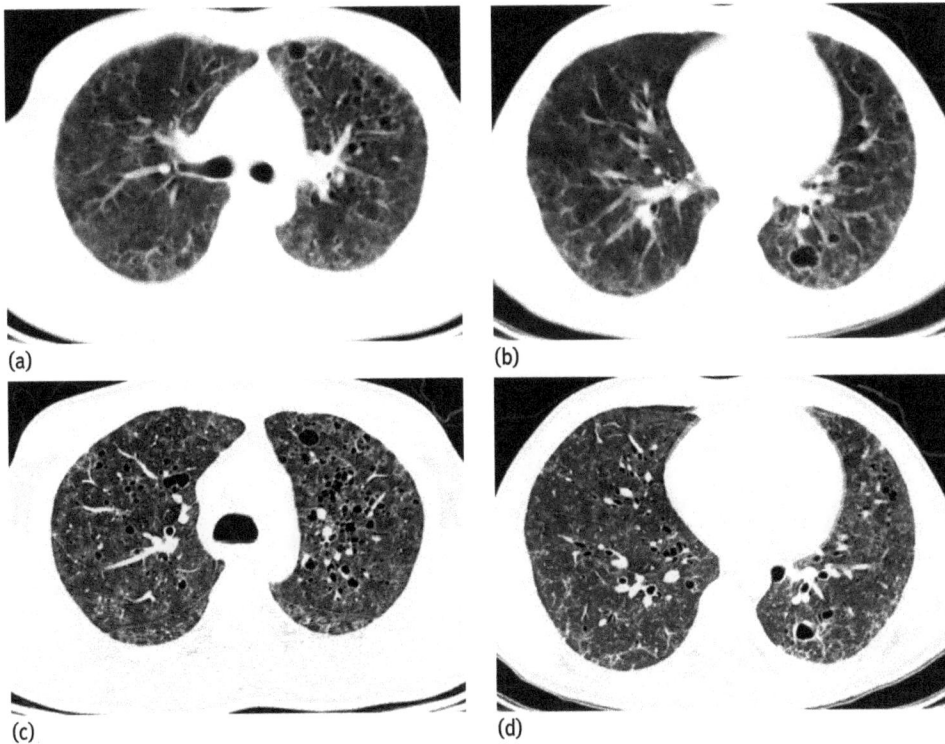

(a)

(b)

(c)

(d)

Fig. 8.7 a–d: Pneumocystis pneumonia (PCP).

CT scans (a, b) and HRCT (c, d) demonstrated widespread ground-glass attenuation associated with the gridding-like thickening of interlobular septa and numerous thin-walled pneumathodes.

8.3 Imaging features

The imaging features include:
1. The typical PCP has such imaging presentations as symmetrical or effusive ground-glass shadow on the bilateral lungs, with symmetrical patchy or only map-like opacities in the bilateral lungs.
2. The thickened interlobular septa due to interstitial pneumonitis is present as reticular shadow, showing a specific "gravel road" sign when the ground-glass attenuated is mixed with reticular shadow.
3. Shadows on thin-walled pneumathode can be seen in some PCP patients with complicated spontaneous pneumothorax. Clinically, the diagnosis of PCP should be chiefly considered when spontaneous pneumothorax is identified.
4. Mediastinal and hilar lymphadenopathies are rarely found on the radiographs and CT scans.

Editors: Bihua Chen, Wanshan Chen, Zhibiao Yin, Yi Liang

9 Imaging findings of pulmonary *Mycobacterium tuberculosis* in AIDS

9.1 Introduction

Pulmonary tuberculosis is a special inflammation caused by *Mycobacterium tuberculosis (MTB)*. It is one of most common opportunistic infections in AIDS patients, accounting for 20 % of pulmonary infections in AIDS patients. AIDS patients contract it mostly due to their impaired immunity of CD4+T lymph cells. For immunocompetent patients, the macrophagocytes in their body engulf the tubercle bacillus (TB) invading the lung and produce the antigen that sensitizes the T lymph cells. In response, the sensitized T lymph cells activate the macrophagocytes to kill more tubercle bacillus. Among these T lymph cells, CD4+T lymph cells play a leading role in cell-mediated immunity. In AIDS patients, HIV cripple the immunity by depleting a number of CD4+T cells significantly, allowing the favorable invasion and spreading of tubercle bacillus into AIDS patients. TB and HIV are mutually coupled in that HIV infection may accelerate TB progression, and TB in response can boost HIV-infection into onset of AIDS.

In pathology, MTB in AIDS patients is highly relevant to HIV infection identified by the CD4+ count. In the early stage of HIV infection, the human immunocytes respond stubborn to inhibit the TB-HIV co-infections or the TB infection following HIV-infection. The evidence can be showed that under pathologic microscope, typical tuberculous granuloma, less caseous necrosis and very few MTB are visible beside and that all the lesions are restricted and even repaired by the surrounding CD4+ cells, epithelioid giant cells and Langhan's giant cells. In the middle stage of HIV infection or TB-AIDS co-infection, the caseous necrosis is viewed to expand together with the increase of MTB counts, against the dramatic decrease of CD4+ cell, pithelioid giant cells and Langhan's giant cell due to weakened response of the immunocytes. In the late-stage of AIDS combined with TB infection, the immunocytes cannot produce immune response to the infections as a result of severe immune impairment. Eventually, in the massive caseous necrosis are full of a huge number of MTB, but no tuberculous granuloma, no epithelioid giant cells, no Langhan's giant cells, together with few CD4+ cells.

Etiologically, bacteriologic test is the exact evidence of pulmonary TB etiology diagnosis. Specimens for the tests can be obtained from sputum, sputum by ultrasonic atomization, and samples from lower respiratory tracts, bronchial alveolar lavage, bronchoalveolar lavage fluid (BALF) and pulmonary and bronchial biopsy.

Smear examinations are done by Ziehl-Neelsen anti-acid dyeing method and fluorescent staining. On smear examination, it is reported that the positive rate by bacteria-collecting sterility test is higher than by direct smear examination. The latter can be used as a routine examination because it boasts of simplicity and rapidness but lower sensibility. The negative results cannot be considered as an evidence for exclusion of PT and consequent examinations for more than three times are suggested for a higher possibility of positive rate. Even though smear dyeing positive is only the evidence of the existing acid-fast bacillus (Color Figure 9.0), but not the evidence of whether it is MTB or nontuberculous mycobacteria (NTM), the acid-fast bacillus positive has great significance in diagnosing TB merely because NTM has a very low morbidity so far in China.

The isolated culture method is considered as the gold standard of tuberculosis diagnosis because it is easy to acquire the bacterial colony in a direct way for its convenience of distinguishing MTB from NTM and importantly it has a higher sensibility higher than smear microscopy. Using this method, a higher isolation rate of tubercule bacillus may be acquired in the patients having never undergoing anti-tuberculosis therapy or those having undergone anti-tuberculosis therapy but having suspended it for 48.72 h. The isolated culture method consists of Lewenstein-Jensen medium and BACTEC. The latter can improve the first generation separation rate by 10%, compared to the former. Moreover, it can differentiate MTB from NTM and shorten detection time significantly.

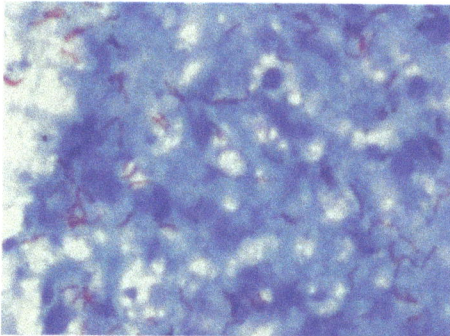

Fig. 9.0: Acid-fast bacillus in lung tissue (acid-fast stain, ×400).

9.2 Radiologic findings

Case 9.1 (Fig. 9.1 a–j)

A 36-year-old female patient presented recurrent fever for 2 months. A tumor was found in the right side of neck 1 month before hospitalized. Body temperature at admission was 39.5 °C. The tumor sized 5 cm × 5 cm was hard in quality, clear with boundary, tender and inactive. The CD4+ cell count was 36/μl. Sputum culture and identification detected *Mycobacterium tuberculosis*. The patient was diagnosed with AIDS (C3) combined with pulmonary TB. After anti-tuberculosis treatment with isoniazide, streptomycin, ethambutol, and pyrazinamide, the patient was discharged with temperature dropping to normal and the enlarged lymph nodes shrunken.

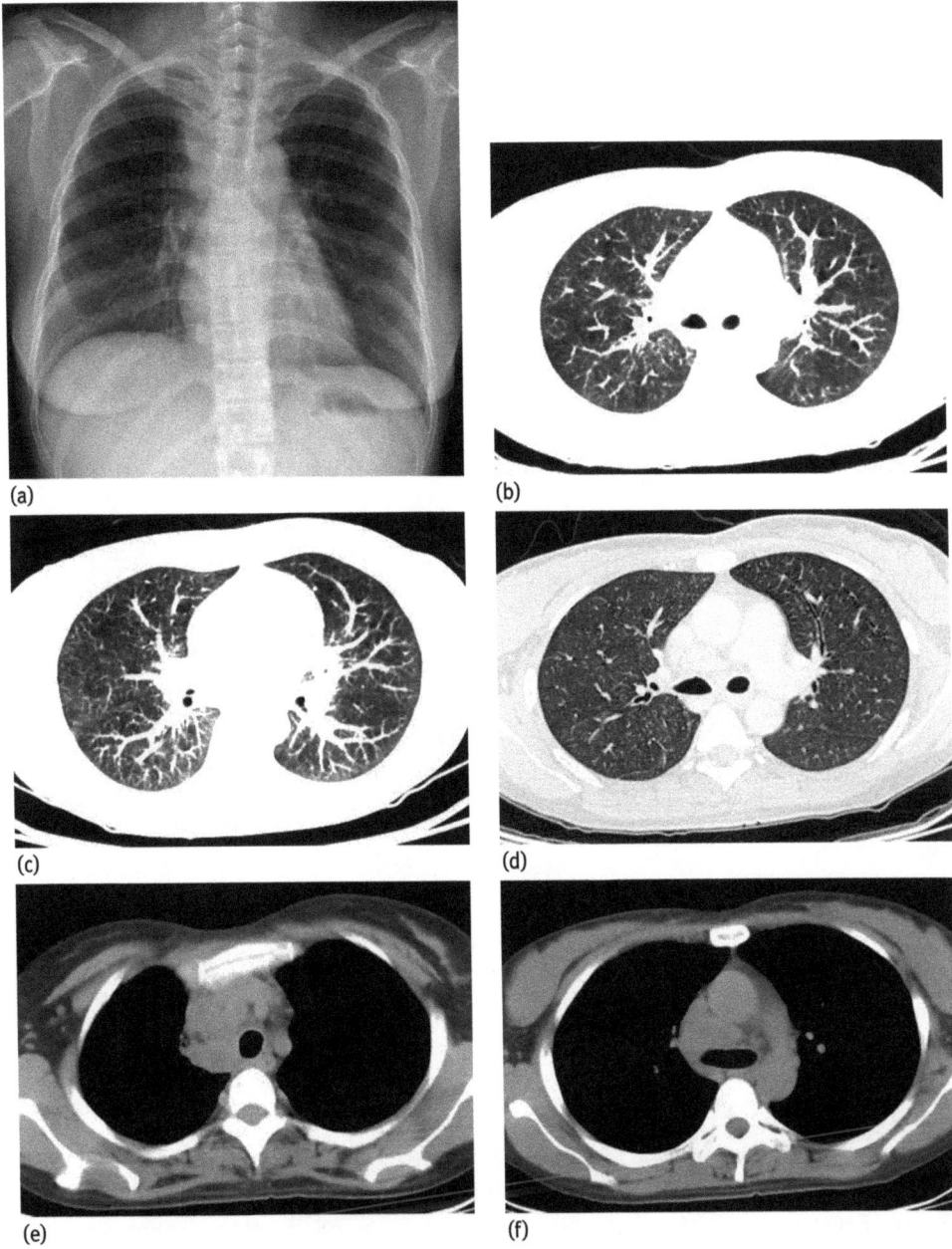

Fig. 9.1 a–j: Pulmonary *Mycobacterium tuberculosis*.

Chest radiographs showed a broadened shadow of right upper mediastinum (a). CT scans with lung window (b–c) and HRCT scan (d) demonstrated slightly thickened markings of bilateral lungs. CT scans with mediastinal window demonstrated the enlarged lymph nodes in the mediastinum and bilateral hilus pulmonis, presented central necrotic low-attenuation of lymph nodes in plain CT scan, and the rim-en-

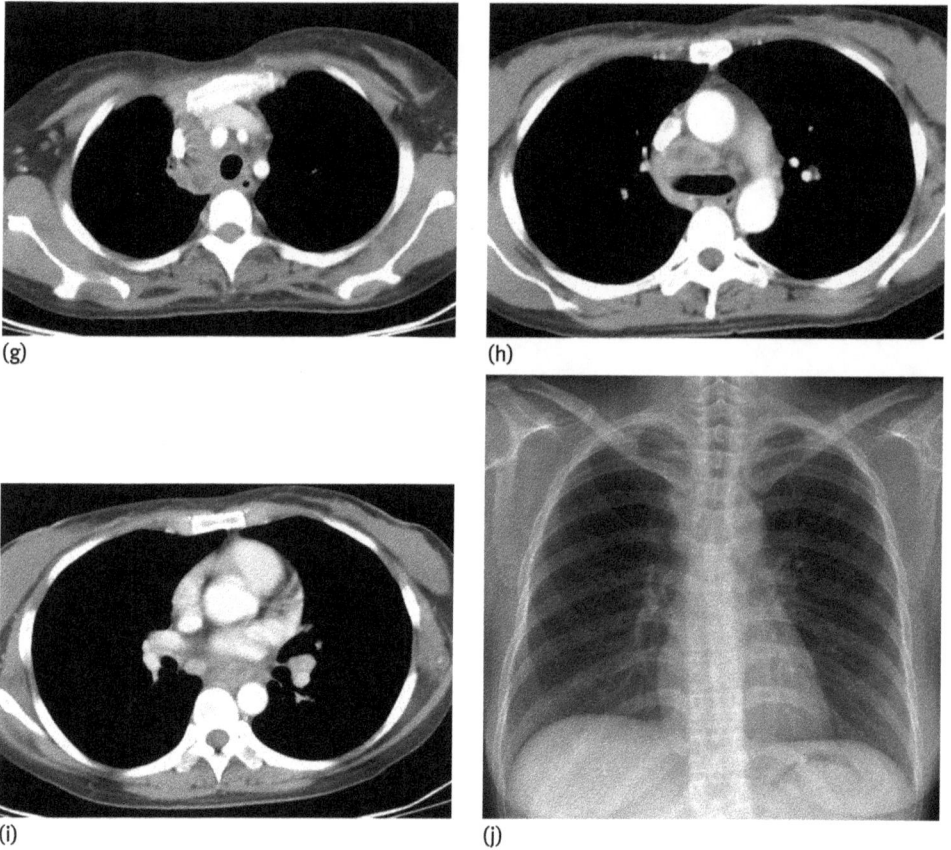

Fig. 9.1: (continuing)

hanced pattern in contrast-enhanced CT scan (e–i). After 19 days treatment, chest radiograph showed that the broadened shadow of right upper mediastinum shrunk than before (j).

Case 9.2 (Fig. 9.2 a–k)

A 31-year-old male patient presented recurrent fever and upper abdominal pain for more than 1 month. Body temperature at admission was 39.2 °C. There were no enlargements of systemic superficial lymph nodes. The CD4+ cell count was 9/µl. Sputum culture: *Mycobacterium tuberculosis* positive. The patient was diagnosed with AIDS (C3) complicated with pulmonary TB. After anti-tuberculosis treatment with isoniazide, streptomycin, ethambutol and rifampicin, the patient was discharged with fever and epigastric pains relieved.

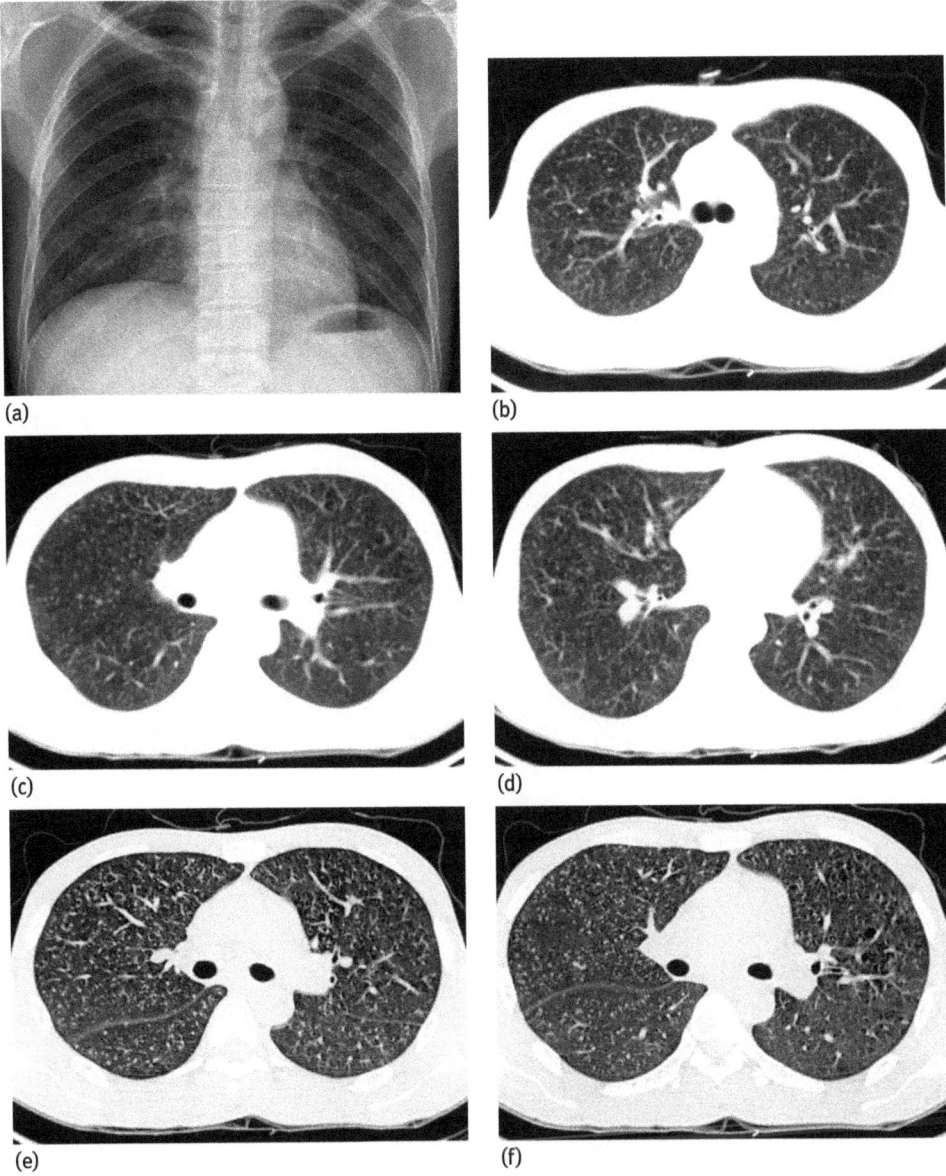

Fig. 9.2 a–k: Pulmonary *Mycobacterium tuberculosis*.

(g)

(h)

(i)

(j)

(k)

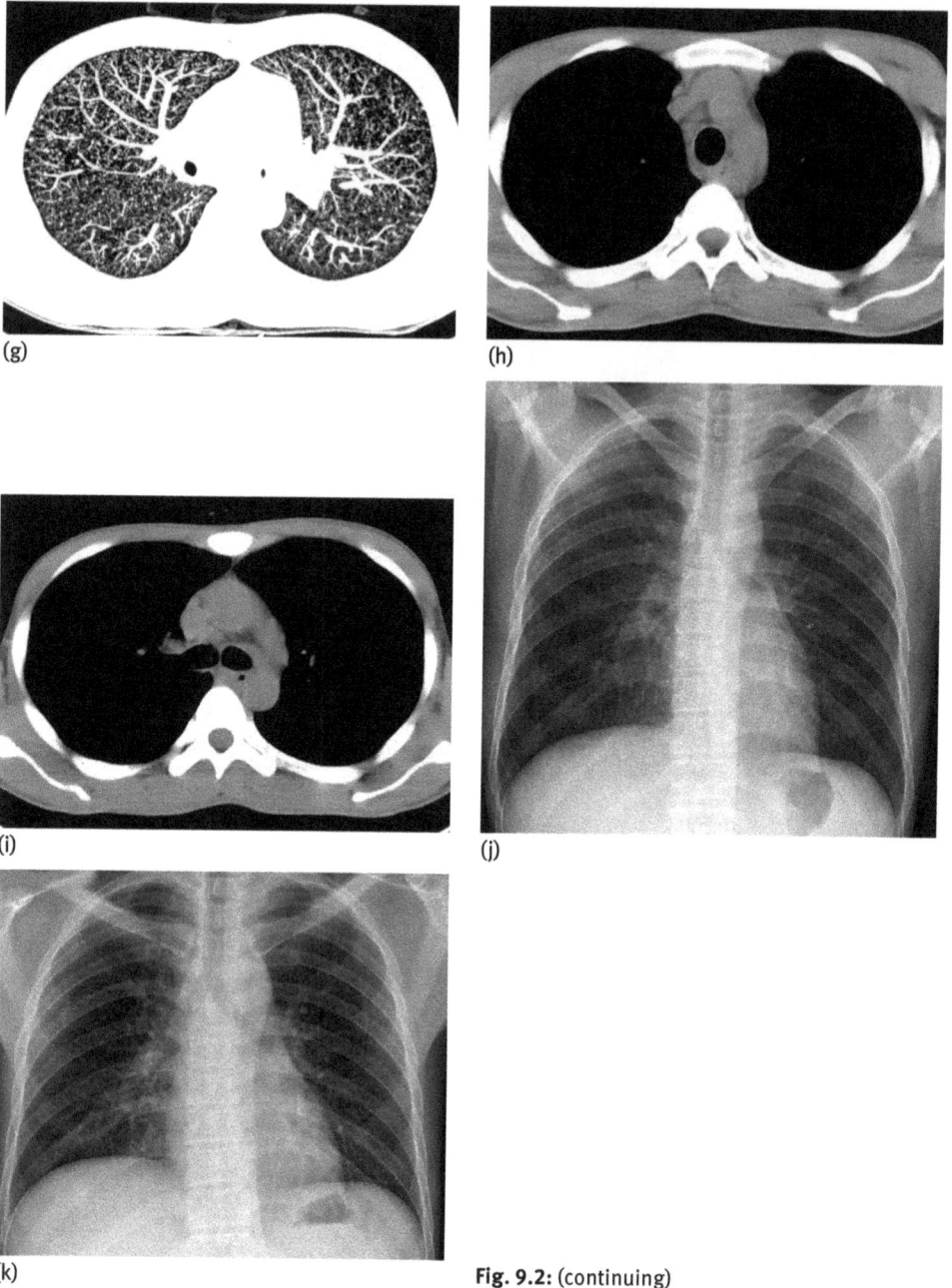

Fig. 9.2: (continuing)

Chest radiograph showed diffuse miliary lesions in bilateral lungs (a). CT scans with lung window showed uniformly distributed lesions with similar sizes and densities (b–g; e and r for HRCT; g for MIP reconstruction image). CT scans with mediastinal window showed the lymphadenectasis in the aortic pulmonic window (h, i). After 30 days and 60 days treatment, chest radiographs showed diffuse miliary lesions of bilateral lungs were gradually absorbed (j, k).

Case 9.3 (Fig. 9.3 a–j)

A 34-year-old male patient found a tumor in the neck more than 9 months before hospitalized. It grew bigger obviously in the recent 2 weeks, accompanied with bdominal pains. Body temperature at admission was 36.6 °C. Examination: a mild soft lymph node with a diameter of about 1.5 cm was palpated in the left submaxilla, ordinary in quality and tender when pressed. Another two tumors sized 7 cm × 10 cm and 5 cm × 6 cm were palpated in the right lateral anterior neck. The CD4+ cell count was 89/μl. Mycobacterium tuberculosis was detected in BALF culture and bacterial culture of pyogenic fluids by cervical lymph node biopsy. The patient was diagnosed with AIDS (C3) and pulmonary TB and tuberculous lymphadenitis. After anti-tuberculosis treatment with isoniazide, streptomycin, ethambutol and rifampicin, the patient was discharged with shrinking of the tumors and vanishing of fever and abdominal pains.

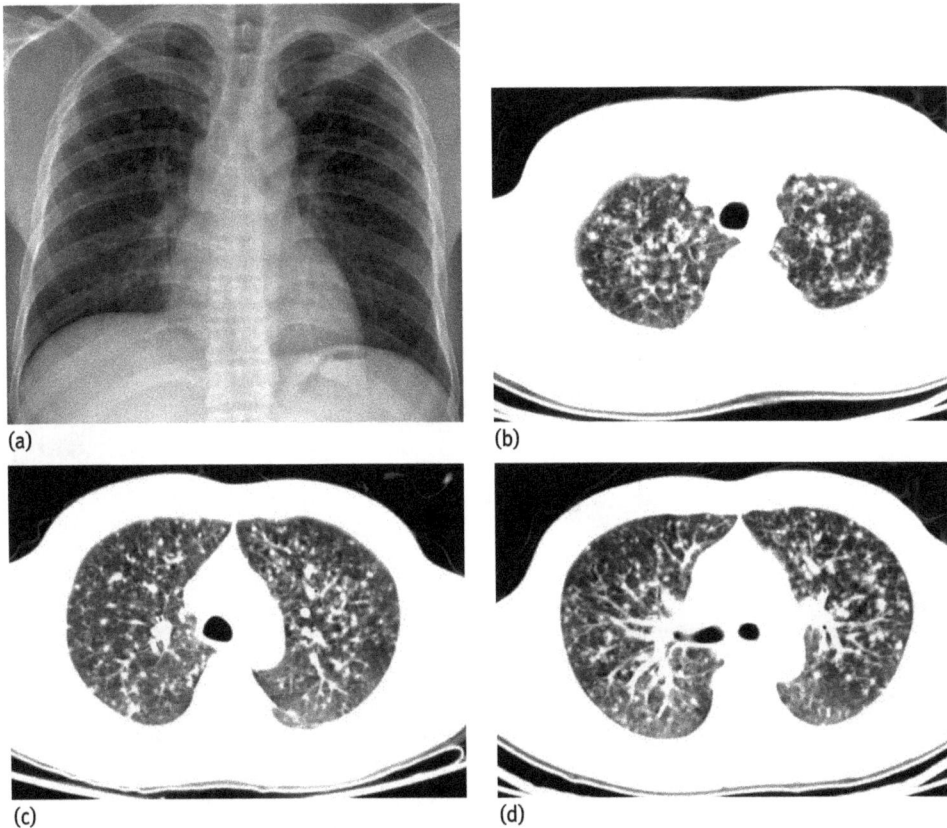

(a)

(b)

(c)

(d)

Fig. 9.3 a–j: Pulmonary *Mycobacterium tuberculosis*, tuberculous lymphadenitis.

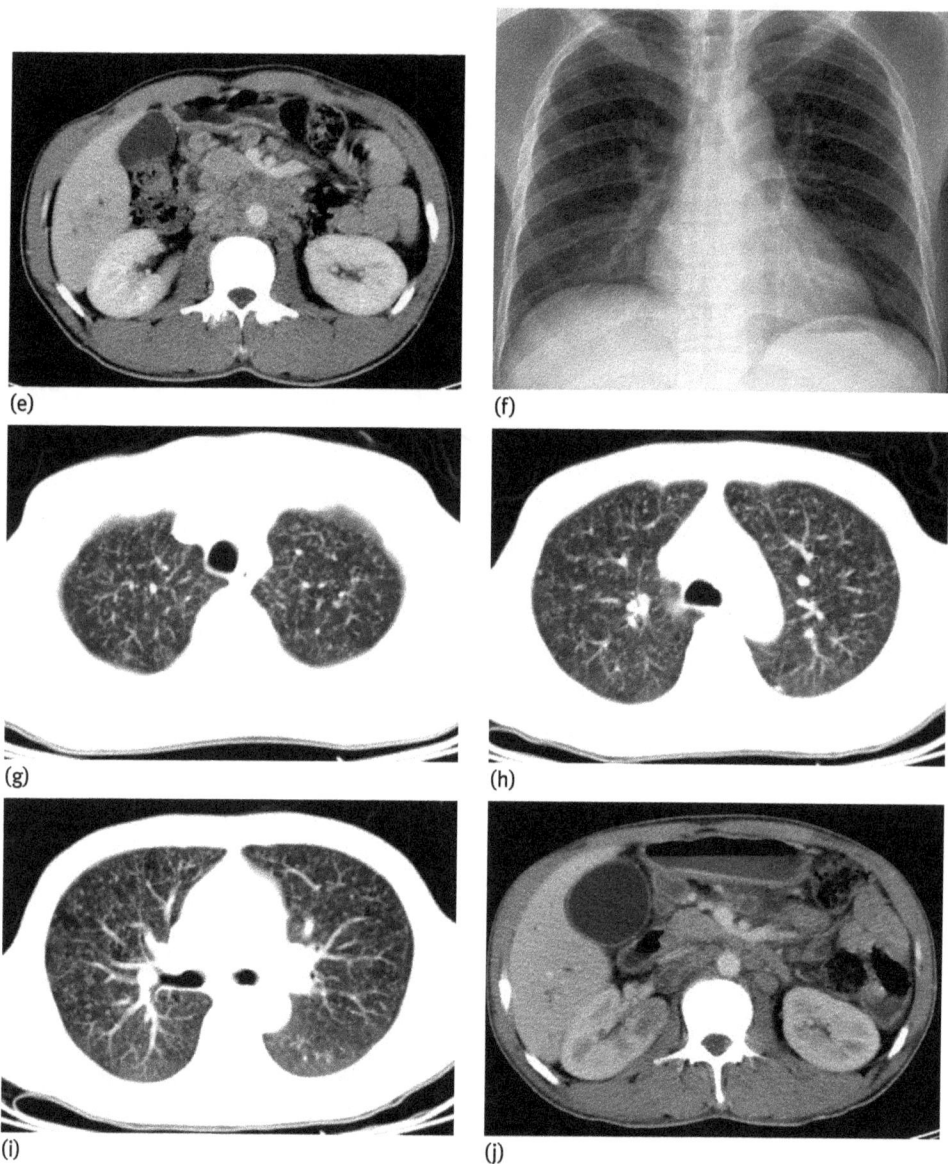

Fig. 9.3: (continuing)

Chest radiograph (a) showed diffuse miliary nodules of different sizes in the bilateral lungs, especially in the upper lobes. CT scans demonstrated diffuse small miliary nodules of various sizes and densities in the bilateral lungs (b–d), low-density patchy lesions in the liver, and lymphadenectasis in the retroperitoneal and mesenteric areas with rim-like enhancement (e). After 11 months treatment, the small nodular lesions were obviously absorbed and shrunk in the bilateral lungs, as showed on the chest radiograph (f) and on the CT scans (g–i). CT showed the liver lesions and enlarged lymph nodes of intrahepatic were shrunken (j).

Case 9.4 (Fig. 9.4 a–k)

A 27-year-old male patient presented prolonged cough and progressive polypena for more than 2 months. Body temperature at admission was 40 °C. The breath sounds of the bilateral lung were weak with slight dry rales in the bilateral middle-lower lungs. The CD4+ cell count was 18/μl. BALF culture detected *Mycobacterium tuberculosis* positive. The patient was diagnosed with AIDS (C3) combined with pulmonary TB. After anti-tuberculosis therapy, the patient was discharged with the symptoms improved.

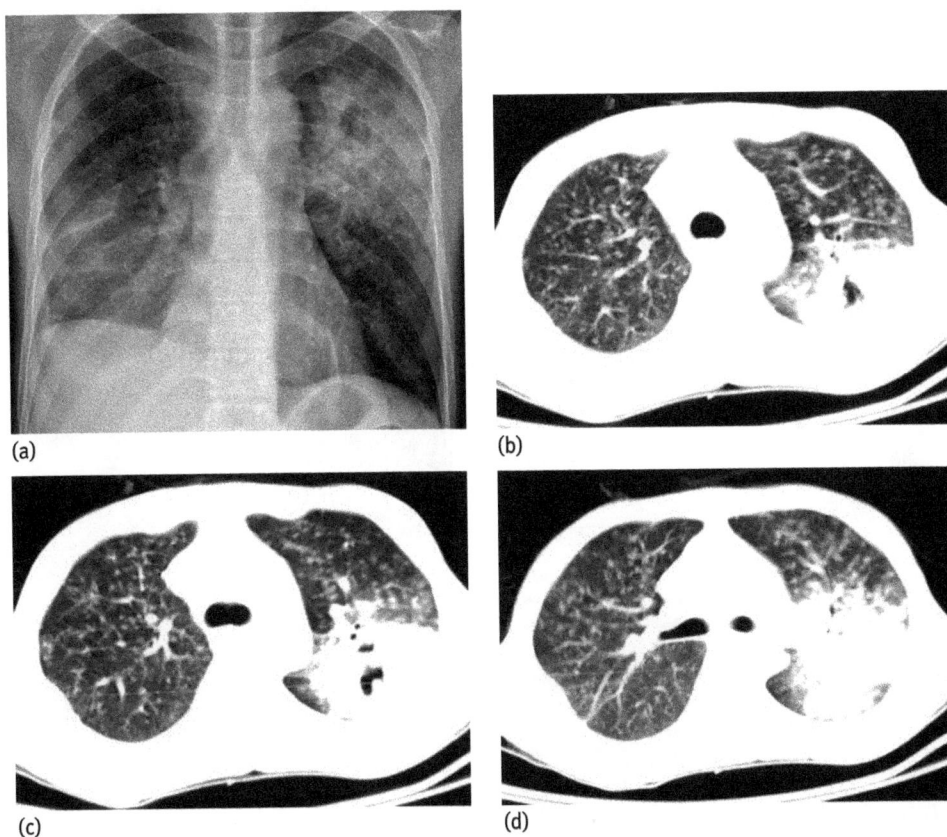

(a)

(b)

(c)

(d)

Fig. 9.4 a–l: Pulmonary *Mycobacterium tuberculosis*.

Chest radiograph (a) showed a massive consolidation with cavities on the left upper lung, slightly high-density patchy opacities in the right lower lung, diffuse miliary opacities in the bilateral lungs, and a few pleural effusions in the right lung (a). CT

(e)

(f)

(g)

(h)

(i)

(j)

(k)

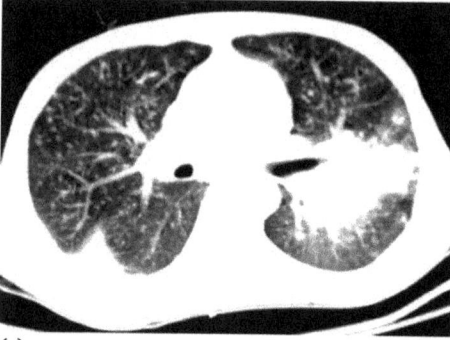

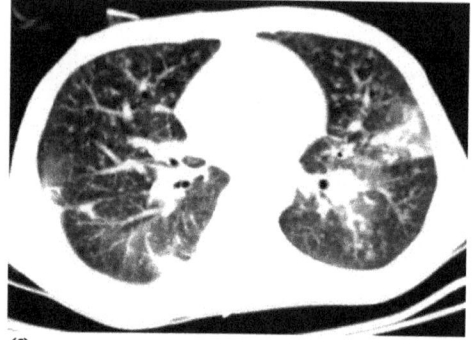

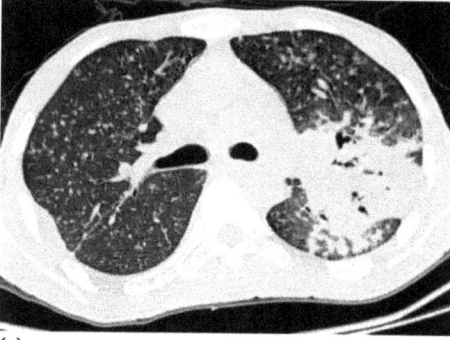

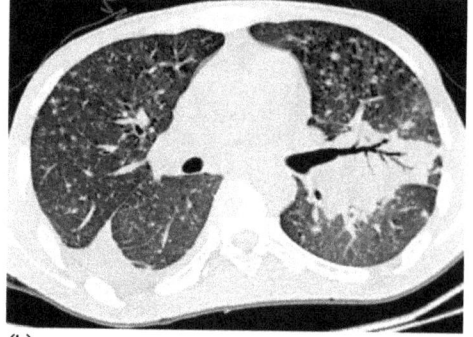

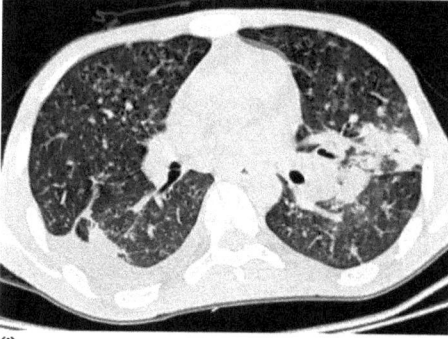

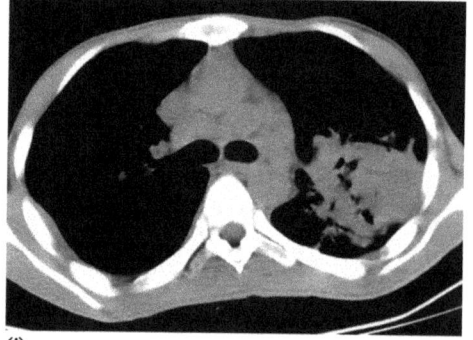

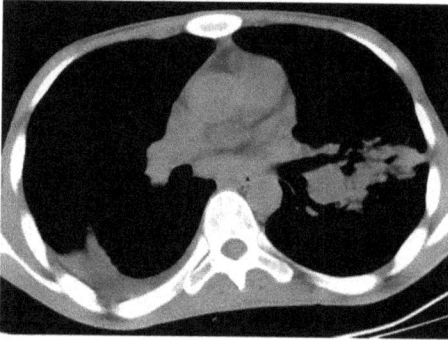

Fig. 9.4: (continuing)

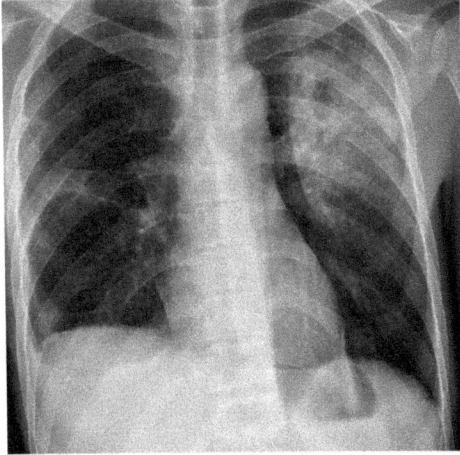

(l)

Fig. 9.4: (continuing)

(b–i) and HRCT (g–i) scans demonstrated a massive consolidation with irregular cavities in the left upper lung, multiple small nodules and scattered patchy lesions in the bilateral lungs. CT scans with mediastinal window (j–k) showed enlarged lymph nodes in the mediastinum and few pleural effusions in the right lung. After a two-month treatment, chest radiograph showed the lesions of both lungs were slightly absorbed, but cavity still can be seen in the lesions of left upper lung (l).

Case 9.5 (Fig. 9.5 a–l)
A 31-year-old male patient presented fatigue and had poor appetites for more than one month, which were aggravated with polypena for 3 weeks. Body temperature at admission was 36.5 °C. The breath sounds of the bilateral lungs were rough, with slight moist sounds in the lower right lung. The CD4+ cell count was 94/μl. BALF smear showed AFB positive (+++). The bronchofiberscopic biopsy detected caseous

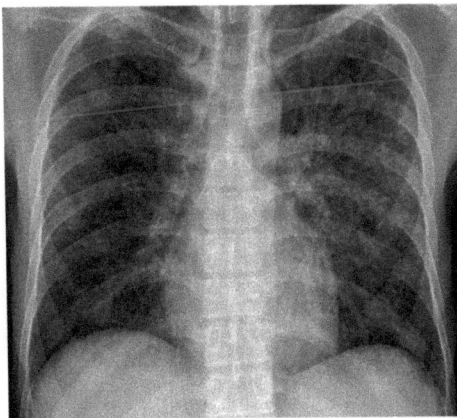

(a)

Fig. 9.5 a–l: Pulmonary *Mycobacterium tuberculosis.*

tuberculous. Eventually, he was diagnosed with AIDS (C3) combined with caseous tuberculous.

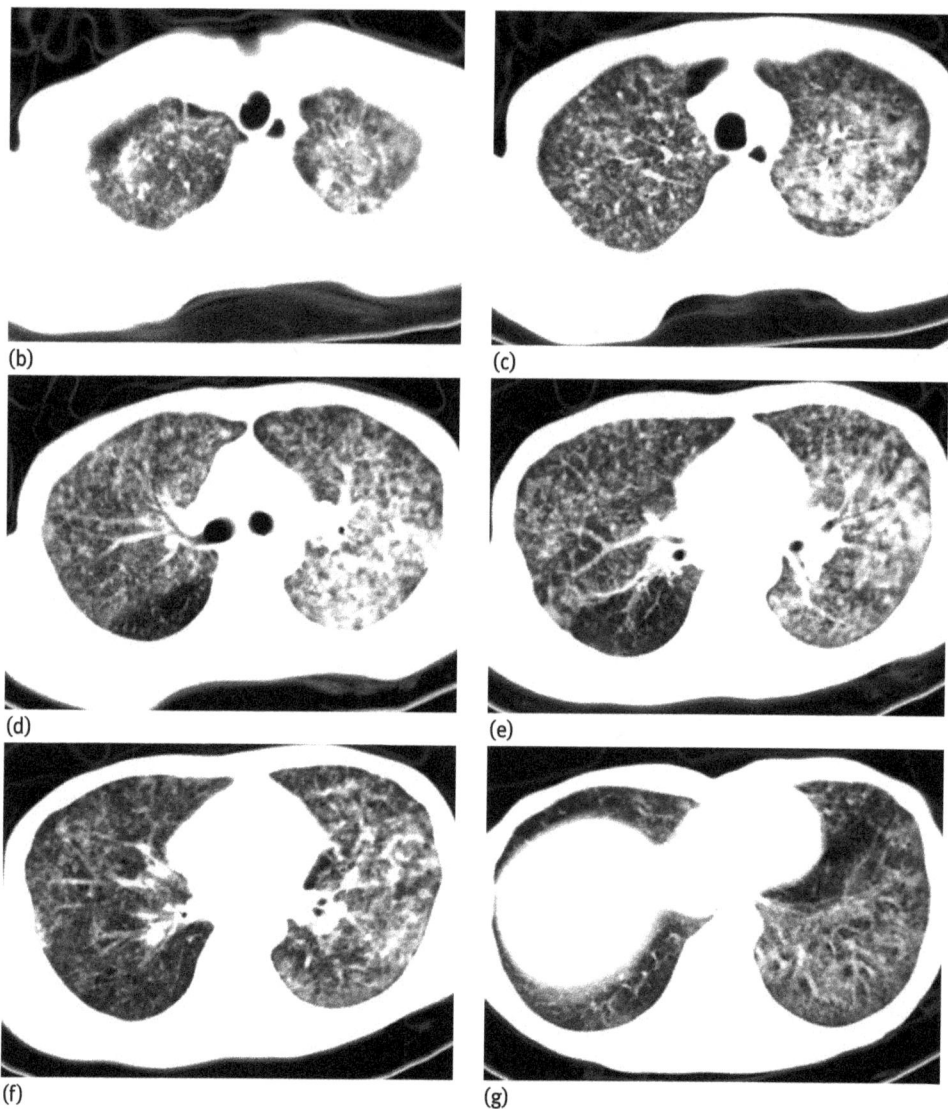

(b)

(c)

(d)

(e)

(f)

(g)

Fig. 9.5: (continuing)

(h)

(i)

(j)

(k)

(l)

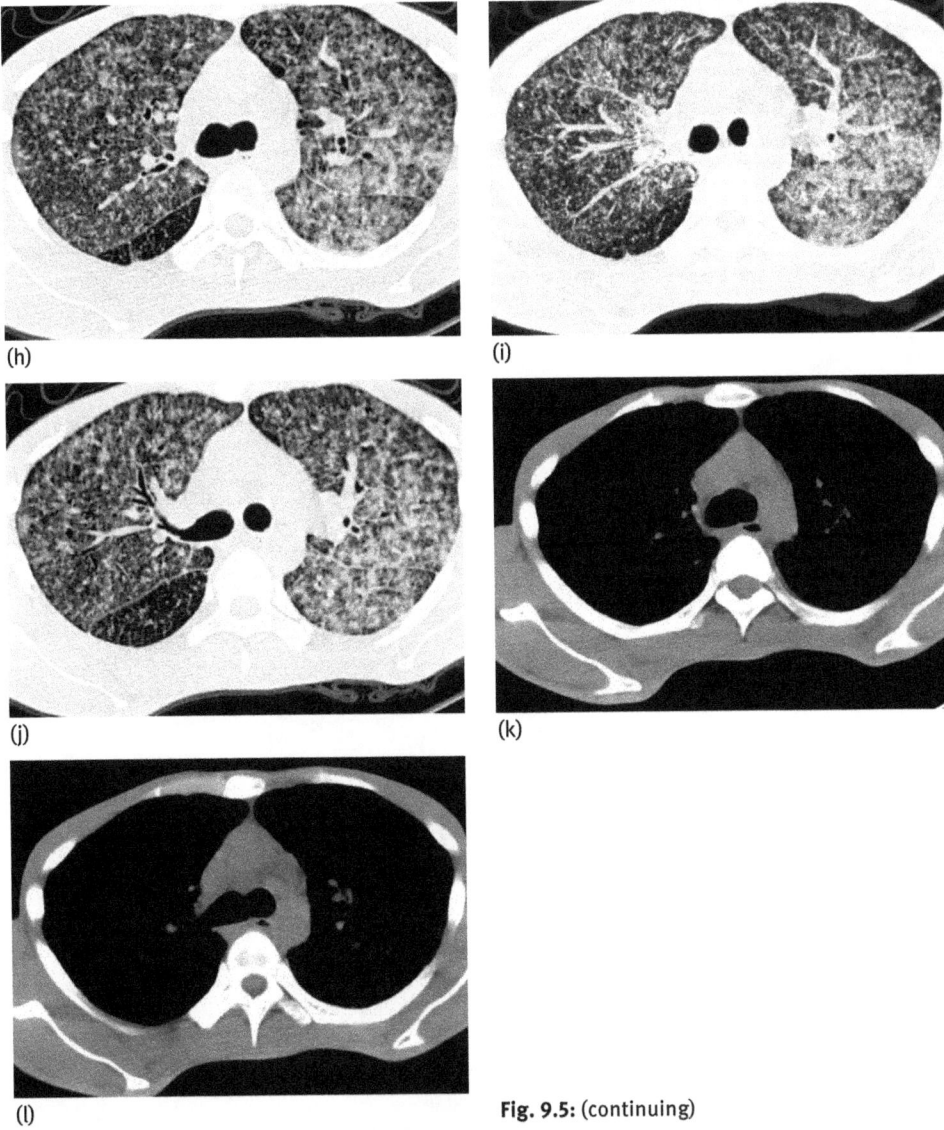

Fig. 9.5: (continuing)

Chest radiograph (a) showed diffuse patchy and miliary lesions in the bilateral lungs, with apparently thickened pulmonary markings. CT (b–j) and HRCT (h–j) scans showed diffuse patchy opacities of high density and miliary opacities in the bilateral lungs, and obviously decreased transparency of pulmonary fields. CT scan with mediastinal window showed no remarkable enlargement in the mediastinal lymph nodes (k, l).

Case 9.6 (Fig. 9.6 a–l)

A 36-year-old male patient presented fever and diarrhea for 2 weeks. Body temperature at admission was 38.5 °C. The CD4+ cell count was 24/μl. BALF culture detected *Mycobacterium tuberculosis* positive. The patient was diagnosed with AIDS (C3) and pulmonary TB.

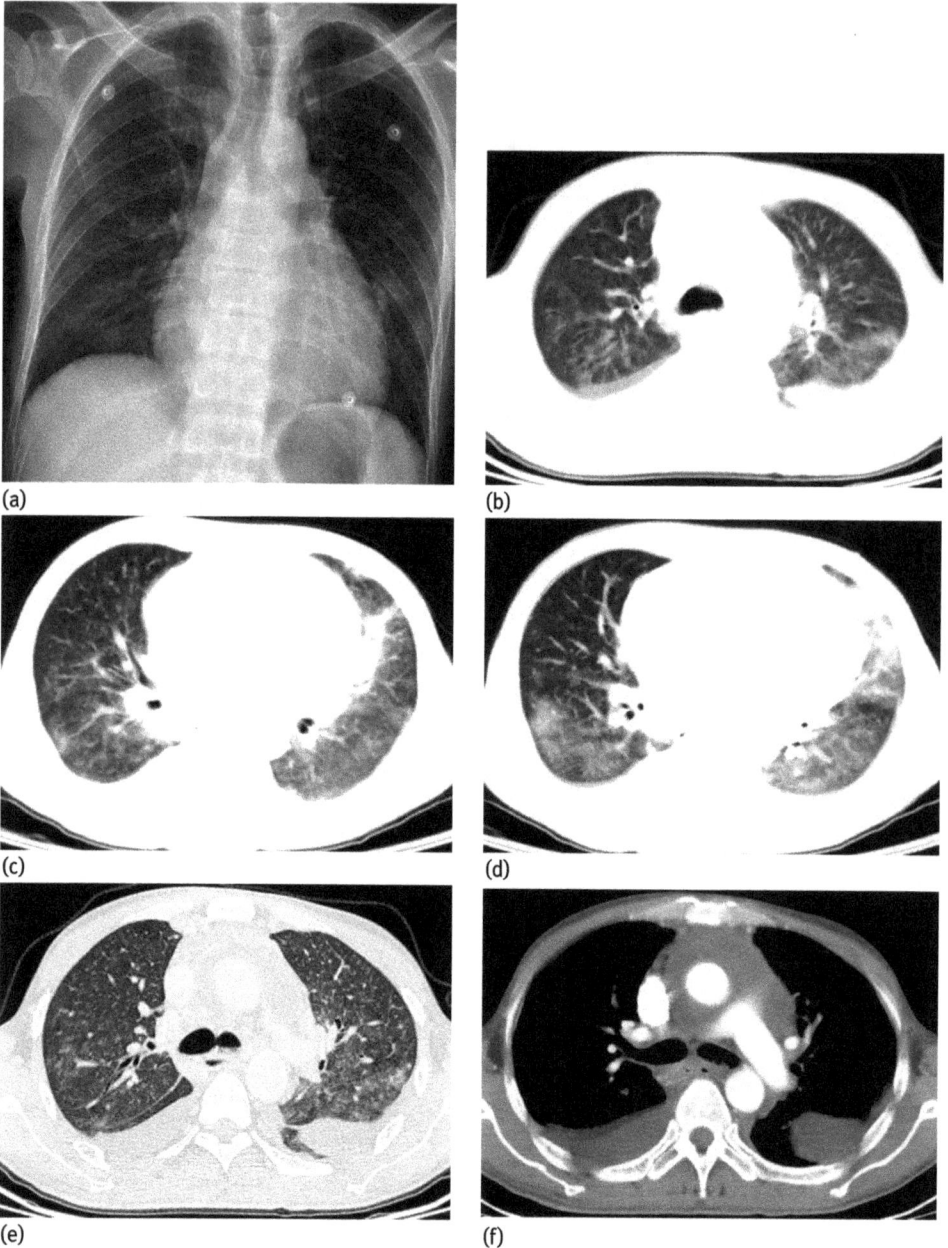

(a)

(b)

(c)

(d)

(e)

(f)

Fig. 9.6 a–l: Pulmonary *Mycobacterium tuberculosis*.

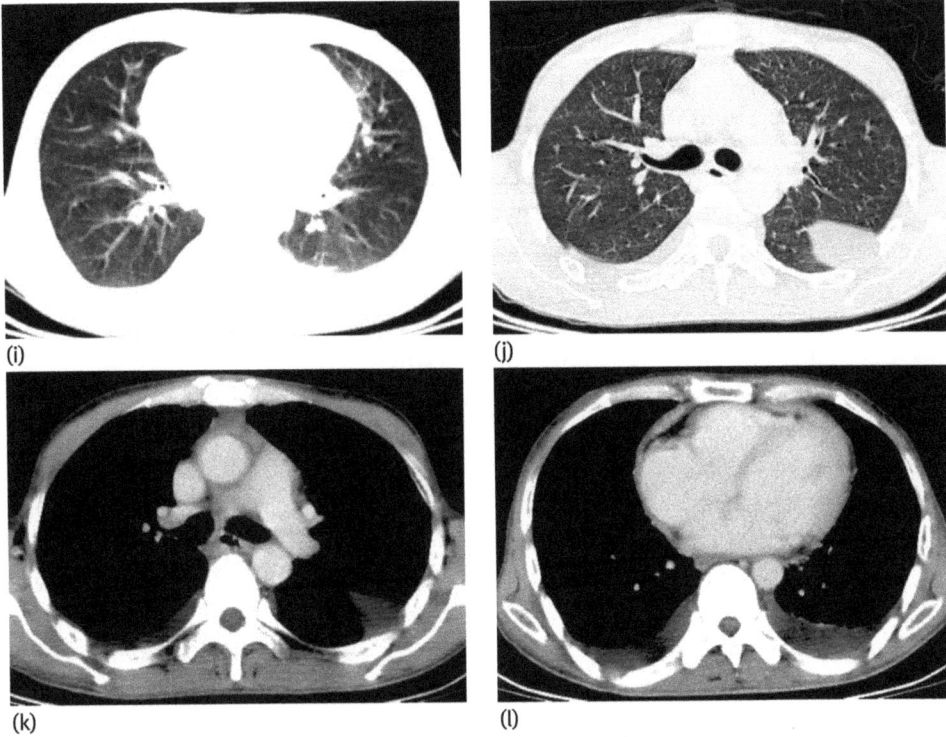

(i)

(j)

(k)

(l)

Fig. 9.6: (continuing)

Chest radiograph (a) showed scattered high-density patchy opacities with blurring edges in the bilateral lungs as well as the significantly enlarged heart shadow. The plain CT (b–d, f and g) and HRCT (e) scans showed scattered high-density patchy opacities in the bilateral lungs, bilateral pleural effusions and pericardial effusions. After three months treatment, the lesions in the bilateral lungs were absorbed to a great extent and eliminated, and the heart shadow became normal, as showed on the radiograph (h). As showed on the CT (h, i, k and l) and HRCT (j) scans, those lesions in the bilateral lungs were significantly absorbed and eliminated, the bilateral pleural effusions were reduced and pericardial effusions were totally absorbed.

9.3 Imaging features

1. Primary pulmonary TB: AIDS patients are more likely to perform with primary tuberculosis type, the imaging feature is multiple widely distributed enlarged lymph nodes which has the trend of conglomeration and occur central necrotic. Plain CT scan show low-attenuation change in enlarged lymph node, enlarged mediastinal and bilateral hilar lymph nodes containing in ordinary scan, enhanced CT scan show enlarged lymph peripheral rim-enhancement which is the typical imaging feature. The calcification rate of mediastinum lymph nodes in AIDS patients is much more lower than PTB in non HIV-infected patient.

2. Secondary pulmonary TB: due to severe depressed of cell immune function in AIDS patients, imaging of patient with PTB demonstrate more widely spread severe atypical lung lesion in both lungs, all segment and lobes can be involved. But typical localized lesion PTB imaging is less common. When CD4+ cell count is at the extremely low level, the lung may appear multiple mixed signs, such as infiltrating lesions, miliary and diffuse small nodes, indicating that hematogenous spread and bronchogenic spread is easy to happen at the same time when AIDS patient immune function is inhibited severely, resulting in wide and severe diffuse lesions.

3. Hematogenous disseminated pulmonary TB: incidence of miliary TB is quite high when the CD4+ cell of AIDS patient is extremely low.

4. Tuberculous pleuritis: It is reported in some literature that AIDS patients with pulmonary TB have a higher rate of pleural effusions than those with single pulmonary TB. Moreover, pleural effusion combined pericardial effusion is common in HIV/AIDS patient.

5. Extrapulmanory tuberculosis: abdominal lymphadenopathy is often involved in AIDS patient with PTB.

The essentials of AIDS tuberculosis imaging diagnosis are concluded as followed: less localized lesion and more diffuse lesion in the lung, presenting atypical infiltration, miliary lesion, mediastinal lymphadenopathy, pleural effusion. On the the other hand, cavity formation, nodules, fibrosis scars and lymph calcification are relatively less common.

The differential diagnosis of AIDS tuberculosis and AIDS NTM pulmonary disease: NTM pulmonary disease is likely to perform with diffuse distributed lesion and/or large cavity consolidation of lobe/segment, nodules, bronchiectasis, mediastinal and hilar lymphadenopathy. NTM pulmonary disease has similar clinical and imaging manifestations to PTB, but has slower progression than TB. NTM pulmonary disease should be considered when long-termed anti-TB treatment is ineffective or relapse of disease, NTM culture should be taken as soon as possible to establish the diagnosis.

The differential diagnosis of AIDS tuberculosis and AIDS-associated diffuse miliary pulmonary disease: the diagnosis of AIDS-associated pulmonary diffuse miliary lesion depend on comprehensive consideration of disease region, history, progression and thoracic-abdominal lymph changes. In Guangdong, Guangxi province of China and southeast Asia, when AIDS patient lung appear with miliary changes, the diagnoses should involve the considerations of pulmonary fungal infections by *Penicillium marneffei* and pulmonary mucormycosis except mililary TB. Miliary lesion of pulmonary fungal infection can be absorbed significantly with 1–3 weeks effective therapy, which is not coincide with mililary TB progression, this point is valuable for the differential diagnosis. Otherwise, AIDS patient with *Penicillium marneffei* pulmonary infection always simultaneously present with obvious mediastinal and retroperitoneal mesenteric lymphadenopathy.

Editors: Bihua Chen, Wanshan Chen, Zhibiao Yin, Wanhua Guan

10 Imaging findings of nontuberculous mycobaterial pulmonary infection in AIDS

10.1 Introduction

The *Nontuberculous mycobacteria* (NTM) are a grouping of all mycobacterium species other than the obligate pathogens like *M. (Mycobacterium) tuberculosis* complex and *M. leprae*. As a kind of opportunistic pathogen, NTM is less virulent than MTB, and has evident differention from MTB in ecology and physiology. As a saprophytic species, NTM resides generally in natural environment and can be isolated from water, soil and dust. As a kind of rapidly growing mycobacteria, NTM has similar bacterial composition and antigenicity with MTB, but its pathogenicity is lower than MTB.

NTM has the same histopathology with MTB, including exudation, proliferation and sclerosis. The pathology of NTM pulmonary disease present with granuloma, epithelioid cell and lymphocyte get gather to form the nodule which is not the typical tuberculous tubercle. Necrosis and cavity also can be seen in the lungs, which is multifocal and multi-room, thin-wall cavity predominantely, thick and sparse soft necrosis in the cavity, that is different from TB cavity.

The prevalence of NTM varies greatly due to the geographic region, race, different isolation and identification. Before AIDS epidemic globally, the pathogen causing NTM infection came from the environment. NTM mainly cause pulmonary infection, regional lymphadenitis and skin infection, rarely cause disseminated infection. The main NTM species caused lung infection is *Mycobacterium kansasii* and *M. aviumand* Intracellulare complex (MAC). With the global prevalence of AIDS, incidence of NTM infection has changed fundamentally, the NTM morbidity increase rapidly. There was a report that 25%–50% AIDS patients in Europe and America affected NTM. At the same time, the clinical manifestations of NTM disease has changed a lot as well. Before AIDS prevalence, the lesion of NTM infection in the immunocompetent patients is usually localized. In AIDS patients and other immunocompromised patients, NTM can cause disseminated infection. Meanwhile, the NTM species composition ratio has changed due to the spread of AIDS epidemic, most NTM infection in AIDS is mainly caused by *Mycobacterium avium complex* (MAC). MAC accounts for the majority of NTM infection in AIDS patients. The NTM infection transmission changed with AIDS epidemic. Transmit from person-to-person rarely happened before AIDS prevalent, with very rare exceptions. Now AIDS allows the transmitability among humans by way of respiratory or gastrointestinal tract.

MAC is the main species that cause AIDS NTM infection currently (MAC accounts for the majority of NTM infection in AIDS). MAC is a kind of achromatic slowly-growing mycobacterium. MAC not only lead to pulmonary infection in AIDS patients, but also cause disseminated infection, lymphadenitis and skin infection. Disseminated MAC infection usually manifest with fever, anemia, spontaneous sweating and diarrhea. Disseminated MAC infection in AIDS patients is closely related with CD4+ count, When the CD4+<100/ul, the morbidity of disseminated MAC infection start to rise, when CD4+<10/ul, the morbidity of disseminated infection reaches the highest.

Testing and identifications of NTM can be done by the conventional method, include chromatography and molecular classification. The conventional method is comprised of microscopic examination, culturing, biochemical identification and histopathology, among which culturing and biochemical identification are always considered as the gold standard for the diagnosis of NTM infections. Due to the lung is the most frequent organ NTM infect, the definite diagnosis of NTM infection usually depend on the sputum culture and bronchoalveolar lavage fluid (BALF) culture and further NTM identification.

10.2 Radiographic findings

Case 10.1 (Fig. 10.1 a–l)
A 25-year-old male patient presented fever for more than one month, accompanied with cough, expectoration and polypena for two weeks, with body temperature high up to 39.5 °C, without chills, shiver or muscular soreness. Examination found no skin rash and no systemic superficial lymph nodes enlargement. CD4+ cell count was 16/μl, with CD4+/CD8+: 0.01. BALF culture was NTM positive. The patient was diagnosed with AIDS (C3) complicated with NTM pulmonary infection.

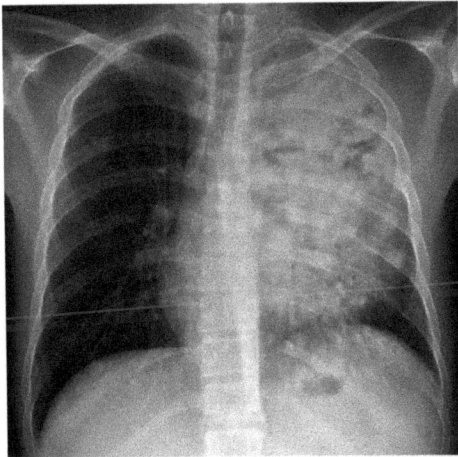

(a)

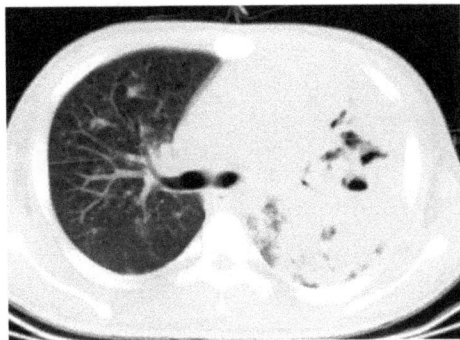

(b)

Fig. 10.1 a–l: Nontuberculous mycobaterial pulmonary disease.

(c)

(d)

(e)

(f)

(g)

(h)

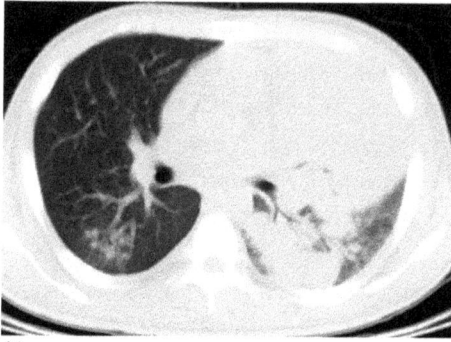

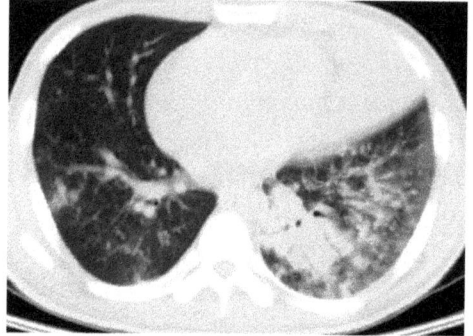

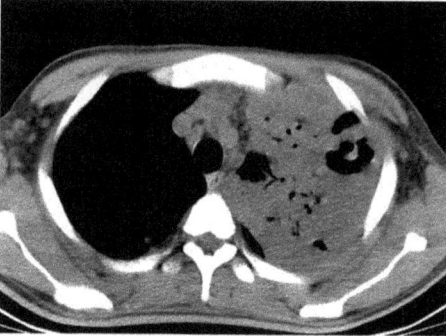

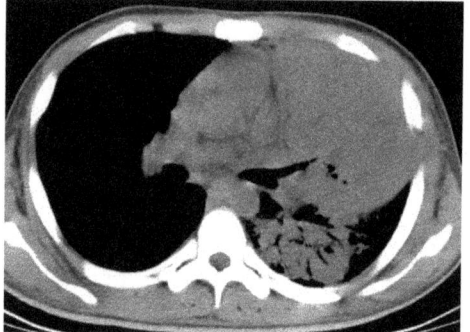

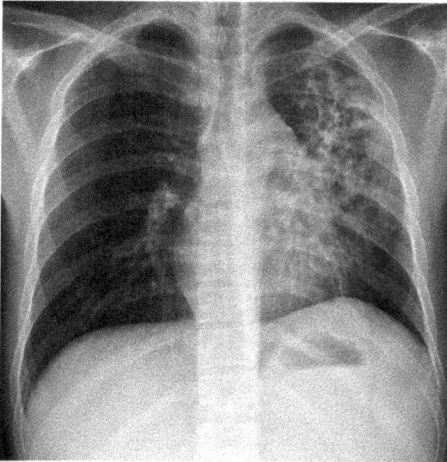

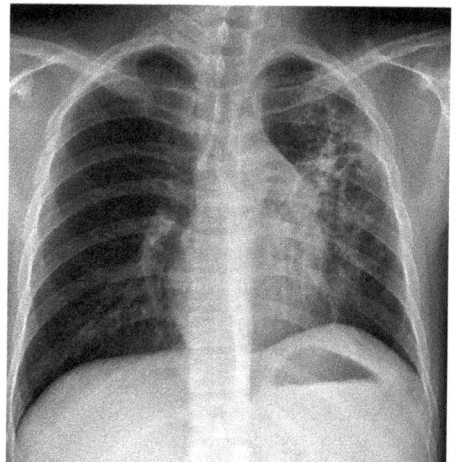

Fig. 10.1: (continuing)

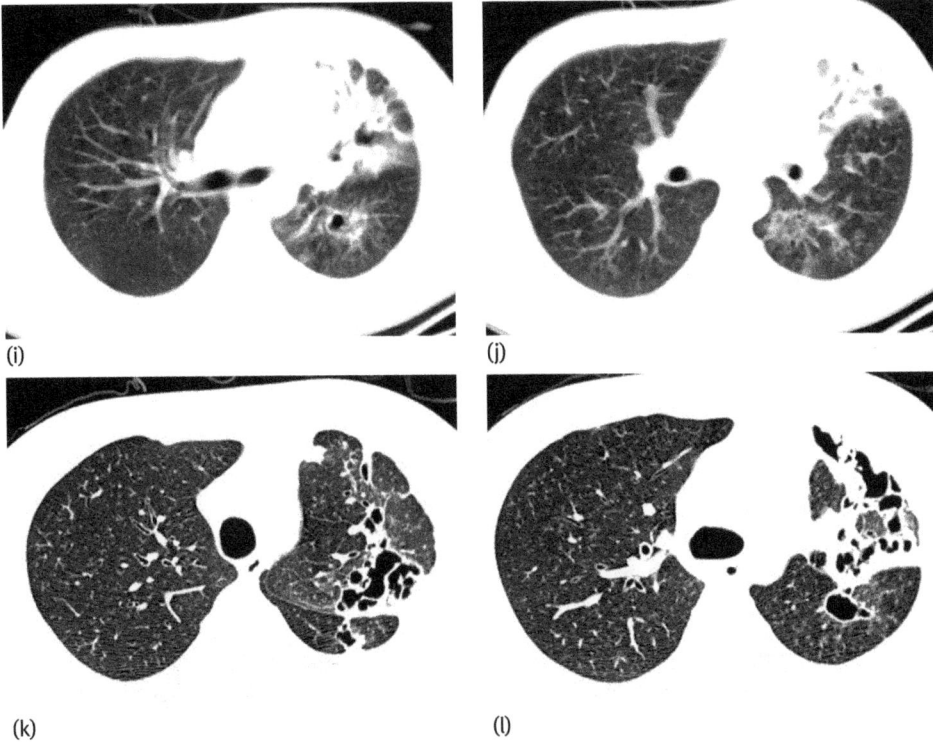

(i)   (j)

(k)   (l)

Fig. 10.1: (continuing)

Chest radiograph (a) showed massive patchy consolidation in the left lung, with air bronchogram and low-density cavity in the lesion, multiple small ill-defined nodules in the right lung. CT scans with lung window (b–d) showed massive patchy consolidation in the left lung, with air bronchogram in it, multiple patchy cavities in the left lung, multiple ill-edged nodules of various size in the posterior basal segment of left lower lobe and right lung. CT scans with the mediastinal window (e–f) demonstrated the massive consolidation and air bronchogram, slightly enlarged lymph nodes in the mediastinum and hilum of left lung. After 5 and 7 weeks treatment, chest radiographs (g, h) respectively showed the lesion of left lung was evidently absorbed, remained a few residual fibering lesions and multiple cavities, accompanied with obviously traction bronchietcasis, and the left lung volume shrunk. CT scans with lung window (i–l) at re-check after 8 weeks treatment showed absorbed markedly lesions in the left lung, remained a few residual fibering lesions and evident bronchietcasis, while nodules in right lung vanished after therapy.

Case 10.2 (Fig. 10.2 a–l)

A 29-year-old female patient presented fever for no definite reasons for more than one month, and no obvious chills with temperature up to 38.5 °C, accompanied by dizziness, spontaneous sweating, cough with yellow phlegm and blood streak sputum, polypena after physical excises but relieved after rest, without chest pain or headache. She had a weight loss of 10 kg. A round mass sized 5 cm in diameter touched hard in the left supraclavicular fossa, with smooth surface and without redness or swelling or tenderness. There were several enlarged lymph nodes in bilateral inguinal, with smooth surface and good mobility, no tenderness at palpation. The CD4+ cell counted 20/µl, CD4+/CD8+: 0.06. BALF culture was NTM positive. The patient was diagnosed with AIDS (C3) combined with NTM pulmonary infection.

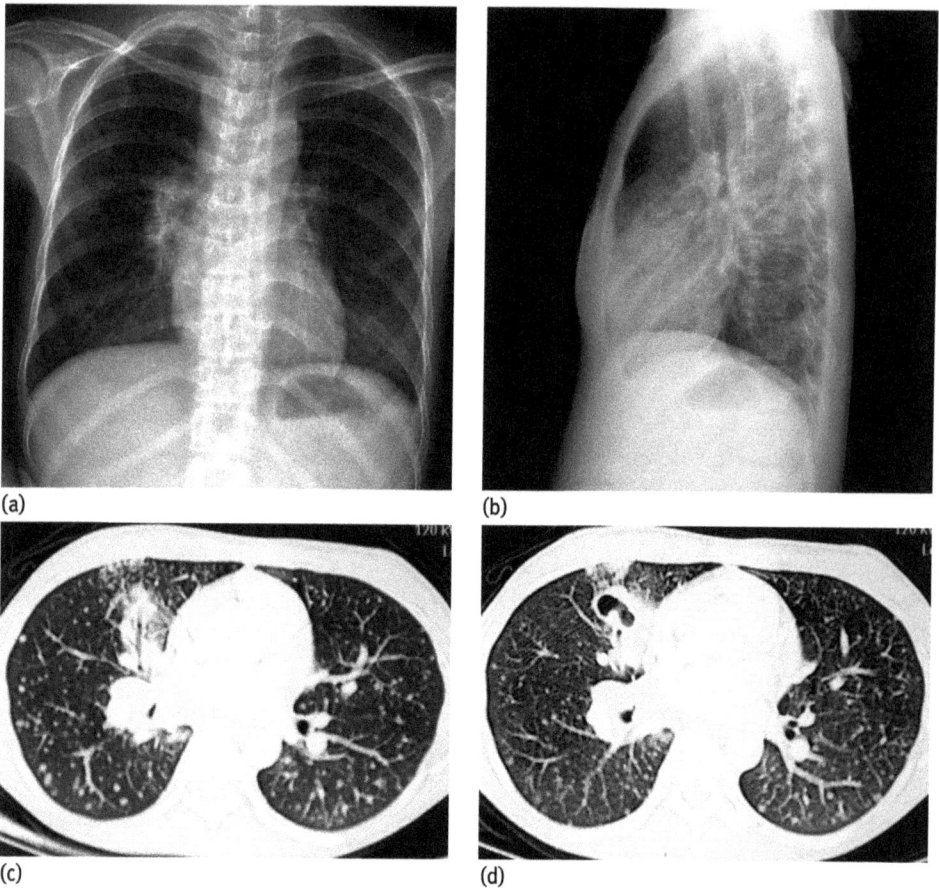

(a)

(b)

(c)

(d)

Fig. 10.2 a–l: Nontuberculous mycobaterial pulmonary disease.

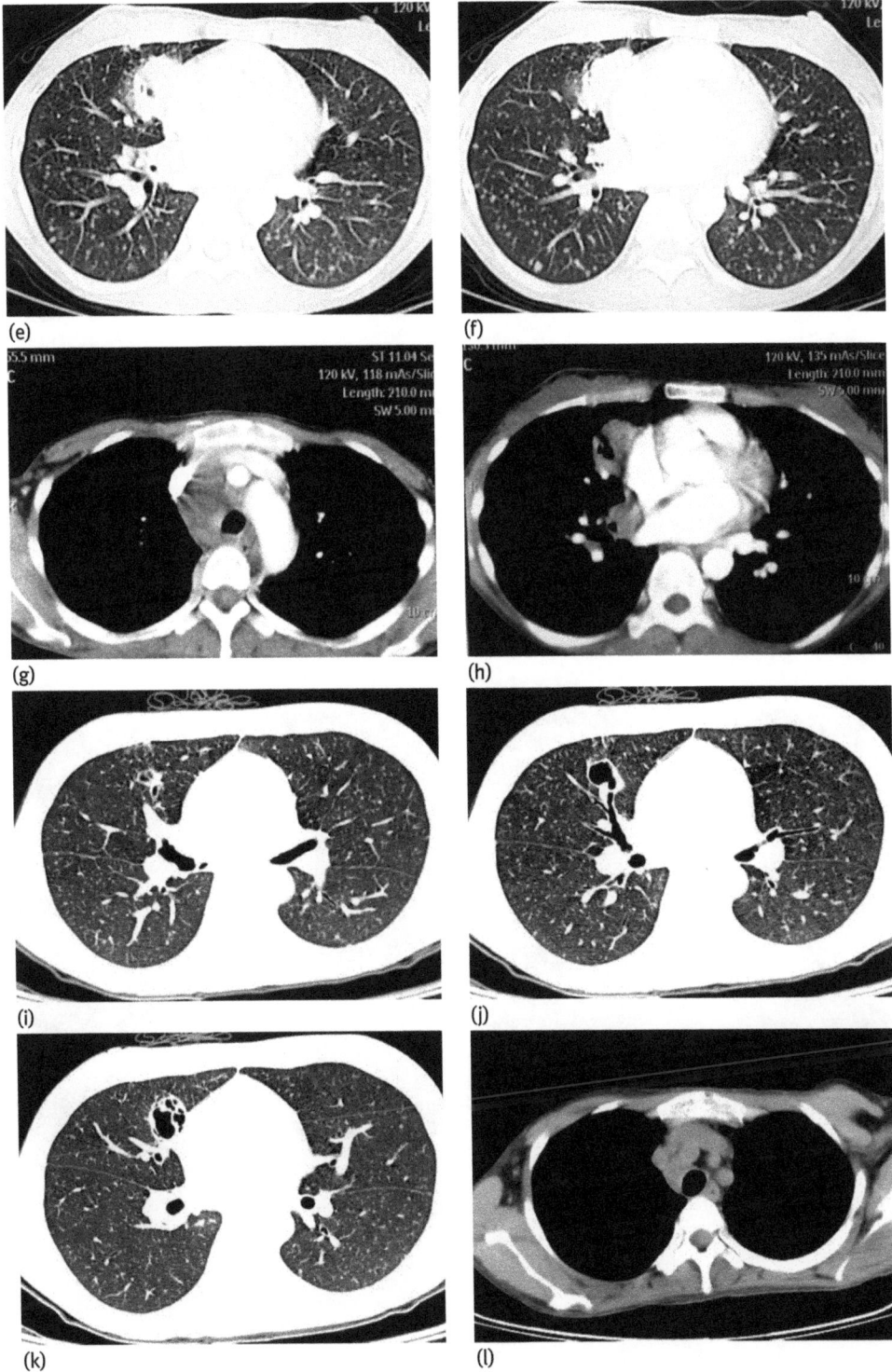

Fig. 10.2: (continuing)

Chest radiographs showed diffusive miliary nodules in the bilateral lungs and the enlarged shadow of the right hilum (a, b). CT scans with lung window (c–f) showed a massive shadow on the right-middle lobe with irregular cavity in it, the diffuse miliary nodules of different sizes in the bilateral lungs and the enlarged right hilum. Enhanced CT scans demonstrated the enlarged lymph nodes in the mediastinum and the right lung hilum (g, h). After 3 months therapy, CT scans showed the lesions in the bilateral lungs dramatically shrank, but significant bronchietcasis and cavities with smooth walls, well-defined edges were seen in the right-middle lobe(i, k). Meanwhile the mediastinal lymph nodes got smaller than before therapy (l).

Case 10.3 (Fig. 10.3 a–j)

A 46-year-old male patient complained of polypena, discomfort and occasional fever for no definite reasons for more than one month. The polypena was aggravated 10 days ago before hospitalized, with body temperature high up to 41 °C, accompanied with chills, shiver and occasional dry cough without expectoration. The lymph nodes seized 1 cm×1 cm were palpable in the bilateral neck, with smooth surface, good mobility but no tenderness at palpation. CD4+ cell counted 15/μl, CD4+/CD8+: 0.04. BALF culture was NTM positive. The patient was diagnosed with AIDS (C3) combined with NTM pulmonary infection.

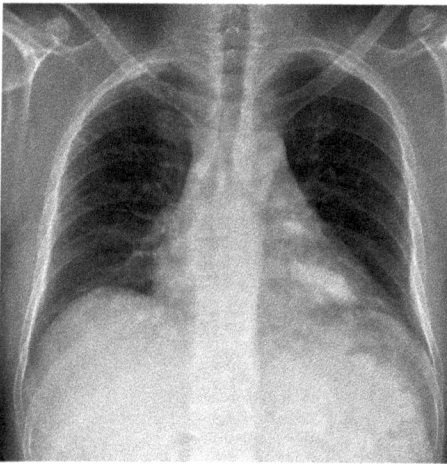 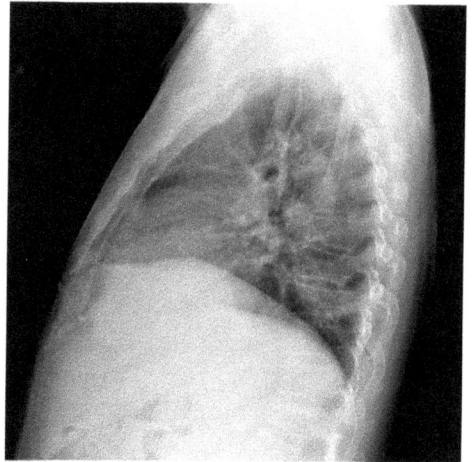

(a) (b)

Fig. 10.3 a–j: Nontuberculous mycobaterial pulmonary disease.

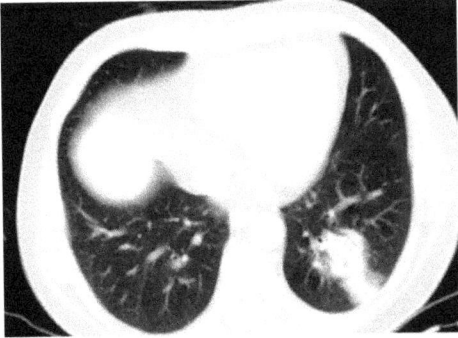
(c)

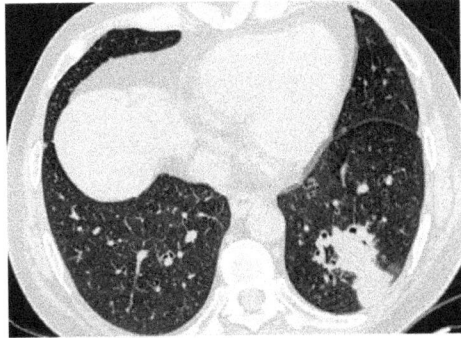
(d)

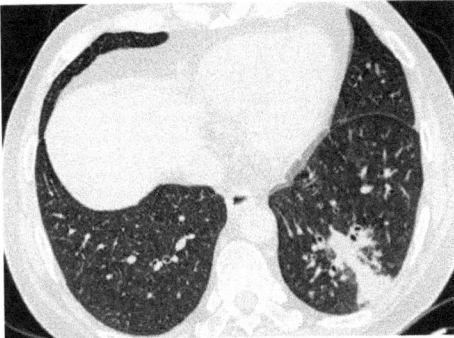
(e)

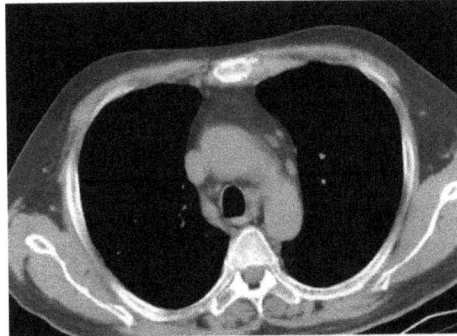
(f)

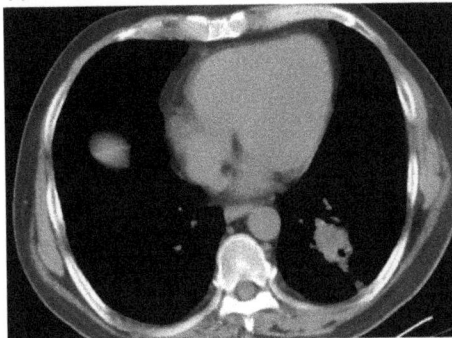
(g)

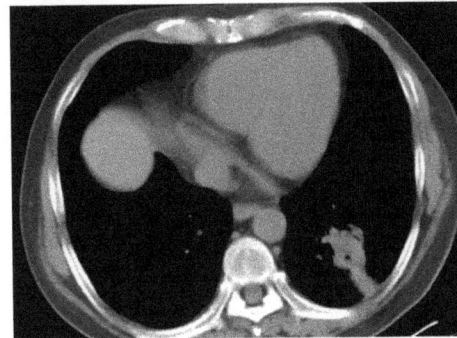
(h)

Fig. 10.3: (continuing)

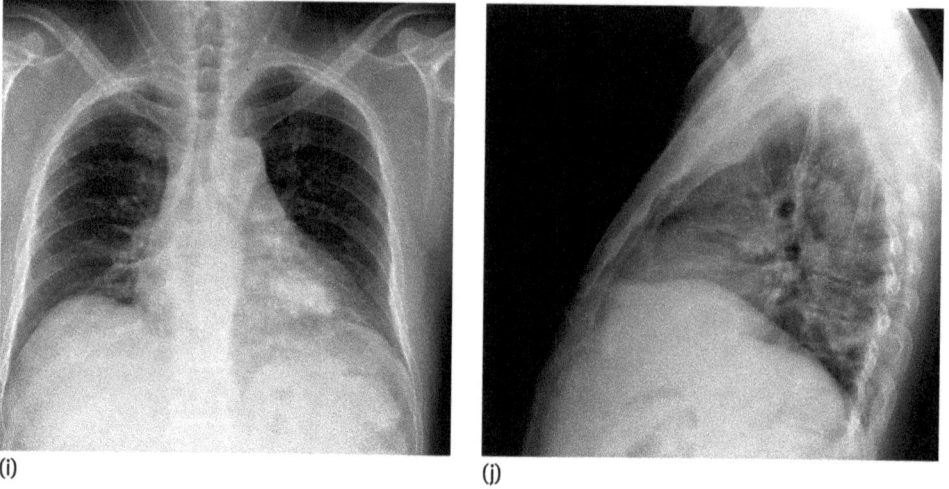

(i)   (j)

Fig. 10.3: (continuing)

Chest radiographs (a, b) show multiple messy pulmonary markings in the bilateral lungs, a high-density patchy shadow with rough edges in the posterior basal segment of left lower lobe. CT scans and HRCT scans (c–e) demonstrated an irregular rough-edged nodular shadow in the posterior basal segment of left lower lobe, with small bronchietcasis and cavities in it. CT scans with mediastinal window (f–h) demonstrated the lower-density lesion with one small cavity in it, and mild enlargements of paratracheal and aortic paraarcus lymph nodes. After 4 weeks therapy, Chest radiographs showed the lesion of left lower lobe grew large, surrounded by multiple patchy opacities with blurring edge (i, j).

10.3 Imaging features

It is reported that CT manifestations of NTM pulmonary disease in non-AIDS patients include air-space consolidations, cavities, multiple nodules and bronchiectasis. It is characterized by simultaneous involvement of multiple lesions in multiple lobes. When NTM affect AIDS patients, it is likely to perform as dissemination, the most common imaging manifestation is mediastinal and hilar lymphadenectasis, while air-space consolidations, miliary nodules and pleural effusion are relatively less common.

Based on continuous observation data of chest imaging of AIDS patients with NTM pulmonary disease in Guangzhou No. 8 people hospital, we conclude some image features of NTM pulmonary disease, as follows:

1. The lesions are of diffuse infiltration and/or massive consolidation in the lobe/segment of lung.

2. Large consolidation accompanied with cavities can be gradually absorbed and improved or vanished with the therapy progression. the lesions shrink but the bronchiectases may significantly increase. Some patients appear with volume reduction in affected lung. This type of NTM relatively has long slowly progression and well prognosis.
3. The diffuse exudative NTM infection is usually seen in the advanced AIDS patients, which is often accompanied with other pathogen co-infection, result in worse condition and rapid aggravation, lead to bad prognosis.
4. Multiple lesion patterns involved in same case.
5. The mediastinal and hilar lymph nodes are slightly enlarged.

In summary, the presences of massive consolidations combined with cavities, nodular lesions, bronchiectasis and mediastinal and hilar lymphadenectases is of significant for the differential diagnosis of NTM pulmonary infection to a certain extent.

Editors: Xiangfeng Guo, Haolan He, Jinxin Liu, Wanhua Guan

11 Imaging findings of CMV pneumonia in AIDS

11.1 Introduction

Cytomegaloviruses (CMV) frequently affect immunocompromised patients, especially those marrow or organ transplant recipients and AIDS patients. Severe CMV infections like CMV pneumonia are characterized by short disease course, rapid aggravation and high mortality.

CMV can be generally passed among people through direct contact with body fluids such as maternal-neonatal transmission, sexual transmission, transplanted organs and blood transfusion. They can stay in a person's body for a lifelong time in case of actual infection, but may be activated in case of immune suppression so as to lead to severe affections. Salivary gland is susceptible to CMV affections, but clinically, identification of CMV from respiratory secretions is even not specific for determination of CMV pneumonia.

In AIDS patients, CMV causes a systemic infection, including pneumonia, amphiblestritis, esophagitis, gastroenteritis, cerebritis, hepatitis and so forth. CMV pneumonia is often seen at AIDS advanced stage and even lead to a larger mortality among AIDS patients. The risk of CMV pneumonia in an AIDS patient increases sharply once the CD4 lymphocyte count drops to less than 50/μl. Most AIDS patients infected with CMV present with unspecific manifestations commonly like fever, sore throat, dyspnea, cyanochroia, and myalgia.

In etiology, CMV pneumonia is identified based on positive cytomegalic cells under microscope. It is very difficult to obtain the specimen from the lesions but it is critical for the affirmative diagnoses, which can be reached by bronchoscopic biopsy and histological tests.

CMV pulmonary infection frequently occurs along with other pathogens.

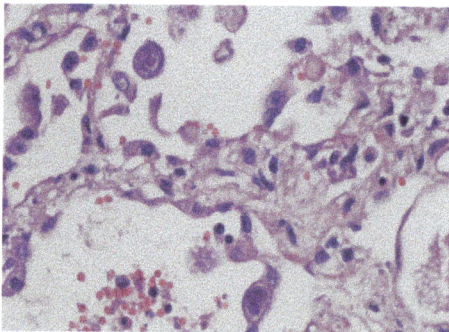

Fig. 11.0: Cytomegalic inclusion in lung tissue (HE stain, ×400).

11.2 Imaging findings

Case 11.1 (Fig 11.1 a–l)

A 36-year-old male patient complained of weight loss for six months, appetite loss and cough for two months, and skin rashes for 1 week. Body temperature at admission was 39.3 °C. Red maculopapules were scattered on his face and extremities, some rash appeared naval-like scabs. The breath sounds of the bilateral lung were rough with the dry rales. There were no enlargements of systemic superficial lymph nodes. CD4+ cell count was 51/μl. Pulmonary tissue biopsy by bronchoscopy identified CMV pneumonia. Bronchoalveolar lavage fluid (BALF) culture was streptococcus mitis positive. Blood culture was *Penicillum marneffei* positive. The patient was diagnosed with AIDS (C3) combined with CMV pneumonia, streptococcus mitis pneumonia and *Penicillum marneffei* infection.

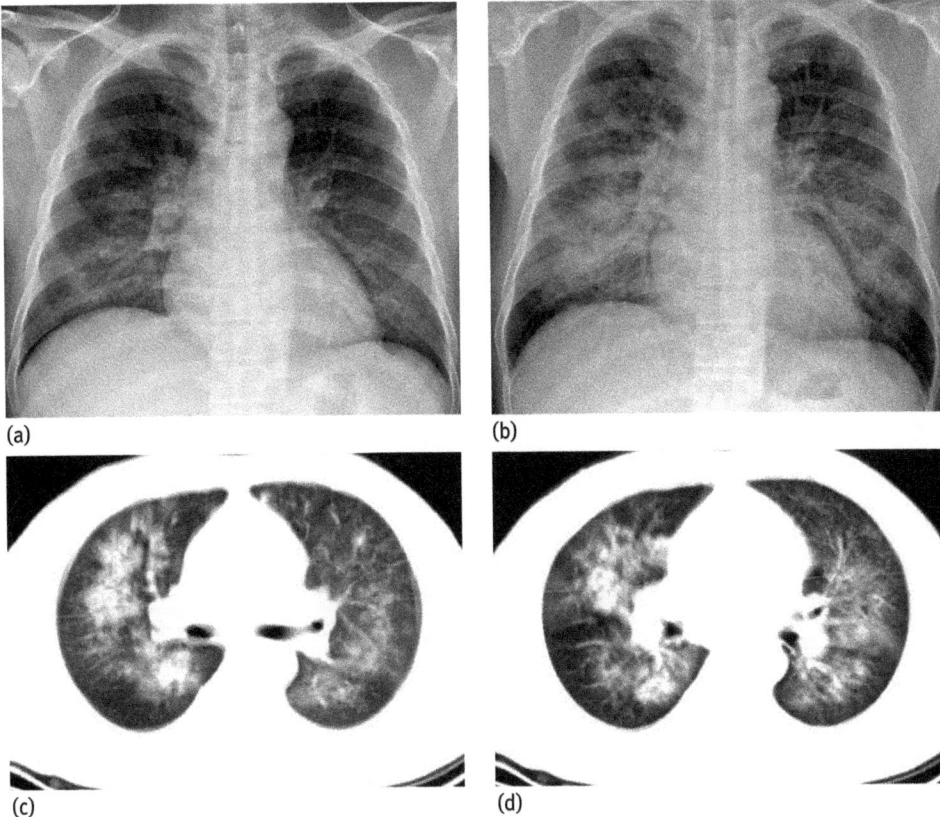

(a) (b) (c) (d)

Fig. 11.1 a–l: CMV pneumonia, streptococcus mitis pneumonia and *Penicillum marneffei* infection.

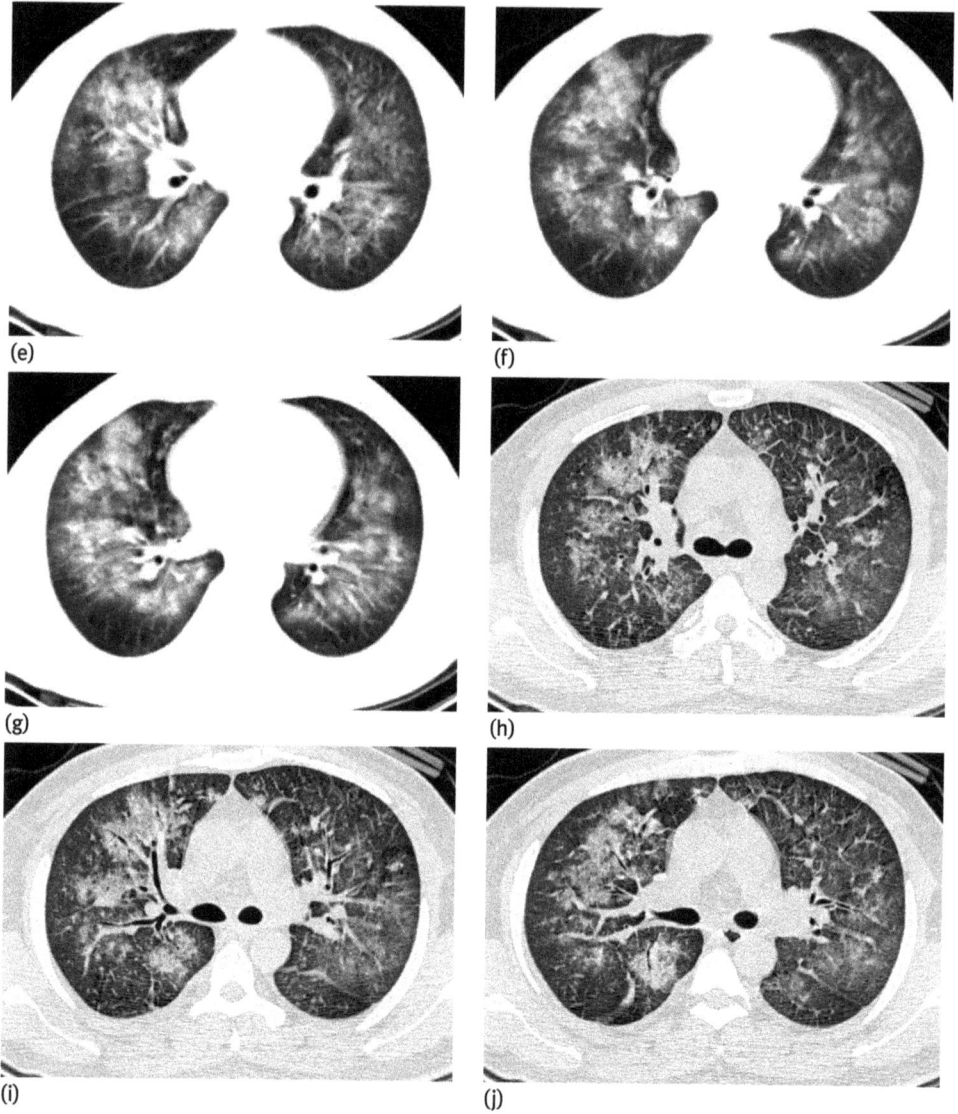

Fig. 11.1: (continuing)

Chest radiographs demonstrated diffuse patchy shadow on the left and right lungs (a) and the radiograph (b) at re-check on the following day shows significant extension and increased density of the lesion shadow on the bilateral lungs. The CT scans (c–g) show high-density effuse patchy opacities with blurring edge mainly in the inner zone of lung field. The HRCT scans (h–j) also confirm the thickened interlobular septae. After 10 days treatment, the bilateral opacities were found to be evidently absorbed, as showed on the radiograph (k). 48 days after treatment, the lesions in the bilateral lungs were fundamentally absorbed as showed on the radiograph (l).

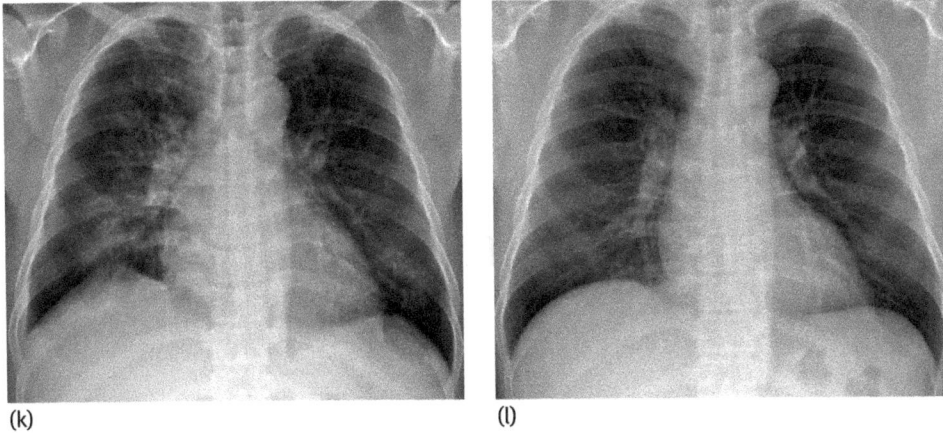

(k)

(l)

Fig. 11.1: (continuing)

Case 11.2 (Fig. 11.2 a–k)

A 37-year-old male patient presented recurrent cough for 4 years, which aggravated and accompanied with fever for 20 days and polypena for 4 days. Body temperature at admission was 37.7 °C. Examination: breath sounds of the bilateral lung were rough with heavy dry rales and slight moist rales. There were no enlargements of systemic superficial lymph nodes. CD4+ cell count was 12/μl. Both lung tissue biopsy by bronchoscopy and the bronchoalveolar lavage fluid (BALF) culture detected *Penicillum marneffei* positive. On the 31st hospital day, the patient died of septic shock. The pathological examination of autopsy on lung specimens identified CMV pneumonia. Diagnosis: AIDS (C3) combined with *Penicillum marneffei* infection and CMV pneumonia.

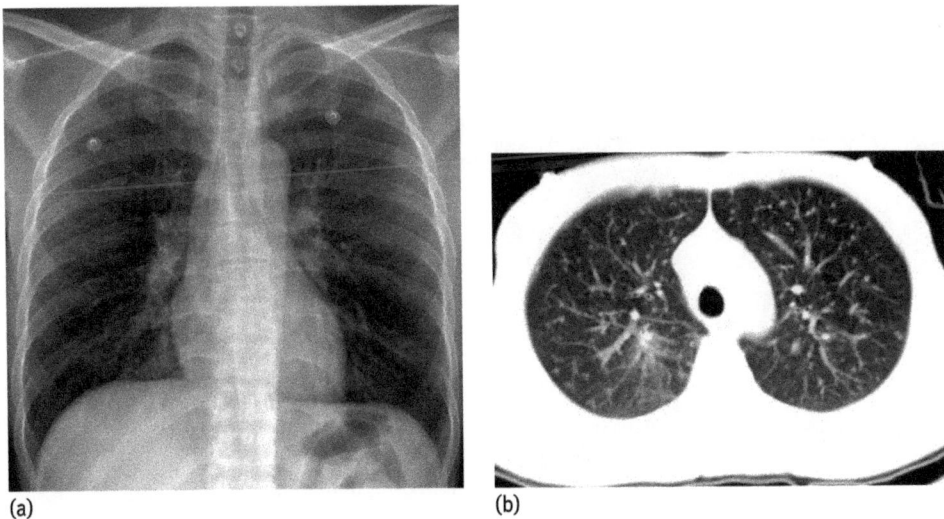

(a)

(b)

Fig. 11.2 a–k: *Penicillum marneffei* infection and CMV pneumonia.

(c)

(d)

(e)

(f)

(g)

(h)

(i)

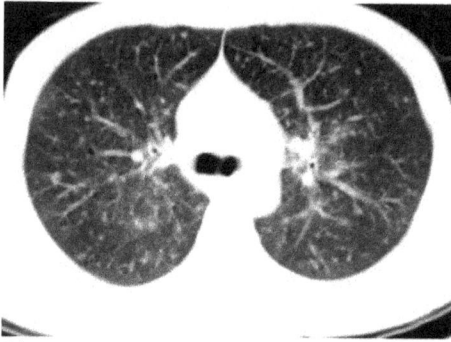

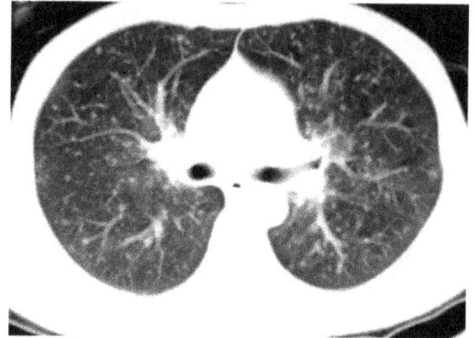

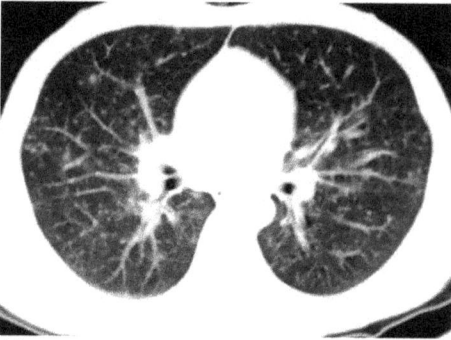

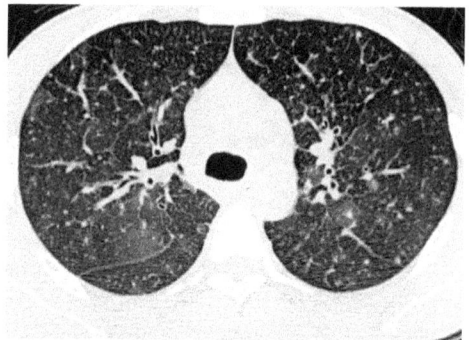

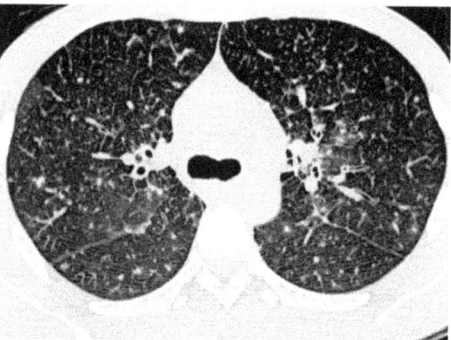

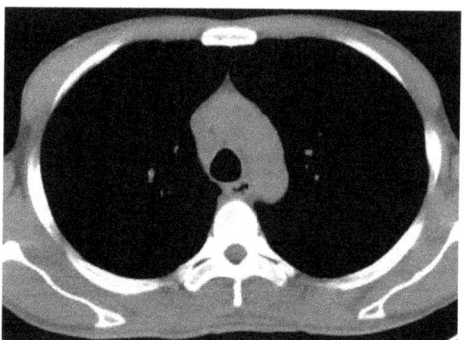

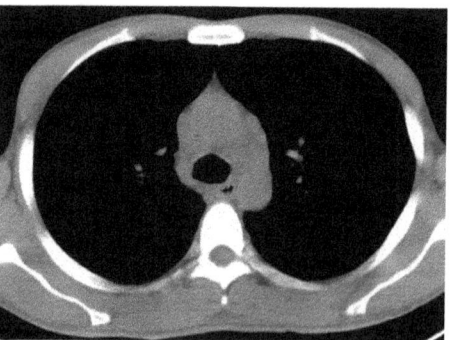

Fig. 11.2: (continuing)

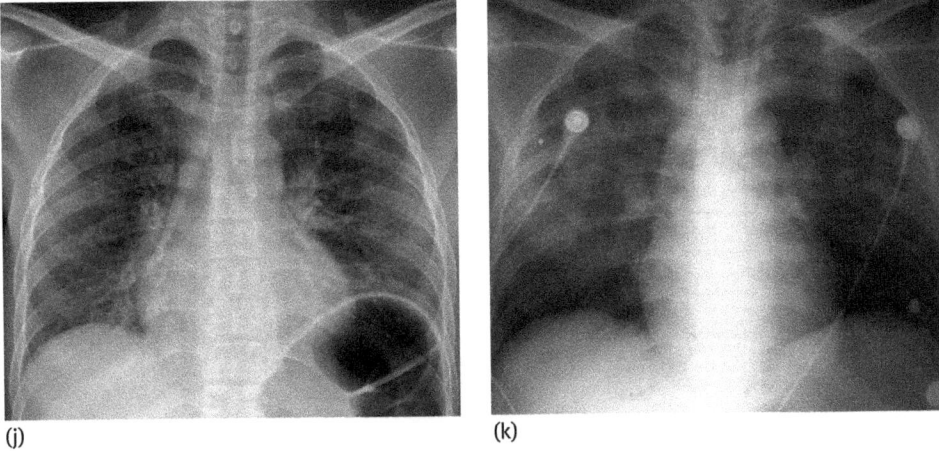

(j)

(k)

Fig. 11.2: (continuing)

Chest radiograph (a) showed multiple rough messy markings and diffusive small miliary nodules in the bilateral lungs. CT scans with lung window (b–e) showed diffuse military nodules and multiple rough messy markings imaging in the bilateral lungs. HRCT scans (f, g) confirmed the thickening of interlobular septae. CT scans with mediastinal window (h, i) showed the mild enlargements of lymph nodes in the mediastinum. At the recheck 10 days after treatment, Chest radiograph showed the lesions in the bilateral lungs were aggravated, with ground-glass-like opacity (j). At the recheck after 27 days treatment, the bed-side film demonstrated infections in the bilateral lungs were evidently aggravated, with high-density massive effuse patchy opacities with blurring edge (k).

Case 11.3 (Fig. 11.3 a–r)

A 41-year-old female patient presented cough and expectoration, fever, polypena for more than one month and rashes for 2 weeks. Body temperature at admission was 38.4 °C. There were no enlargements of systemic superficial lymph nodes. The breath sounds of the bilateral lung were rough without dry or moist rales. The CD4+ cell count was 2/μl. The biopsy by bronchoscopy confirmed CMV pneumonia and pulmonary alveolar proteinosis. Diagnosis: AIDS (C3) combined with CMV pneumonia and pulmonary alveolar proteinosis.

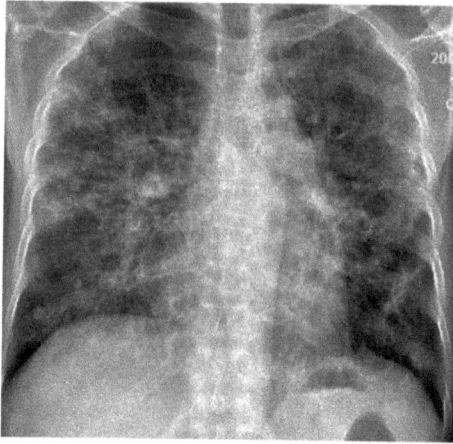
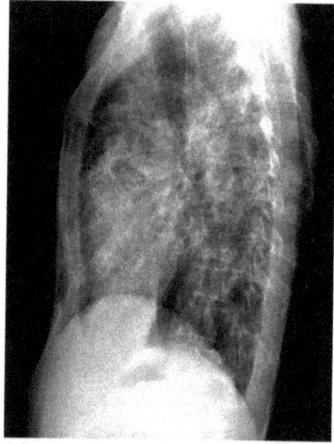

(a)

(b)

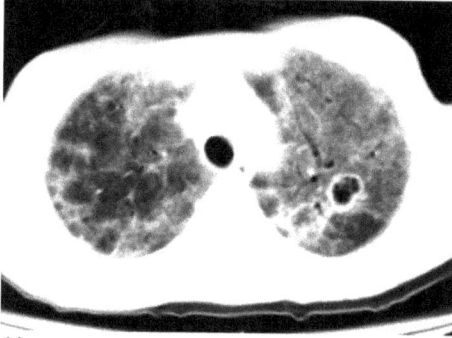
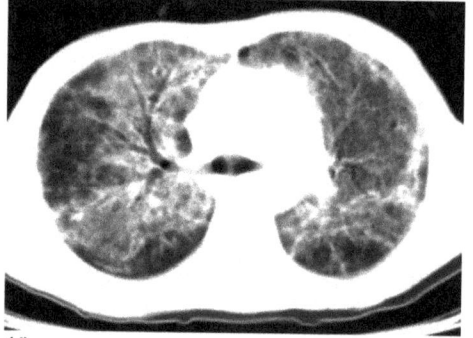

(c)

(d)

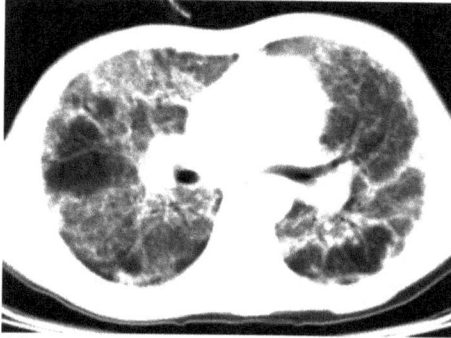
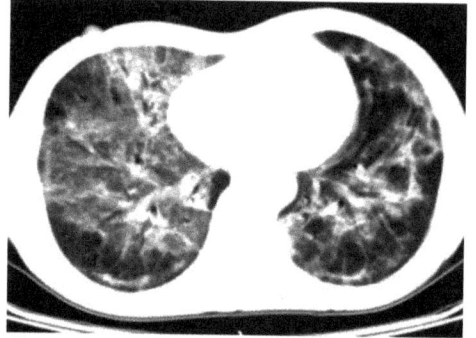

(e)

(f)

Fig. 11.3 a–r: CMV pneumonia and pulmonary alveolar proteinosis.

(g)

(h)

(i)

(j)

(k)

(l)

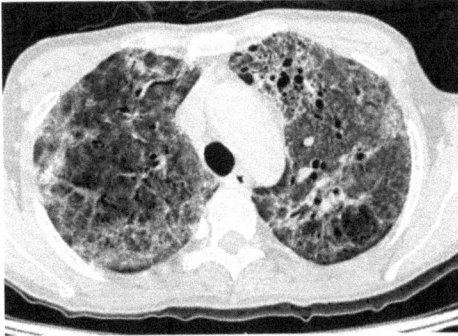

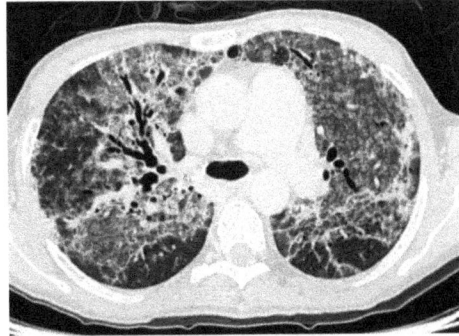

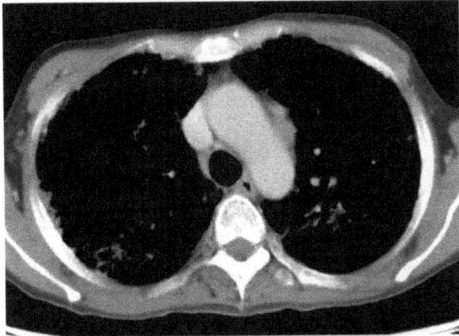

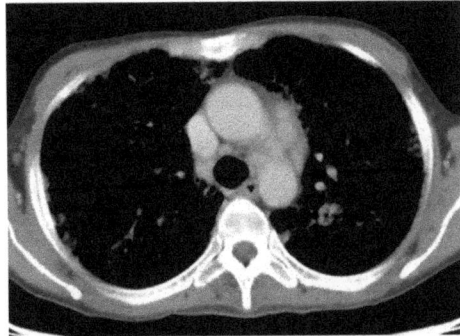

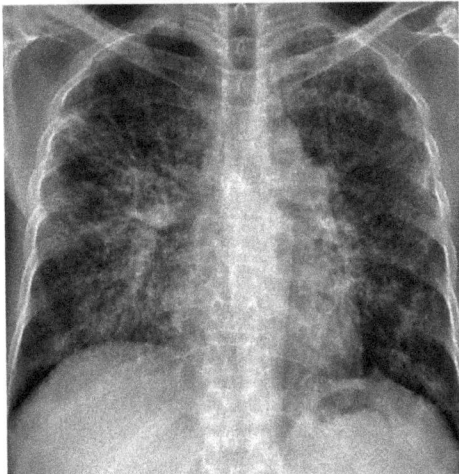

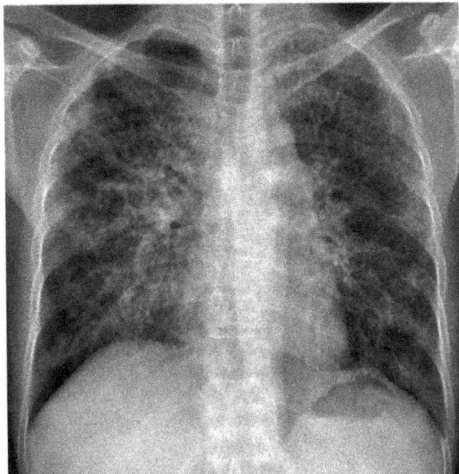

Fig. 11.3: (continuing)

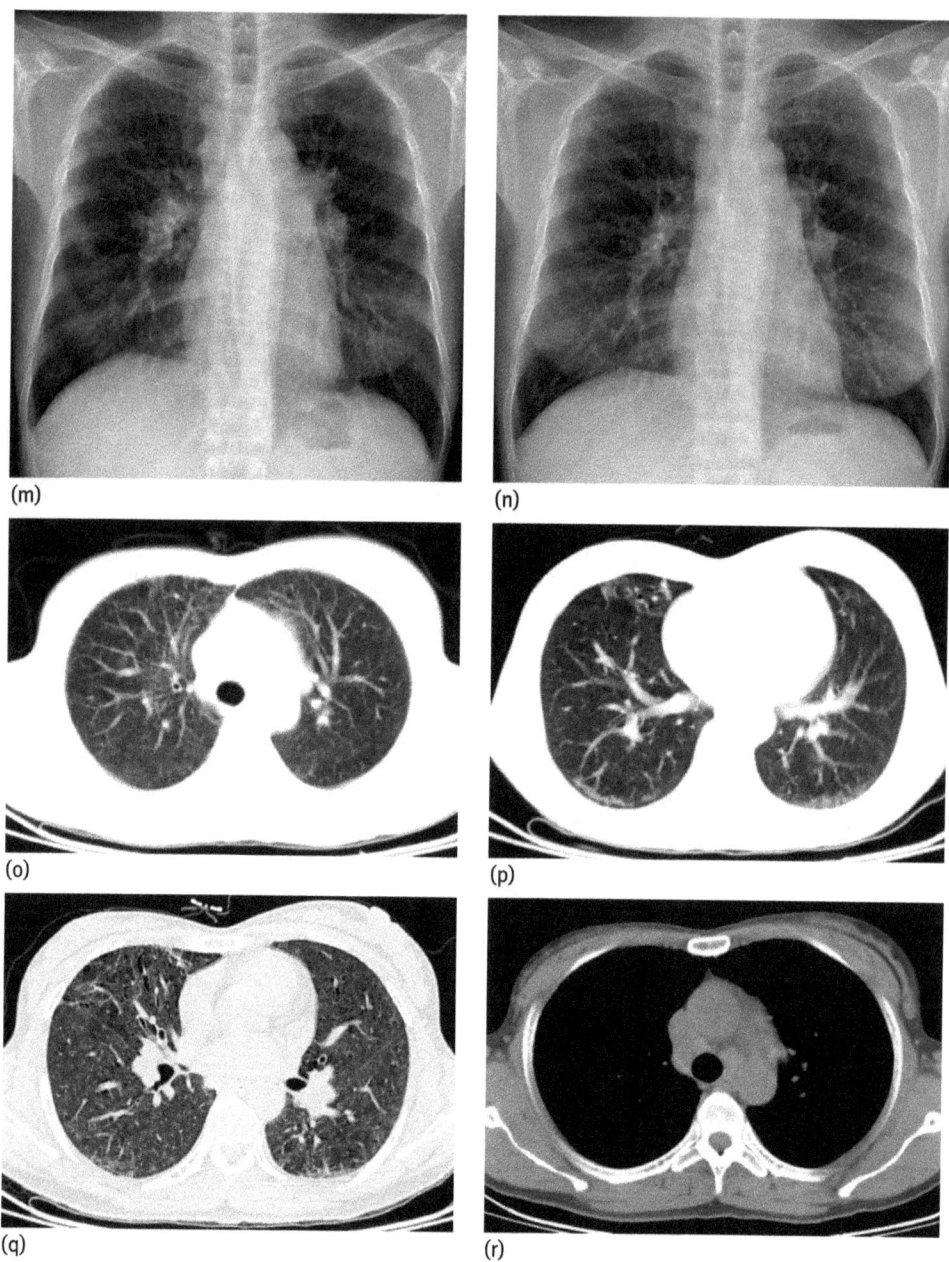

(m)

(n)

(o)

(p)

(q)

(r)

Fig. 11.3: (continuing)

Chest radiographs (a, b) showed diffuse ground-glass-like opacity in the bilateral lungs. CT scans (c, f) revealed diffuse ground-glass-like uneven opacities in the bilateral lungs, a thin-walled cavity in the upper lobe of the left lung and subpleural curvilinear shadow in the bilateral lower lobe. HRCT scans (g, h) presented the diffuse thickened interstitium in the bilateral lungs, focal bronchiectasis and the scans with mediastinal window the enlarged lymph nodes in the mediastinum (i, j). At recheck after 14 and 54 days treatment respectively (k, l), Chest radiographs showed the opacities in the bilateral lungs were gradually absorbed (k, l). At recheck after 7 months treatment, the lesions in the bilateral lungs were fundamentally absorbed (m). At the recheck after 2 years, the appearances in both lung fields were clearer than before (n), CT scans showed interlobular septal thickening, the local bronchiectasis and the subpleural curvilinear shadow were all improved (o–q), and the lymph nodes in the mediastinum shrunk (r).

Case 11.4 (Fig. 11.4 a–n)
A 32-year-old male patient presented fever for 40 days and scattered skin rashes with a sign of umbilical fossa for 1 week. Body temperature at admission was 40 °C. Scattered herpes with central umbilication were seen all over the body. The breath sounds of the bilateral lungs were clear without dry or moist rales. There were no enlargements of the systemic superficial lymph nodes. CD4+ cell count was 4/μl. The blood and bone marrow cultures were *Penicillum marneffei* positive. After 56 days treatment, sadly the patient died of respiratory failure. The pathological examination of autopsy on the lung specimens revealed CMV pneumonia. The patient was diagnosed with AIDS (C3), accompanied by *Penicillum marneffei* infection and CMV pneumonia.

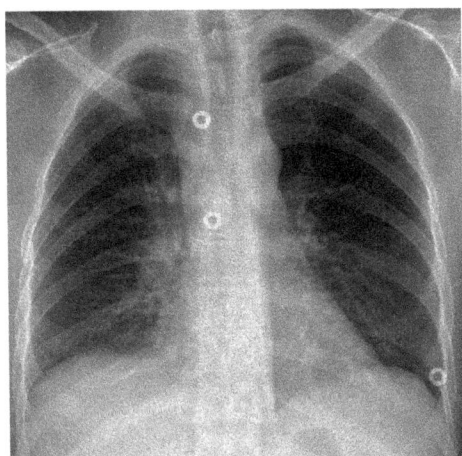 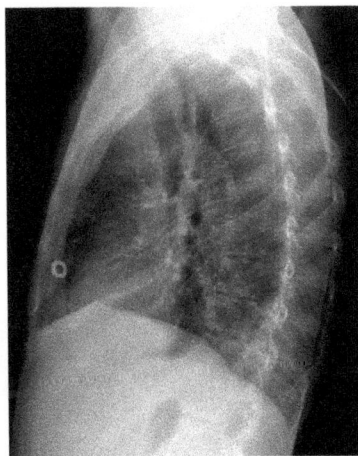

(a) (b)

Fig. 11.4 a–n: *Penicillum marneffei* infection and CMV pneumonia.

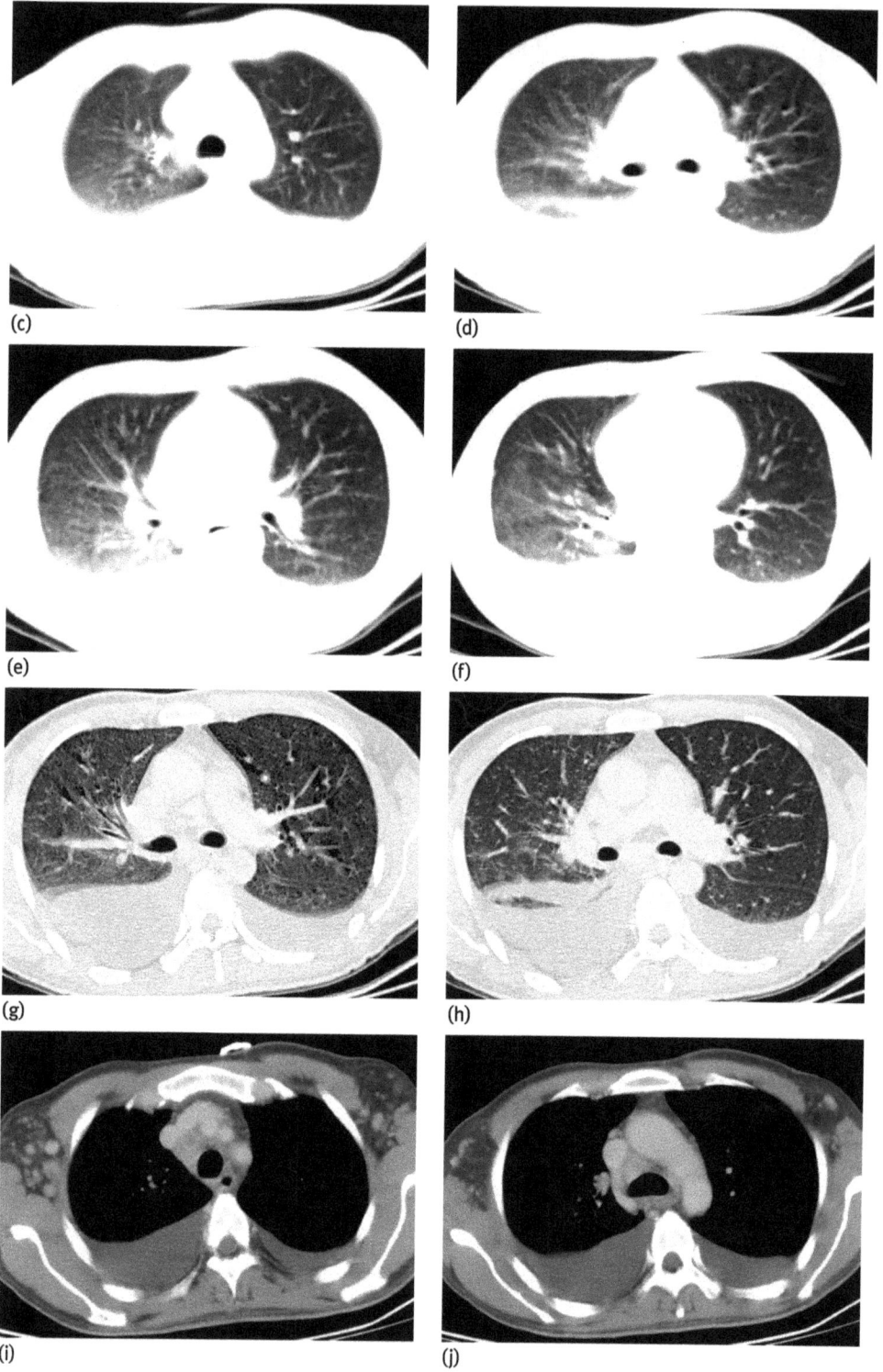

(c)

(d)

(e)

(f)

(g)

(h)

(i)

(j)

Fig. 11.4: (continuing)

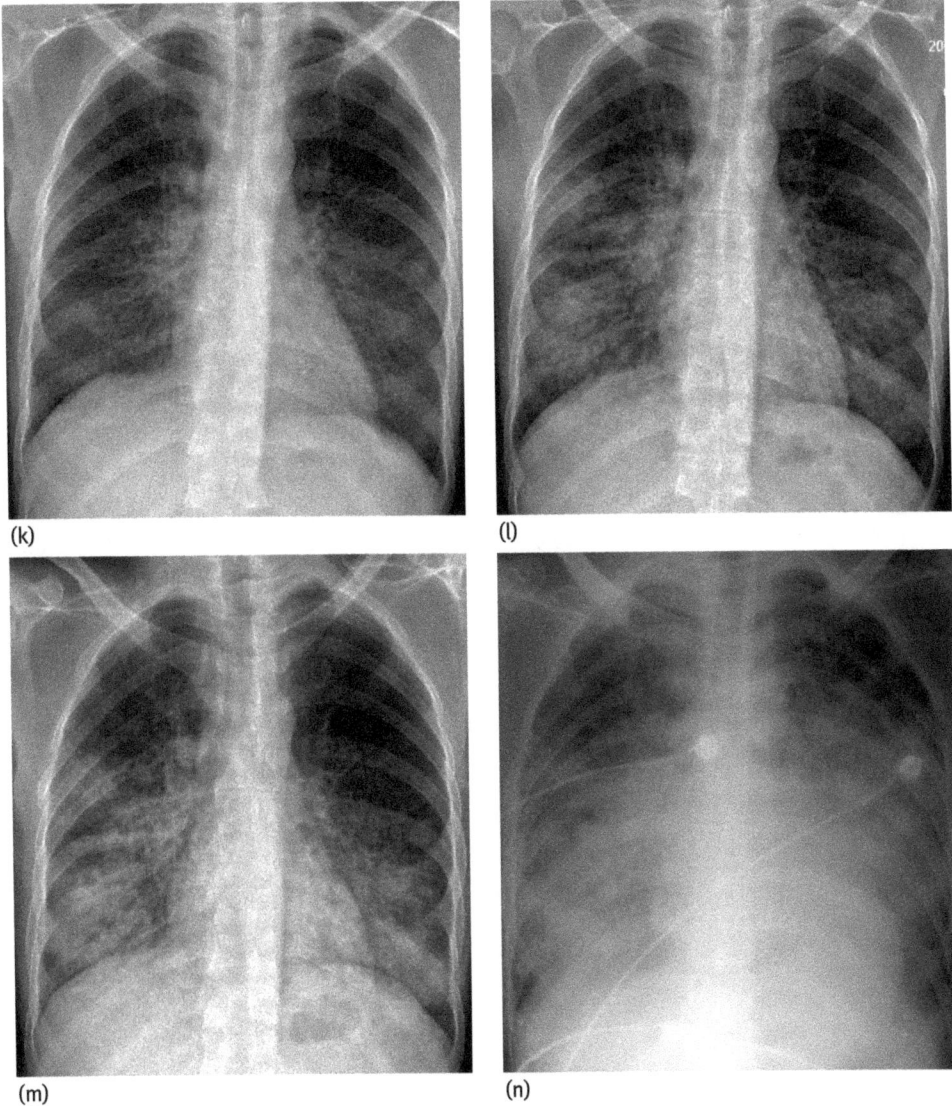

Fig. 11.4: (continuing)

Chest radiographs (a, b) showed multiple markings and cloudiness of the bilateral lungs. CT scans (c–f) showed multiple markings and cloudiness of the bilateral lungs but no solid lesions in them. HRCT scans (g, h) demonstrated thickening of interlobular septum. CT scans with mediastinal window (i, j) showed lymph nodular enlargements in the bilateral axillary and mediastinum as well as bilateral pleural effusions. At the recheck after 13 days treatment, chest radiographs showed the lesions in the bilateral lungs were exacerbated and the markings in the bilateral lungs grew in size and more obscure, with diffuse spotty flaky opacities (k). At the respective recheck after 16 and 17 days treatment, the lesions in the bilateral lungs grew in number and at range, many fusing into high-density massive opacities with blurring edge (l, m). After 20 days treatment (two days before death), the lesions in the bilateral lungs were found with further aggravation, presenting a shadow of "white lung" (n).

11.3 Imaging features

The main thoracic imaging manifestations of CMV pneumonia in AIDS patients hospitalized in Guangzhou No. 8 People's Hospital are characterized as: ground-glass-like diffuse opacities, thickened interstitiums (thickened interlobular septa, thickened lobular interstitium, thickened central lobular interstitium and thickened interstitium along the bronchial blood vessels), diffusive obscure nodules, massive consolidation from lesions fusion, rapid progression of lesions and pleural effusions in some cases. Hormone therapy used to control opportunistic infections in AIDS patients may reactivate the latent CMV infections and eventually result in CMV pneumonia. Although the enlarged lymph nodes in the mediastinum are found in most AIDS patients with CMV pneumonia, the differential diagnosis of CMV pneumonia only in imageology needs further investigation due to limited cases.

Editors: Xiangfeng Guo, Haolan He, Yan Ding, Jinxin Liu

12 Imaging features of multiple microbial pulmonary infections in AIDS

12.1 Introduction

Multiple pathogenic infections are common among patients with advanced AIDS because of their severe immunosuppression. The opportunistic infections by multiple pathogens contribute to their diversity in infection, susceptibility to dissemination and intractability in clinical practice. In imageology, they are characterized as complexity, disseminated and non-specificity due to the overlapping imaging signs, which allow more difficulties in imaging diagnosis. For this reason, the definite diagnoses of multiple infections are dependent on both the clinical data as well as the experimental results, especially on the biopsy by bronchoscopy and cultures of bronchoalveolar lavage fluid (BALF).

Case 12.1 (Fig. 12.1 a–l)
A 34-year-old female patient presented fever and tachypnea for three months. Body temperature at admission was 40 °C. There were bean-curd-like materials on the surface of the tongue and hairy leukoplakia on both sides of the tongue. The breath sounds of the bilateral lung were rough with dry and moist rales in the lower parts. There were no enlargements of systemic superficial lymph nodes. CD4+ cell count was 128/μl. Culture of bronchoalveolar lavage fluid (BALF) was aspergillus positive. The pathological obtained from lung tissues detected pneumocystis jiroveci pneumonia (PCP). Culture of sputum specimen was candida glabrata positive. For the reason,

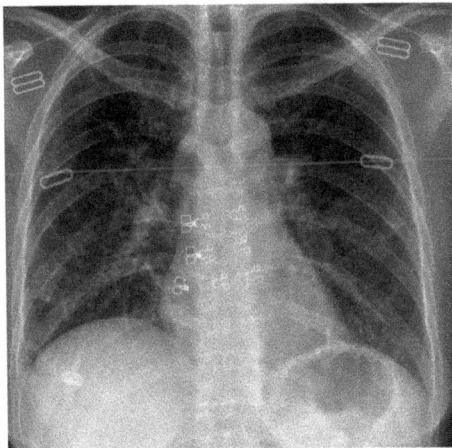
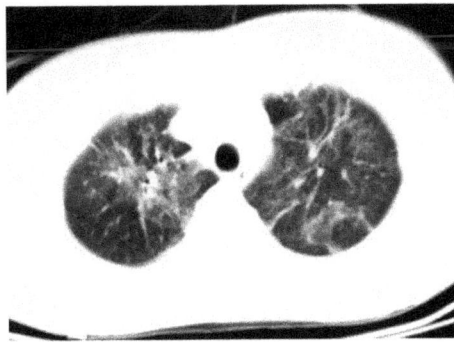

(a)   (b)

Fig. 12.1 a–l: Pulmonary infection *(Klebsiella, Penicillum marneffei)* in AIDS, *Penicillum marneffei* septicaemia.

the patient was diagnosed with AIDS (C3) accompanied by pulmonary infection (PCP, aspergillus), oral fungi infections.

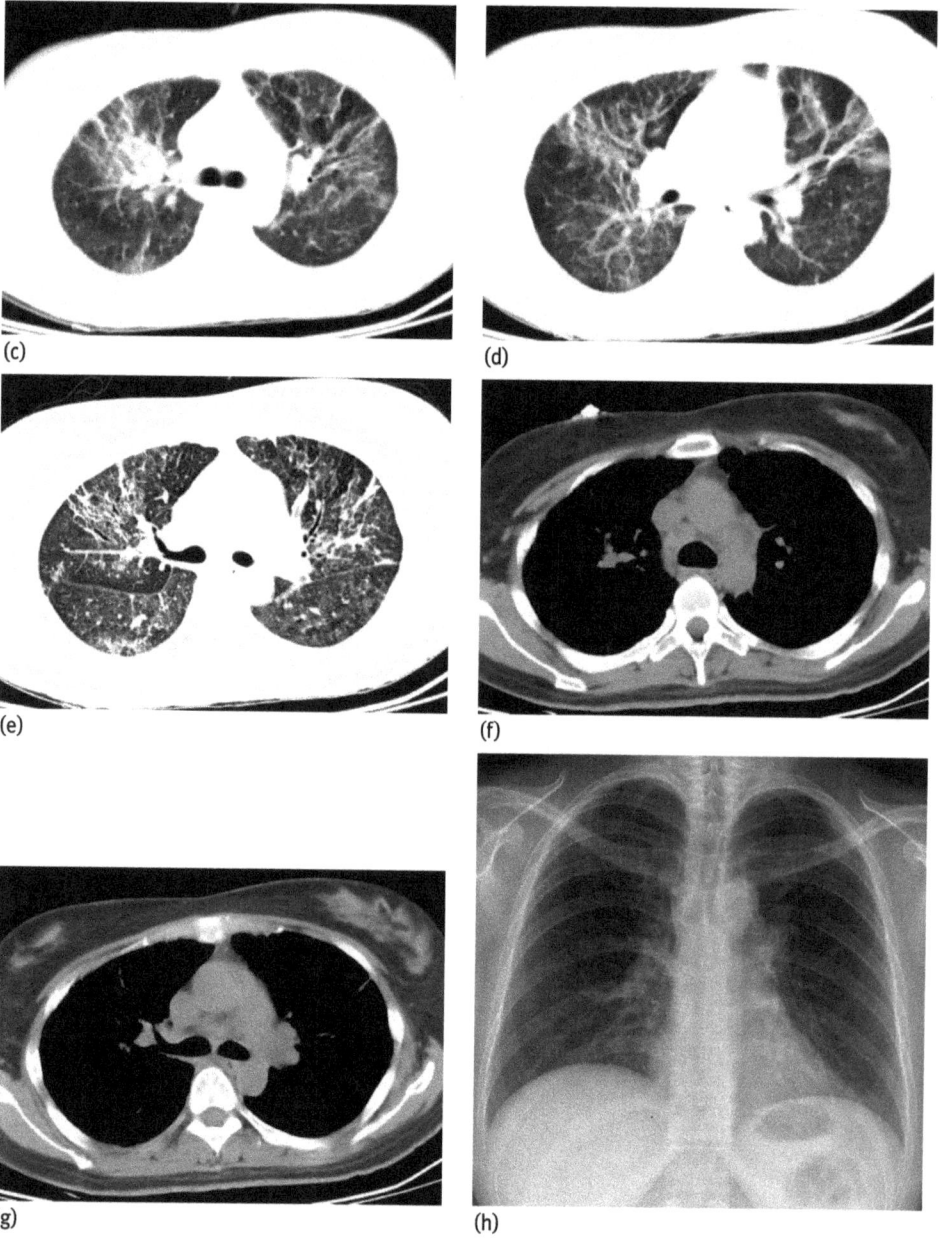

Fig. 12.1: (continuing)

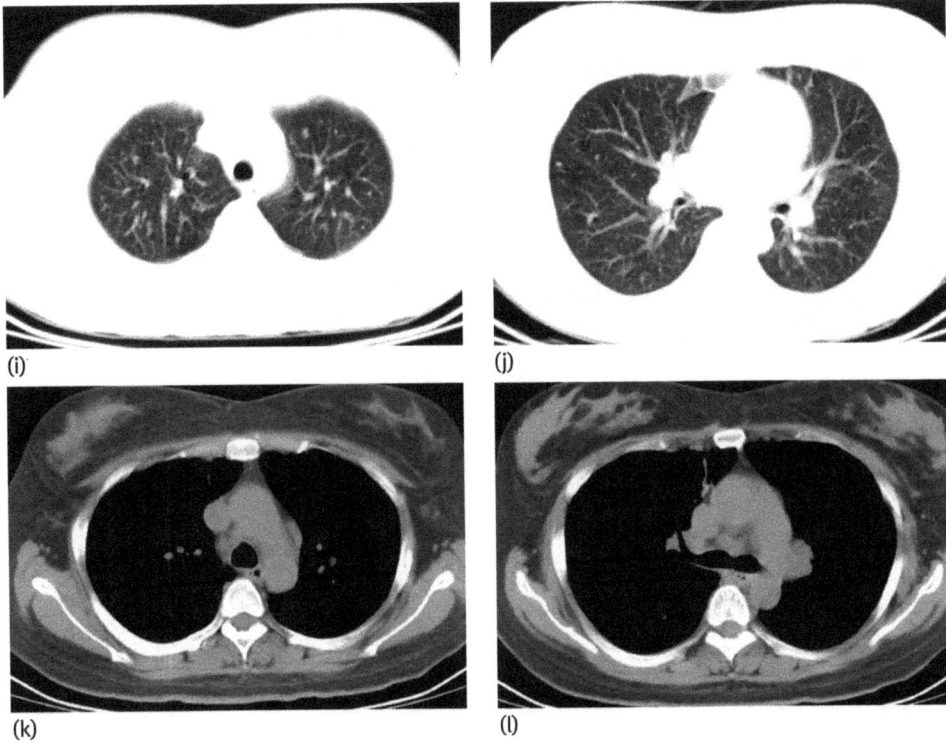

(i) (j)

(k) (l)

Fig. 12.1: (continuing)

Chest radiograph (a) showed thickened markings in the bilateral lungs with asystematic and reticular shadows, and ground-glass-like opacities in the lungs fields. CT scans with lung window (b–d) showed significantly thickened markings of bilateral lungs with cable shadows, ground-glass-like opacities in the lungs fields, and a small patchy consolidation in the anterior segment of the right upper lobe. HRCT (e) scan showed thickened interstitium in the bilateral lungs. CT scans with mediastinal window (f, g) showed the enlarged lymph nodes in the mediastinum. After a month treatment, CT scans showed the lesions were basically absorbed with those slightly thickened markings in the bilateral lungs (h, j) and the lymph nodes in the mediastinum were obviously shrunken (k, l).

Case 12.2 (Fig. 12.2 a–j)

A 26-year-old male patient occurred fever for 20 days and tachypnea for more than 10 days. Body temperature at admission was 36.4 °C. The breath sounds were rough with dry rales. There were no enlargements of systemic superficial lymph nodes. CD4+ cell count was 6/μl. The biopsy by bronchoscopy confirmed CMV, aspergillus, pneumocystis jiroveci pneumonia (PCP) positive. Culture of bronchoalveolar lavage fluid (BALF) was aspergillus positive. Culture of sputum confirmed *Staphylococcus saprophyticus*. After 32 days treatment in the hospital, the patient died of respiratory

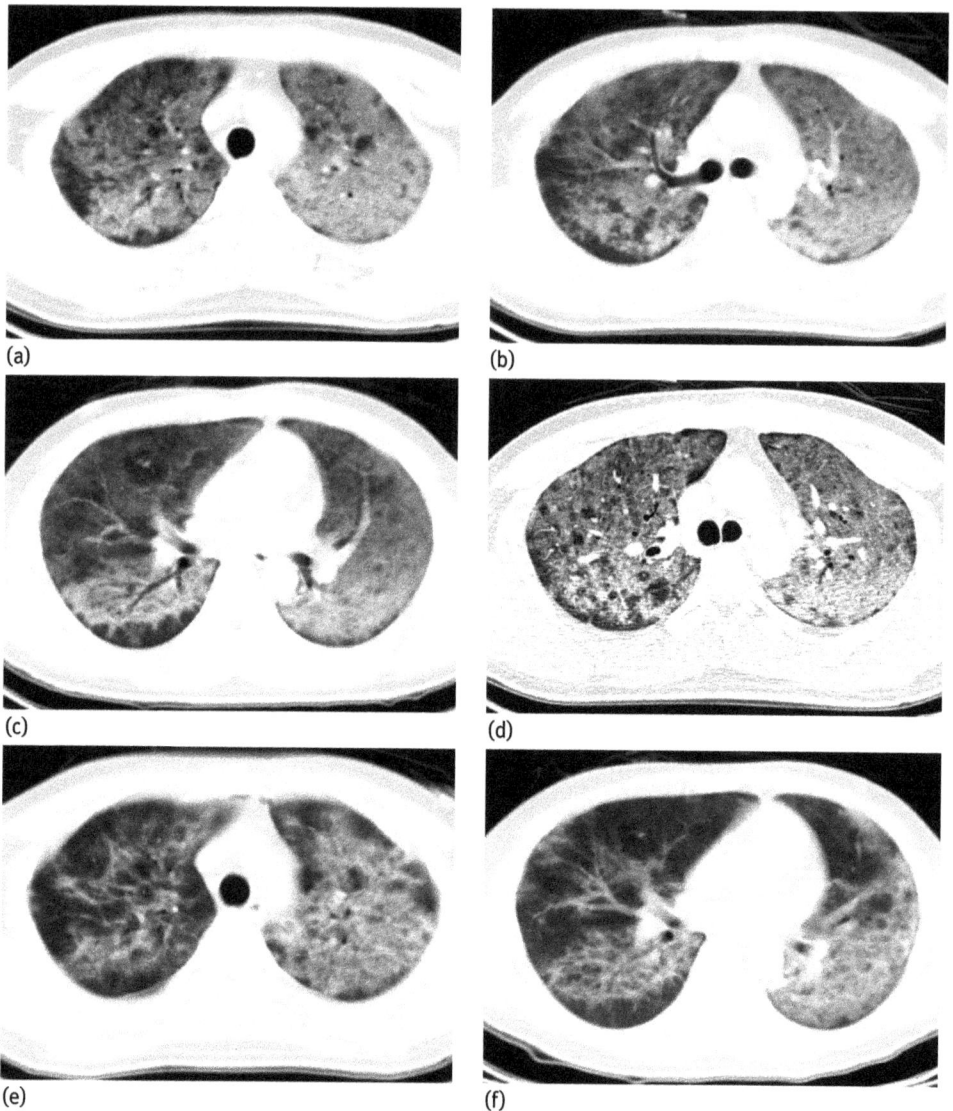

Fig. 12.2 a–j: Pulmonary infections caused by PCP and aspergillus in AIDS.

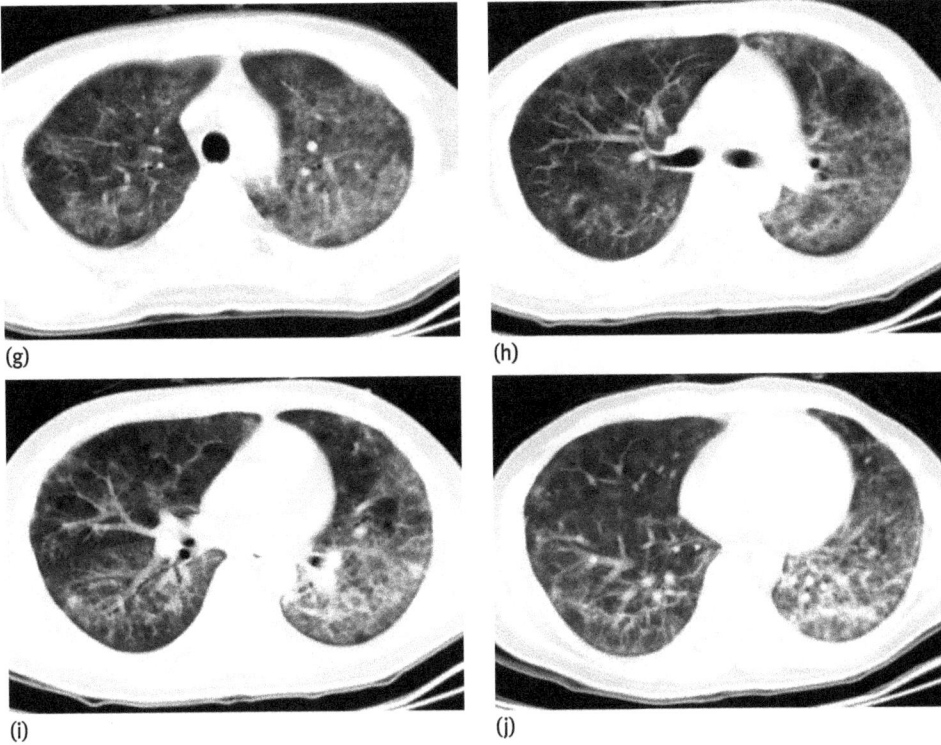

(g)

(h)

(i)

(j)

Fig. 12.2: (continuing)

failure eventually. The patient was diagnosed with AIDS (C3) accompanied by severe pneumonia (CMV, aspergillus, PCP and *Staphylococcus saprophyticus*).

CT scans (a, d) showed diffuse ground-glass opacities in the bilateral lungs. After two weeks treatment, the ground-glass-like opacities were slightly absorbed but the reticular fiber shadows increased in number (e, f). After three weeks treatment, both the ground glass opacities and reticular and linear shadows in bilateral lung were partly absorbed.

Case 12.3 (Fig. 12.3 a–j)

A 45-year-old male presented cough and fever for 2 months, rashes for 1 month and hematochezia for 1 week. Body temperature at admission was 40 °C. The skin rashes scattered on the face and body were hard in quality, navel-like changes central umbilication and painless at palpation. There were no enlargements of systemic superficial lymph nodes. CD4+ cell count was 56/µl. Culture of sputum specimen was *Klebsiella pneumonia* positive. Cultures of blood and bone marrow were *Penicillum marneffei* positive. The patient was diagnosed with AIDS (C3) complicated with pneumonia caused by *Klebsiella* and *Penicillum marneffei*.

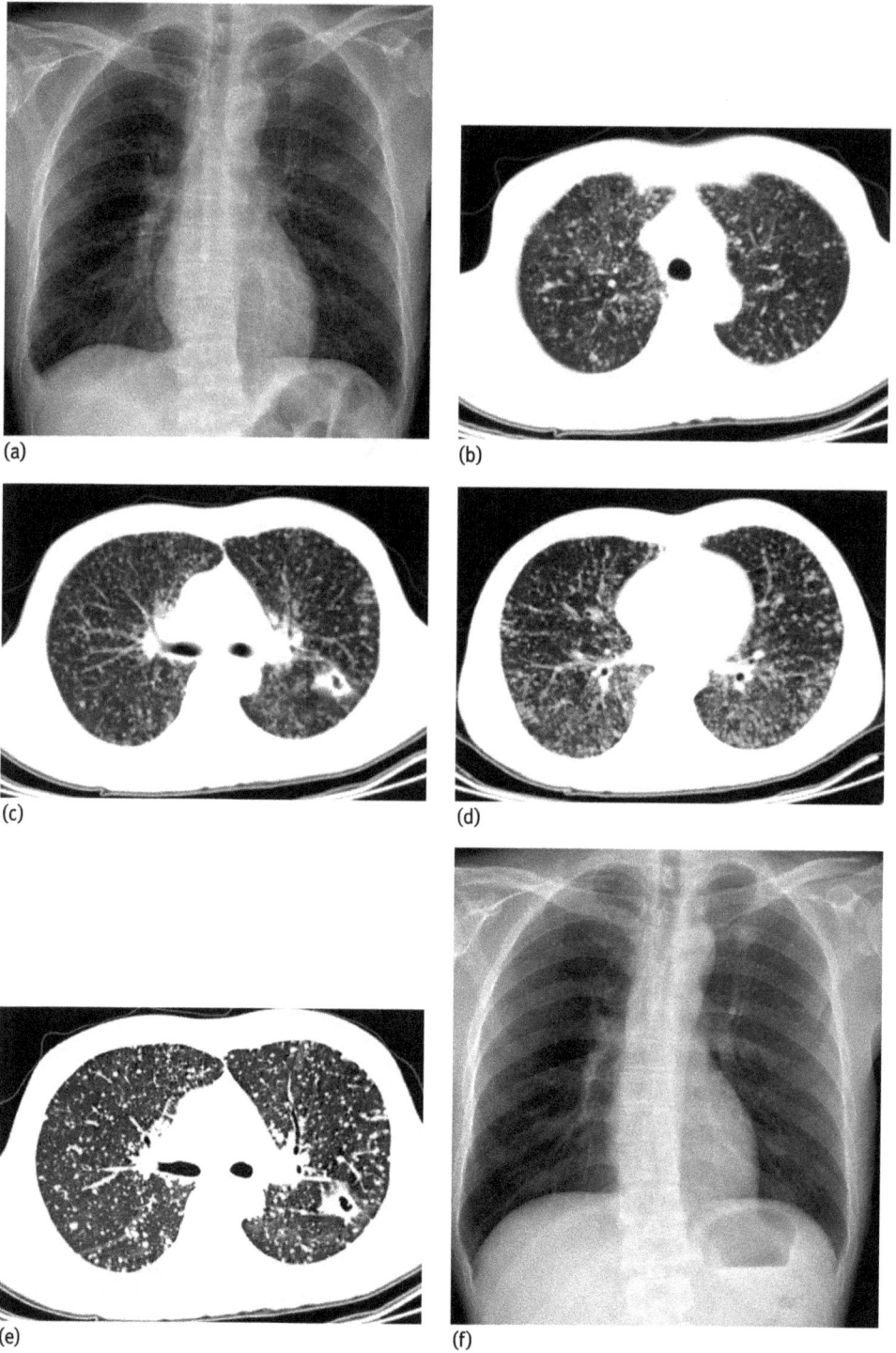

Fig. 12.3 a–j: Severe pneumonia caused by CMV, aspergillus, PCP and *Staphylococcus saprophyticus* in AIDS (C3) patients.

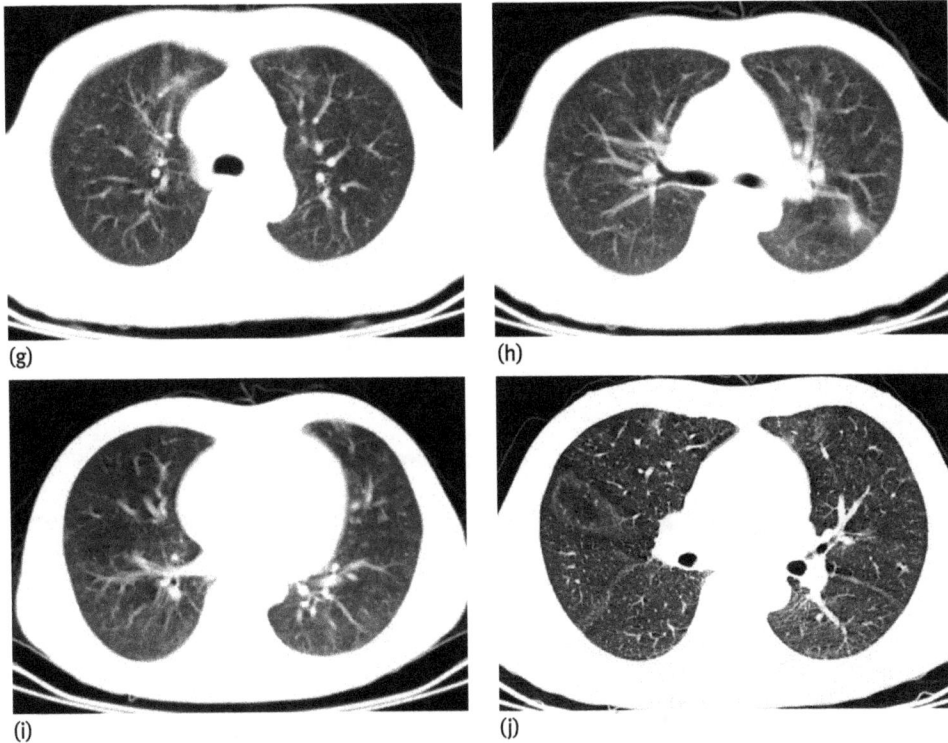

Fig. 12.3: (continuing)

Chest radiograph (a) showed diffuse miliary nodules in the bilateral lungs with a nodular lesion in the left upper lobe, and a few pleural effusions in the right lung. CT scans (b–d) demonstrated diffuse miliary nodules, with a cavity in the lesion of the left upper lobe (b–d). HRCT (e) scan showed uneven inner walls of the cavity. After five weeks treatment, the lesions were basically absorbed in the bilateral lungs (f–j).

Case 12.4 (Fig. 12.4 a–k)

A 41-year-old male presented cough and fever for one month. Body temperature at admission was 38.9 °C. The breath sounds of the bilateral lung were rough. The lymph nodes in the cervix and axillary fossa were palpated soft and smooth. Hepatomegaly was palpable 2 cm below the right costal margin. CD4+ cell count was 93/μl. Cultures of blood and bone marrow were *Penicillum marneffei* positive. Culture of bronchoalveolar lavage fluid (BALF) was aspergillus positive. The patient was diagnosed with AIDS (C3) complicated with pneumonia caused by *Penicillum marneffei* and aspergillus.

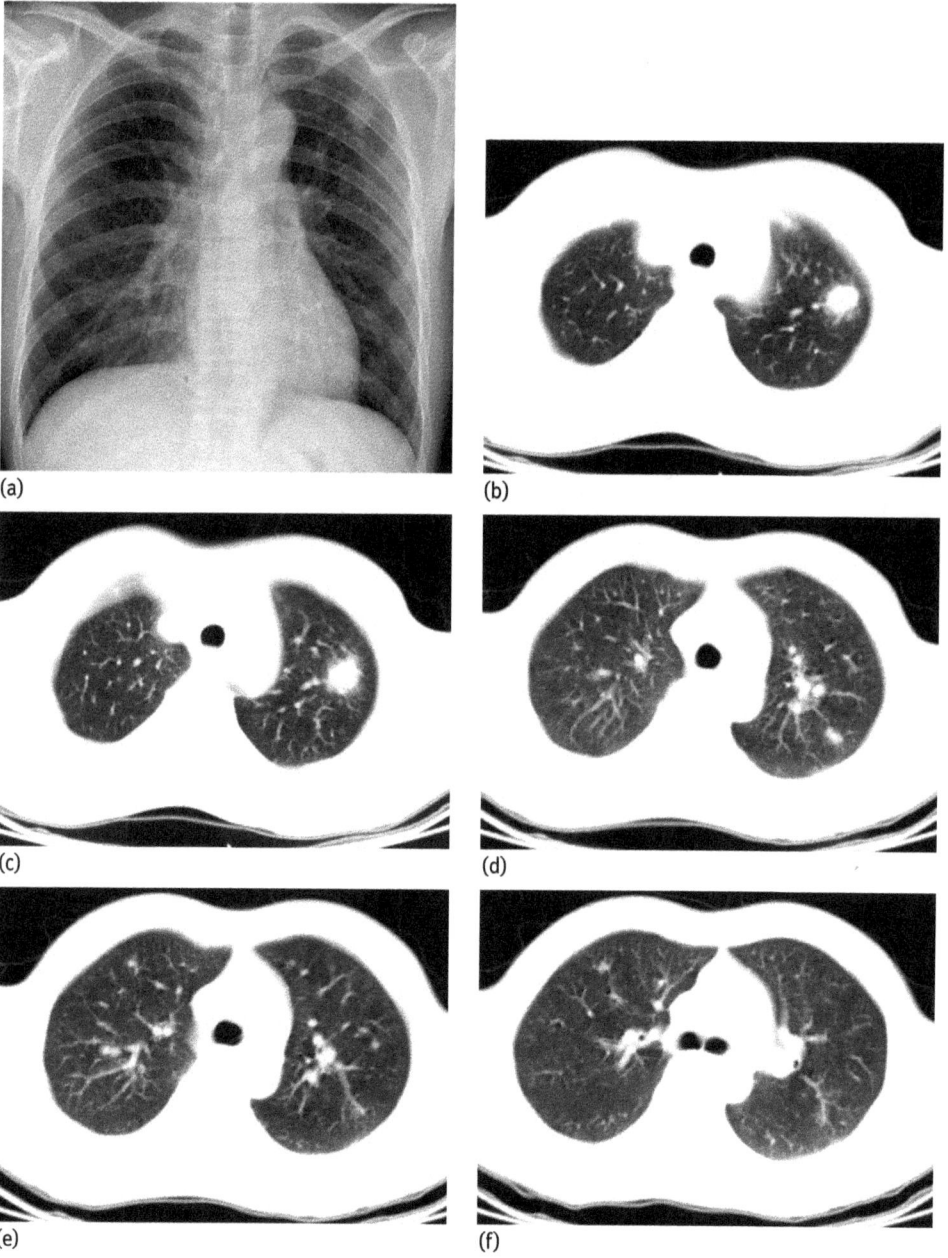

Fig. 12.4 a–k: Pneumonia caused by *Klebsiella* and *Penicillum marneffei.*

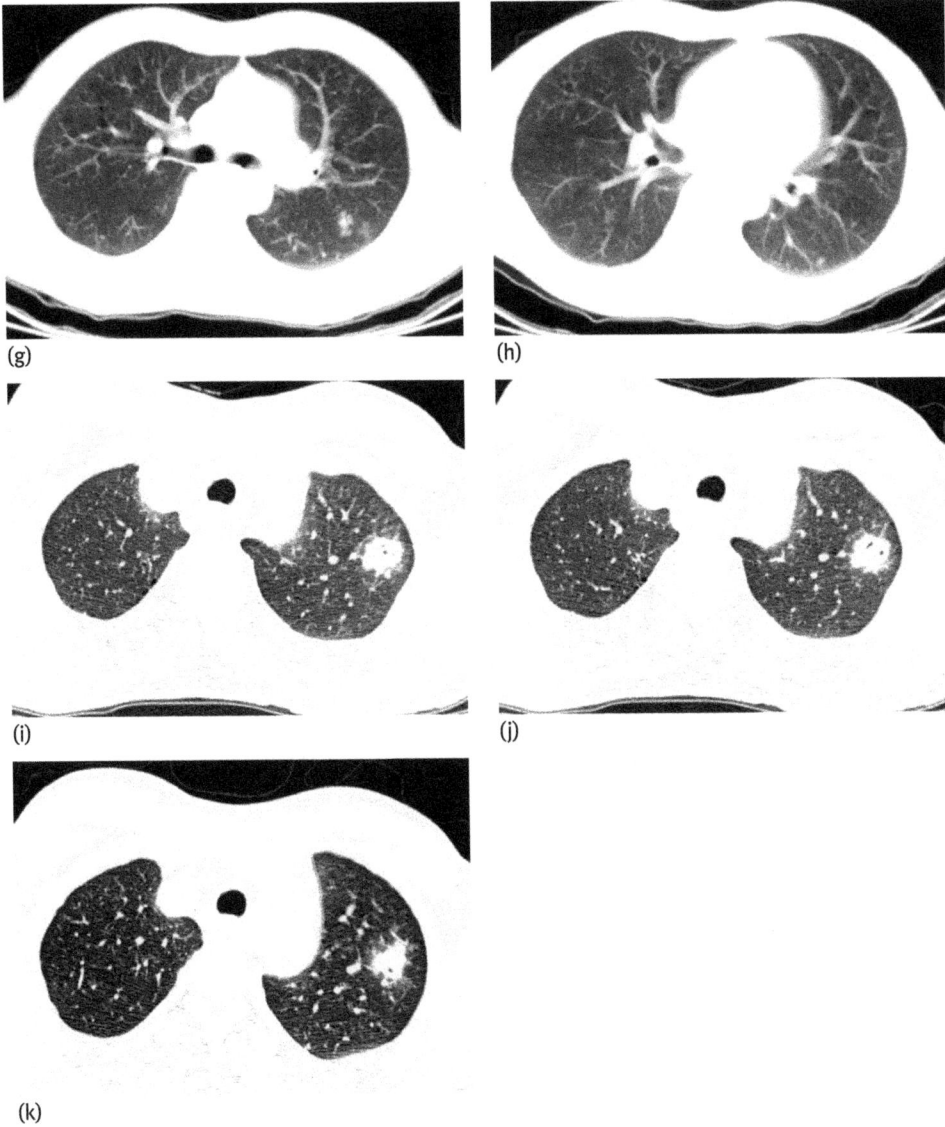

(g)

(h)

(i)

(j)

(k)

Fig. 12.4: (continuing)

Chest radiograph (a) showed high-density nodular opacities with rough edge in the left upper lobe. CT scans (b–h) showed a nodular lesion with rough edge located in the apicoposterior segment of left upper lobe, its rim presented with halo sign, besides with a cavity within it, scattered nodular lesions in the rest part of the bilateral lungs. HRCT (i–k) showed multiple small cavities in the nodule lesion of left upper lobe.

Case 12.5 (Fig. 12.5 a–k)

A 47-year-old male presented fever, cough and tachypnea for more than one month. Body temperature at admission was 40 °C. There were bean-curb-like materials on the surface of his tongue. The breath sounds of the bilateral lung were clear. CD4+ cell count was 95/μl. Culture of sputum was *Candida albicans* positive. Cultures of blood and bone marrow were *Penicillum marneffei* positive, culture of bronchoalveolar lavage fluid (BALF) were for *Penicillum marneffei* and *Klebsiella pneumonia* positive. The biopsy by bronchoscopy confirmed pneumocystis jiroveci pneumonia (PCP) and CMV pneumonia. The patient was diagnosed with AIDS (C3) complicated with pneumonia from PCP, CMV, *Penicillum marneffei* and bacteria, oral infections caused by *Candida albicans*, cytomegalovirus retinitis (CMVR) and disseminated *penincillum marneffei*.

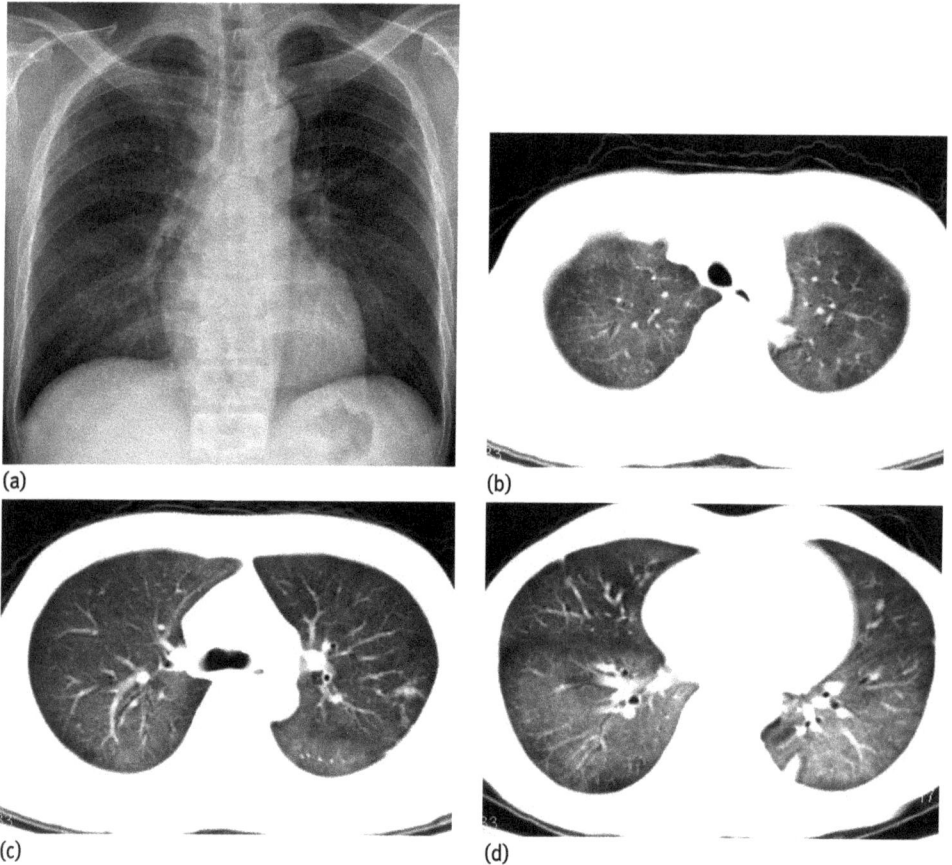

(a) (b) (c) (d)

Fig. 12.5 a–k: Pneumonia *(Penicillum marneffei,* aspergillus*)* in AIDS.

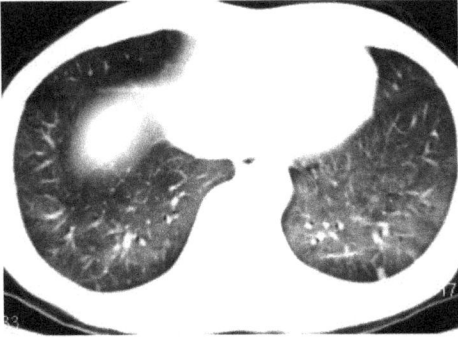

(e)

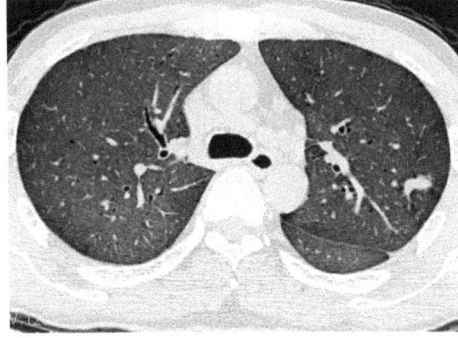

(f)

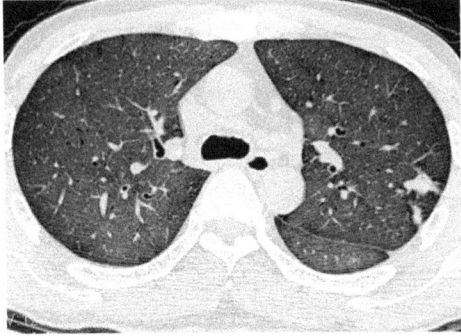

(g)

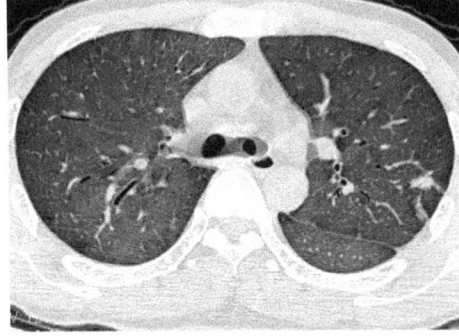

(h)

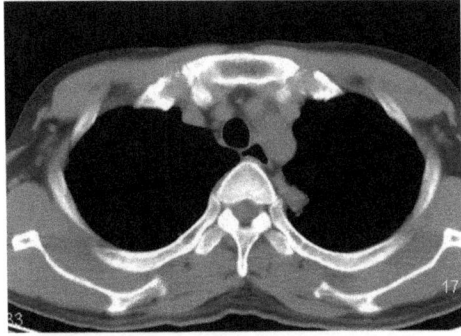

(i)

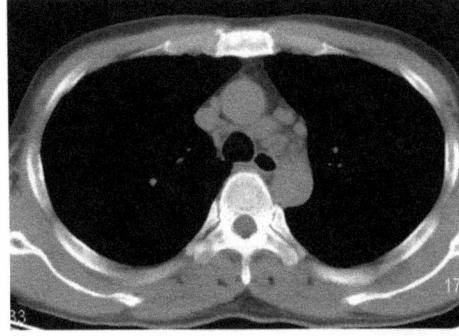

(j)

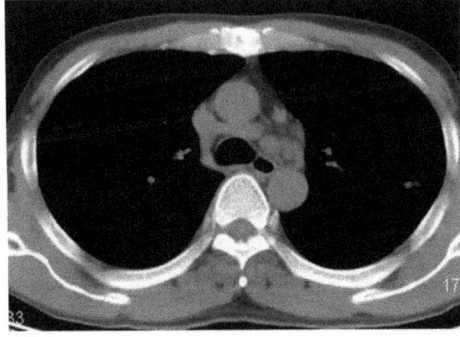

(k)

Fig. 12.5: (continuing)

Chest radiograph (a) showed the slightly decreased transparency of the bilateral lungs with thickened markings, and a vague patchy opacity both in the lateral regions of the left upper lobe and beside the left upper mediastinum. CT scans (b–e) showed diffuse ground-glass-like opacities in bilateral lungs, vague nodular shadows on the left upper lobe (behind arch of aorta), apicoposterior segment of the left upper lobe and posterior basal segment of the left lower lobe respectively. HRCT scans (f–h) showed ground-glass-like lesions with the irregular nodules in the lateral regions of the left upper lobe. The lesions behind the arch of aorta was notable in the soft tissue window, with enlarged lymph nodes in the mediastinum, as showed on the CT scans with mediastinal window (i–k).

Case 12.6 (Fig. 12.6 a–l)

A 45-year-old male presented tachypnea for more than one month, the symptoms aggravated accompanied with fever for half a month. Body temperature at admission was 39 °C. There were fine moist rales throughout the bilateral lung, especially in the middle and lower parts. There were no enlargements of systemic superficial lymph nodes. CD4+ cell count was 2/μl and HCMV-DNA was 1.16×10^5. Sputum culture: *Acinetobacter baumannii* and *Staphylococcus haemolyticus* (MRSH) positive. Cultures of bronchoalveolar lavage fluid (BALF) were non-tuberculous mycobacteria and aspergillus positive. The biopsy by bronchoscopy confirmed pneumocystis jiroveci pneumonia (PCP). The patient was diagnosed with AIDS (C3) complicated with severe pneumonia (PCP, CMV, fungi, non-tuberculous mycobacteria and bacteria).

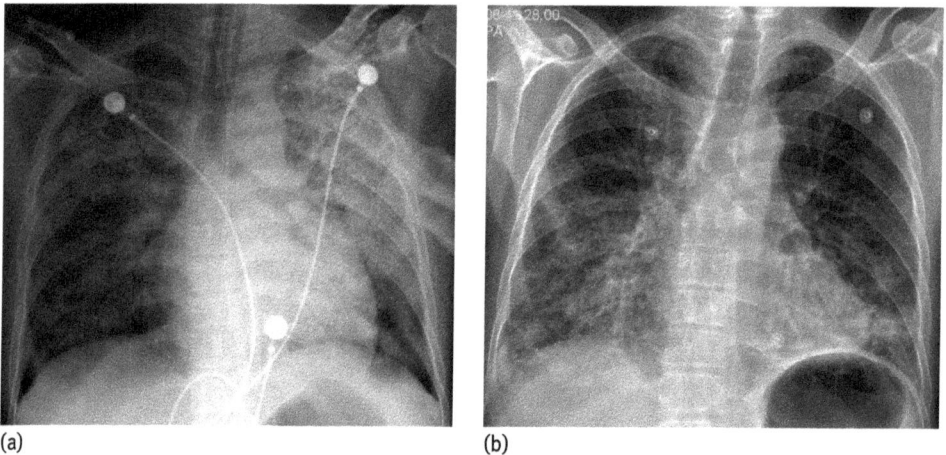

(a)

(b)

Fig. 12.6 a–l: Pneumonia by PCP, CMV, *Penicillum marneffei* and bacterium in AIDS.

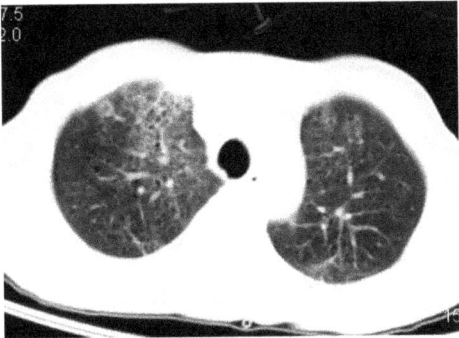

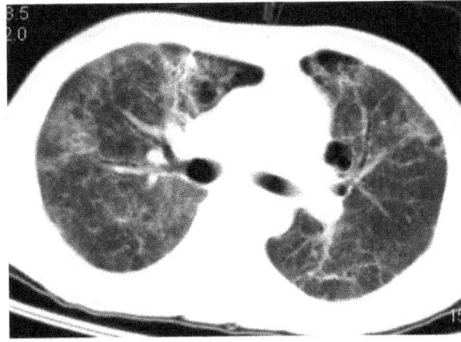

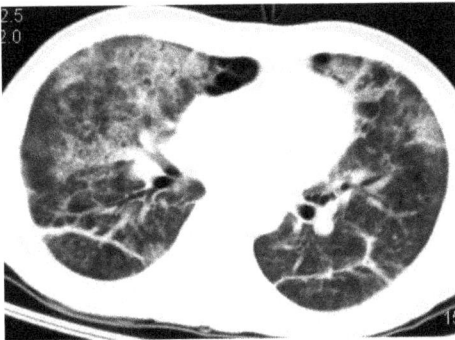

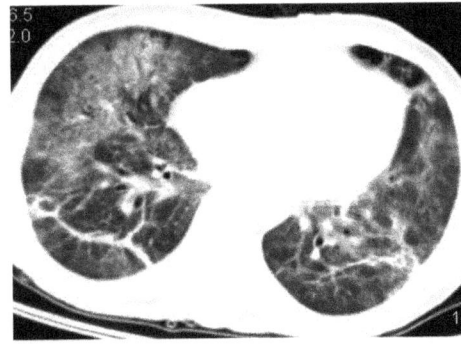

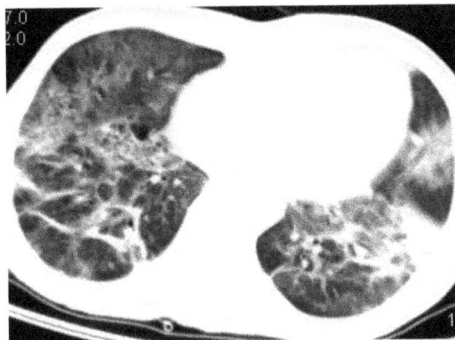

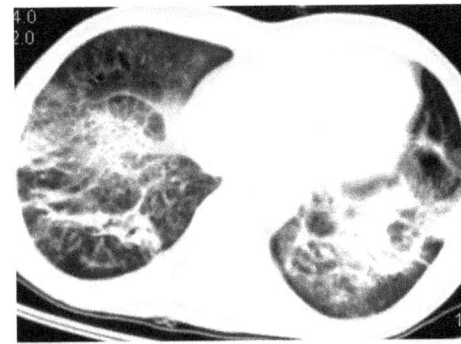

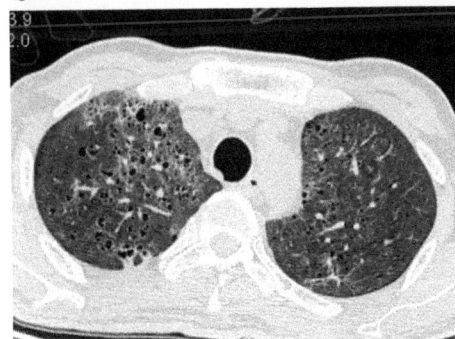

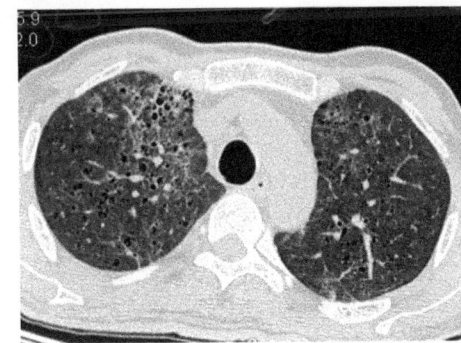

Fig. 12.6: (continuing)

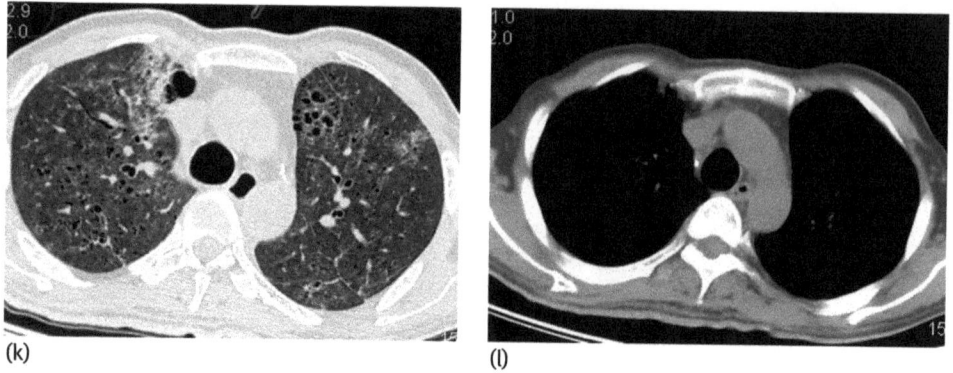

(k)   (l)

Fig. 12.6: (continuing)

Chest radiograph showed obviously decreased transparency of the bilateral lungs with severe ground-glass opacities, air-bronchogram can be seen in it (a). After 15 days treatment, the lung fields were clearer, but the diffuse ground-glass opacities, multiple patchy opacities and stripy fibrous opacities in the bilateral lungs remained with fewer changes than before treatment (b). CT scans (c–h) demonstrated diffuse ground-glass opacities, multiple vague patchy opacities and stripy fibrous opacities as showed in chest radiograph. HRCT (i–k) showed ground-glass-like opacities on the bilateral lungs with multiple cystic shadows and thickened inerstitinum. CT scan (l) showed no enlargement of the mediastinum lymph node.

Case 12.7 (Fig. 12.7 a–k)

A 41-year-old male presented tachypnea for half a month, worsened when he stepped upstairs. Body temperature at admission was 38 °C. There was bean-curd-like materials on the surface of the tongue and hairy leukoplakia on the lateral surface of his tongue. The breath sounds of the bilateral tongue were rough, with small amount of moist rales, especially from the middle and lower parts of the lung. CD4+ cell count was 27/μl. The serum antigens were aspergillus positive. Culture of bronchoalveolar lavage fluid (BALF) were aspergillus positive. BALF smear was Gram bacteria positive. The biopsy by bronchoscopy confirmed pneumocystis jiroveci pneumonia (PCP). The patient was diagnosed with AIDS (C3) complicated with pneumonia (PCP, aspergillus and bacterium), oral fungal infection.

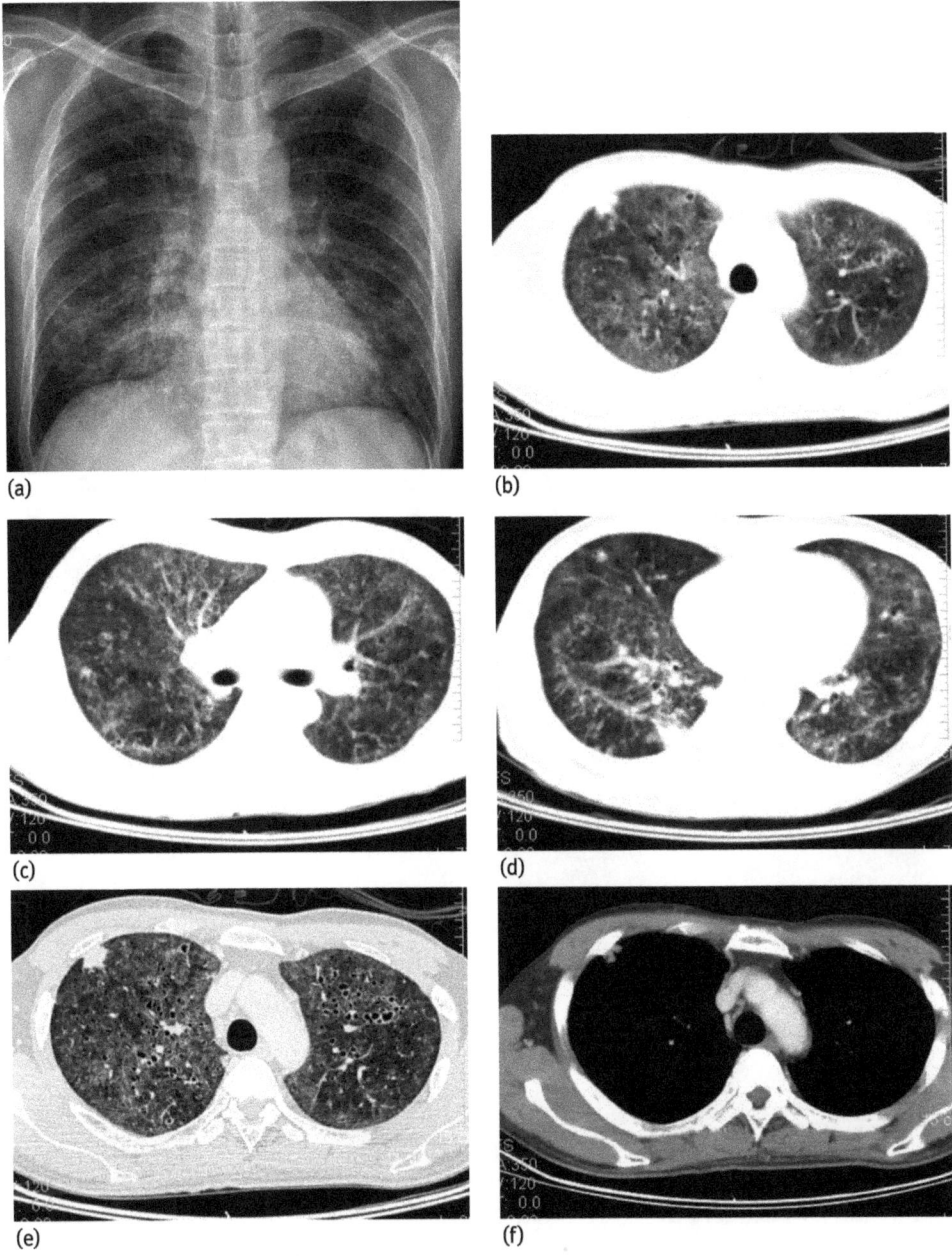

Fig. 12.7 a–k: Severe pneumonia (PCP, CMV, fungi, non-tuberculous mycobacteria and bacterium).

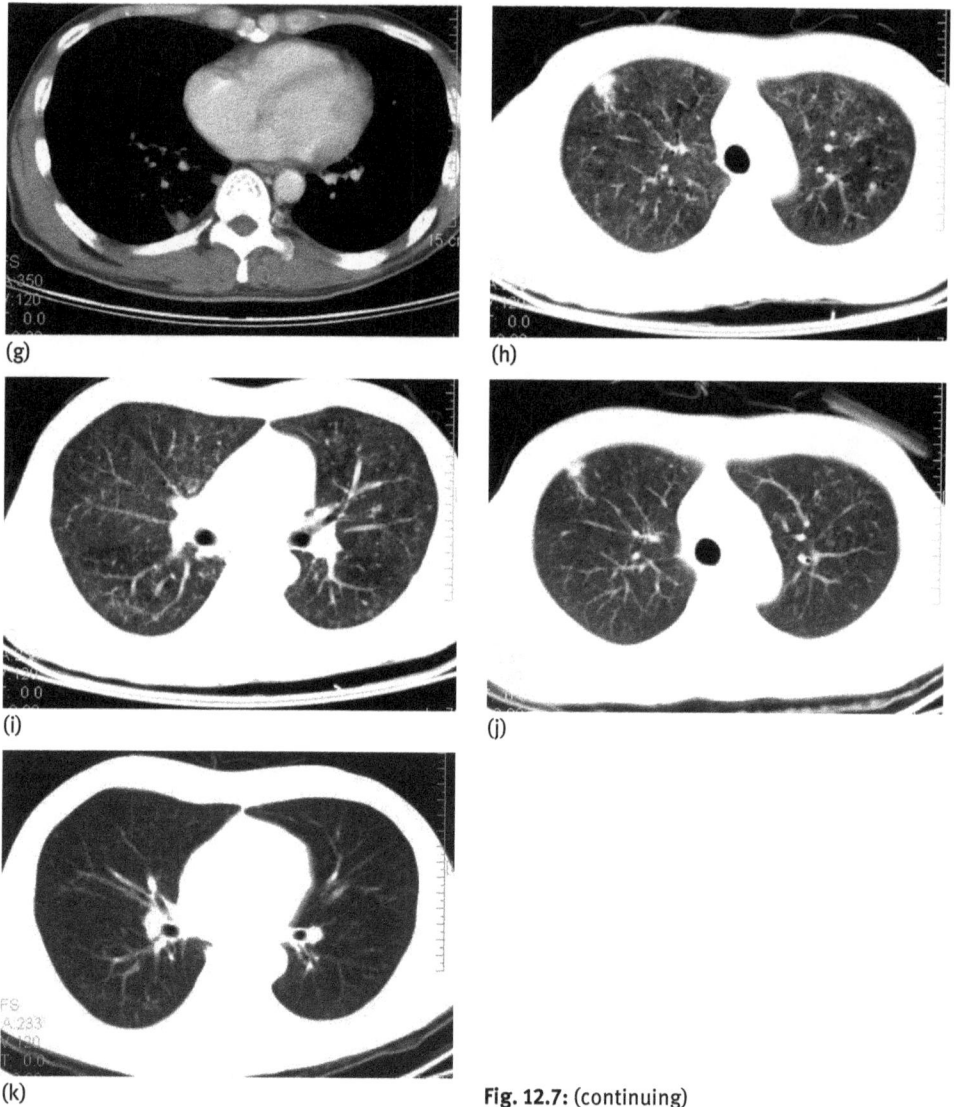

Fig. 12.7: (continuing)

Chest radiograph (a) showed declined transparency of the bilateral lungs, with multiple vague nodules and diffuse ground-glass-like opacities. CT scans (b–d) showed diffuse ground-glass-like opacities, accompanied with multiple ill-edged nodules and stripy fibrous lesions, and the largest nodule in the anterior segment of the right upper lobe (about 1 cm in diameter). HRCT (e) showed ground-glass-like opacities with multiple cystic shadows on both upper lobes, nodules in the right upper lobe with blurring edges and glitches around them. Enhanced CT scans with mediastinal window (f, g) showed mild enhancement of the large nodules in the lung, adjacent pleural thickening mildly, and no enlarged lymph nodes of the mediastinum. Two weeks after anti-PCP treatment of tabellae sulfamethoxazoli composite (TSC), the diffuse ground-glass-like opacities were absorbed evidently, multiple small miliary nodules were seen in the bilateral lung fields, part nodules of the right upper lobe were slightly absorbed, with small cavities formed in it. After 6 weeks, CT scans showed the small miliary nodules in bilateral lungs were remarkably reduced and the lung field was clearer than before (j, k).

Case 12.8 (Fig 12.8 a–l)

A 41-year-old male presented recurrent fever and tachypnea for two months and visual blurring and skin rashes for one week. CD4+ cell count was 38/μl. The tachypnea was remarkably improved after anti-PCP treatment. CSF smear was cryptococcus positive. Cultures of CSF and hemoculture confirmed cryptococcus positive. Sputum culture was *Acinetobacter baumannii* positive. The patient was diagnosed with AIDS (C3) complicated with intracal or hematal cryptococcosis infections, pulmonary infections (PCP, *Acinetobacter baumannii*), cytomegalovirus retinitis (CMVR) and oral fugal infections.

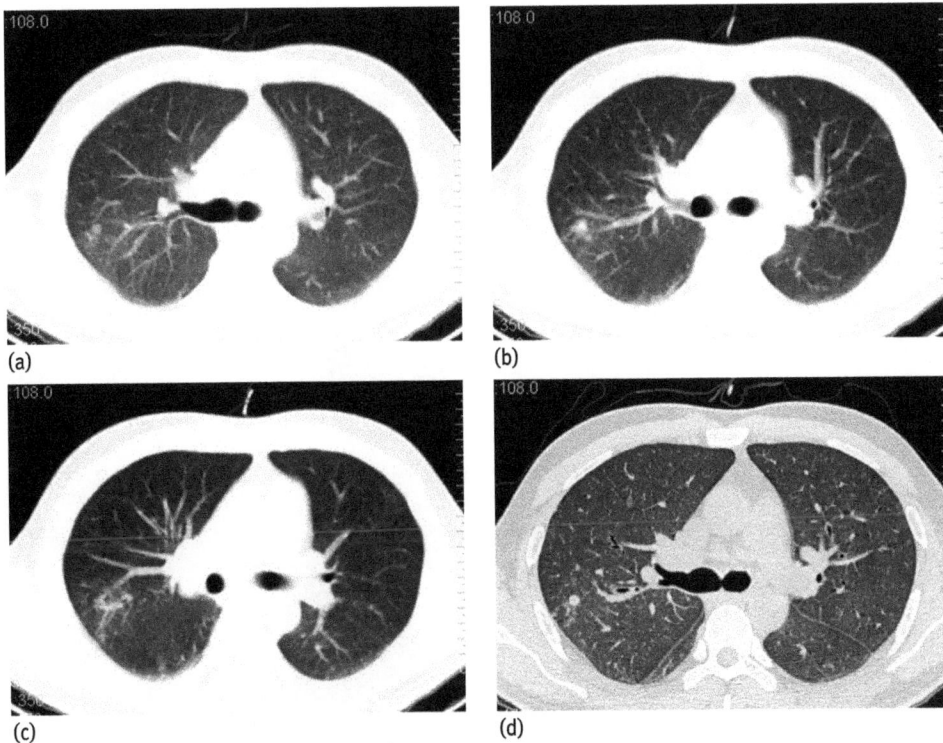

Fig. 12.8 a–l: Pneumonia (PCP, aspergillus and bacteria) in AIDS.

(e)

(f)

(g)

(h)

(i)

(j)

(k)

(l)

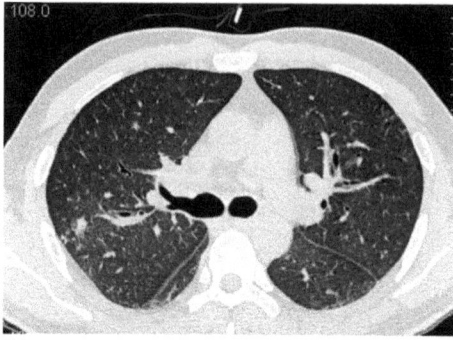

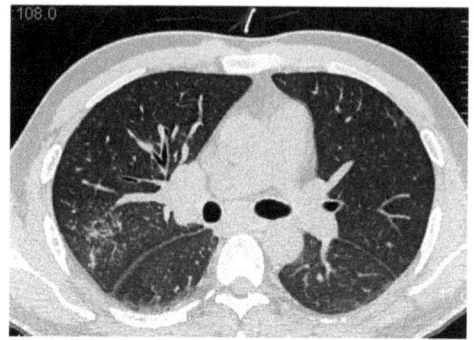

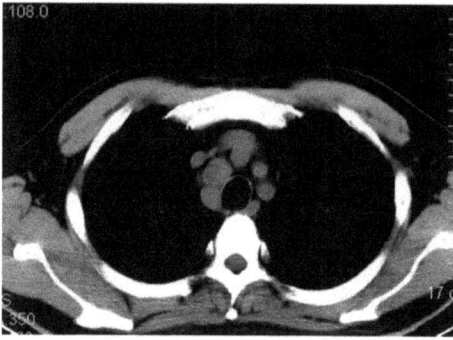

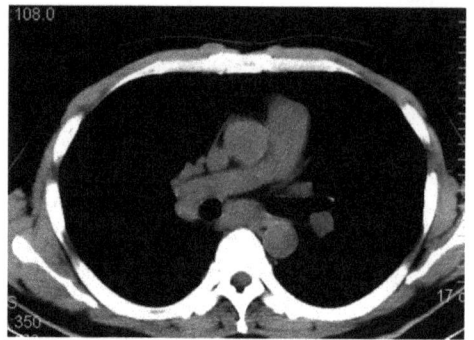

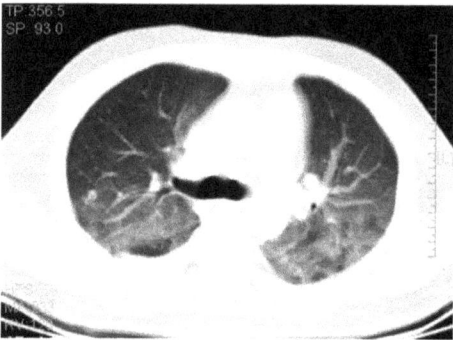

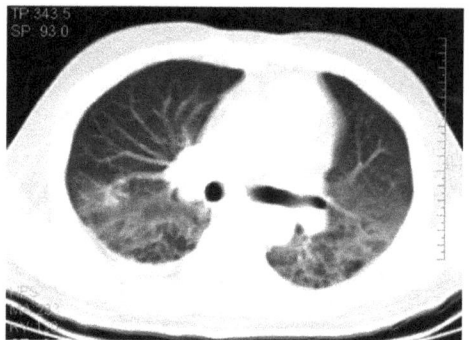

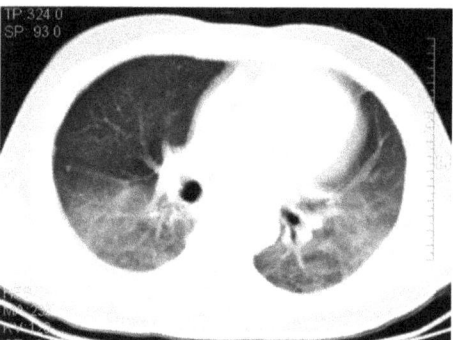

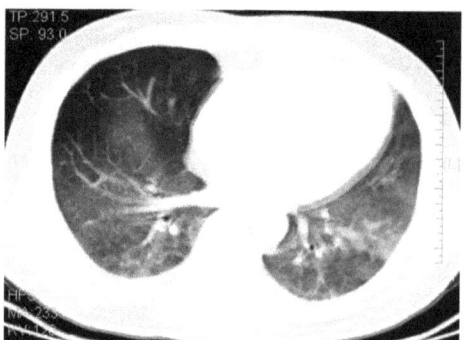

Fig. 12.8: (continuing)

CT scans (a–f) showed an oval nodule in the posterior segment of the right upper lobe surrounded by blurring patchy opacities and multiple small nodules in the lesion showing a tree-in-bud sign. HRCT scans (d–f) showed nodules with a faintly visible small cavity in the right upper lobe. CT scans with mediastinal window (g, h) showed enlarged lymph nodes in the mediastinum. After 4 weeks treatment, CT scans showed new lesion like diffuse ground-glass-like opacities were added in the bilateral lungs, and the lesions of the right lung were still remained(i–l).

Case 12.9 (Fig. 12.9 a–k)

A 58-year-old male presented fever, cough and tachypnea for more than 20 days with temperature up to 39.2 °C, accompanied by aversion to cold and chills. No sputum, hemoptysis or bloody sputum was noted in cough. He experienced chest distress and anhelation when coughing hard, walking for long time and stepping upstairs, and appetite lose. CD4+ cell count was 75/µl. Culture of bronchoalveolar lavage fluid (BALF) was *Klebsiella* positive. The biopsy by bronchoscopy confirmed CMV pneumonia and PCP. The patient was diagnosed with AIDS (C3) complicated by severe pneumonia (PCP, *Klebsiella* and CMV).

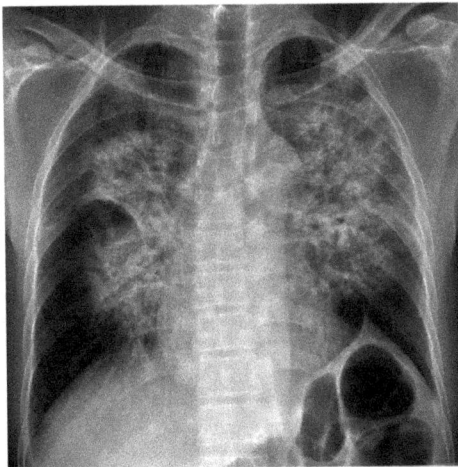

(a)

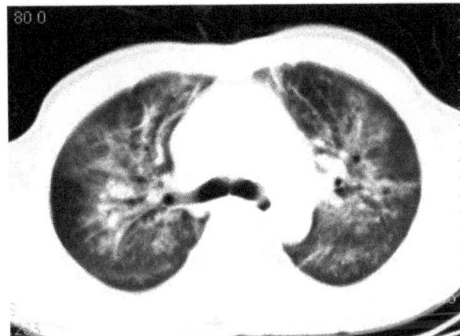

(b)

Fig. 12.9 a–k: Pneumonia (PCP, cryptococcus and *Acinetobacter baumannii)* in AIDS.

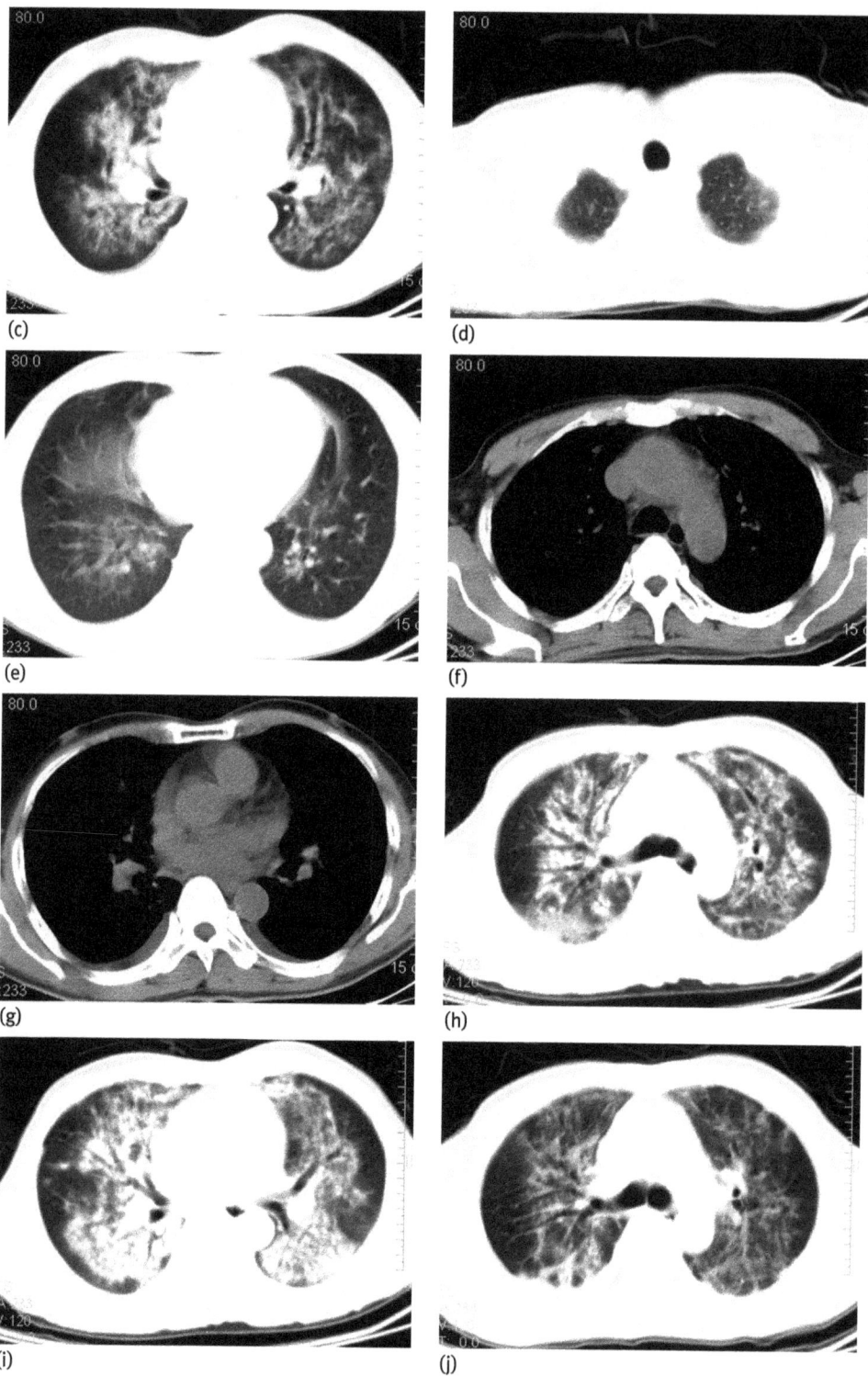

(c)

(d)

(e)

(f)

(g)

(h)

(i)

(j)

Fig. 12.9: (continuing)

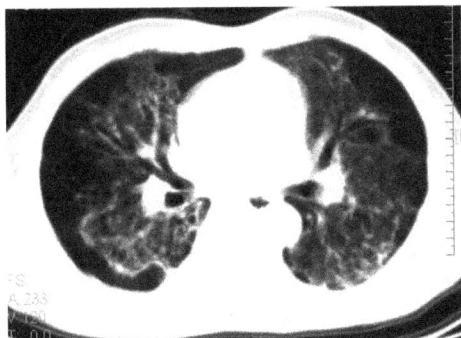

(k)

Fig. 12.9: (continuing)

Chest radiograph (a) showed extensive flaky opacities throughout both lungs, more prominent in bilateral pulmonary hilar, which were ill-defined, and the lateral fields looked approximately normal. CT scans (b–e) revealed multiple segmental, patchy, veiling ground-glass opacities throughout both lungs, which was more obvious in bilateral lung hilar. Soft tissue window showed minimal bilateral pleural effusions, and no enlarged lymph nodes in the mediastinum. After 2 weeks treatment, CT scans (h, i) showed diffuse ground-glass opacities which had become more confluent and dense with air bronchograms, while the lateral fields relatively normal. After 5 weeks treatment, the lesion of bilateral lungs were obviously absorbed, with reticular fibrous shadows forming(j, k).

Case 12.10 (Fig. 12.10 a–j)

A 50-year-old male presented fever without any obvious causes one week before, especially in the afternoon. He complained of spontaneous sweating, with no cough and expectorations and the body temperature up to 39 °C, accompanied with aversion to cold and chills. CD4+ cell count was 27/μl. Sputum smear detected Gram cocci positive. Culture of sputum was *Klebsiella* positive. Blood and bone marrow cultures were *Penicillum marneffei* positive. The patient was diagnosed with AIDS (C3) with pulmonary infections (*Klebsiella* and *Penicillum marneffei*), *Penicillum marneffei* septicaemia.

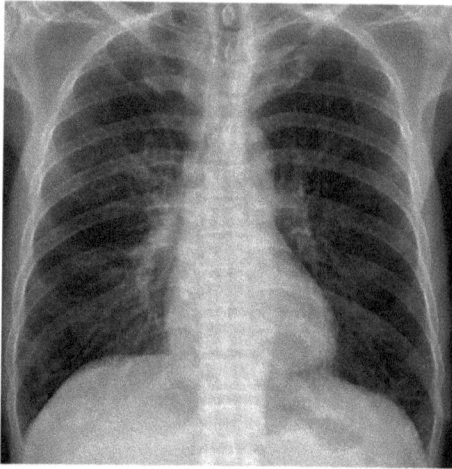

(a)

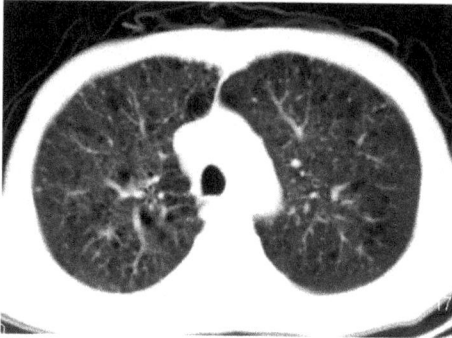

(b)

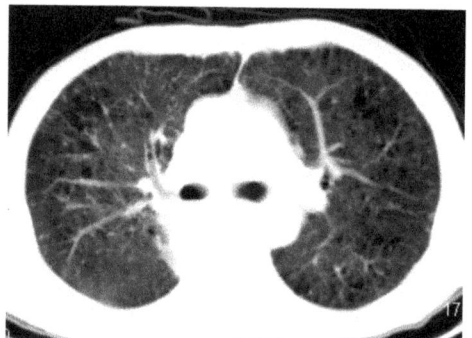

(c)

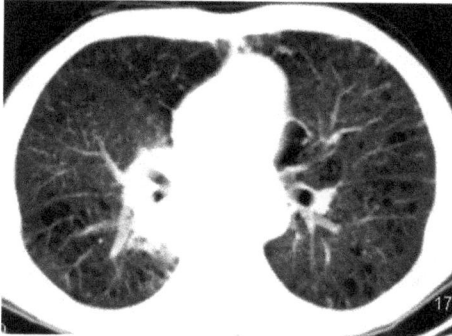

(d)

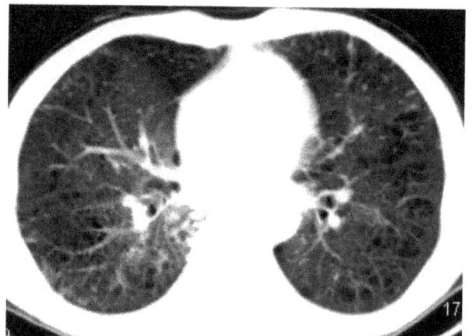

(e)

Fig. 12.10 a–j: Severe pneumonia (PCP, *Klebsiella*, CMV) in AIDS.

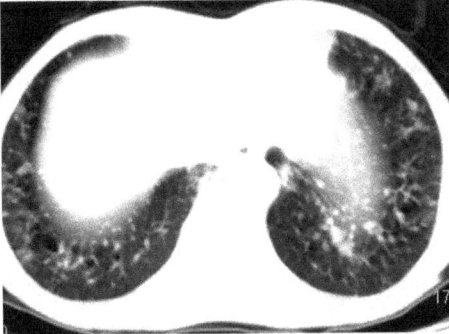
(f)

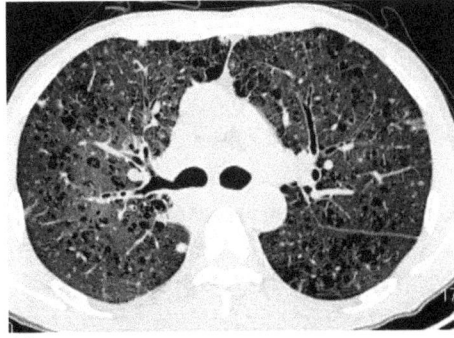
(g)

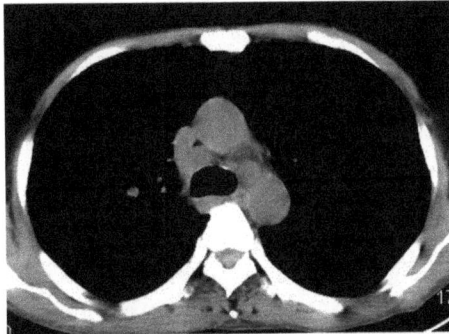
(h)

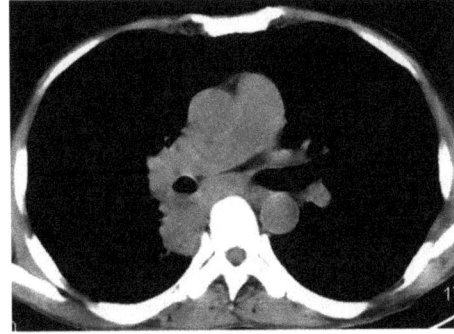
(i)

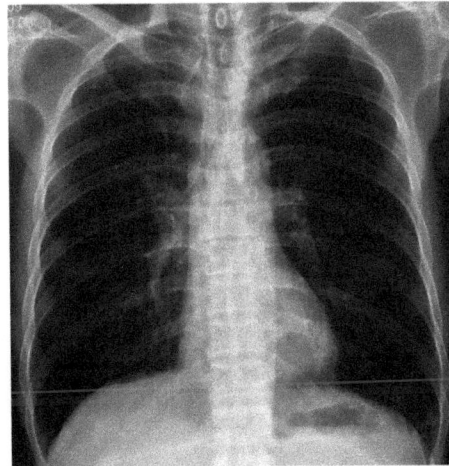
(j)

Fig. 12.10: (continuing)

Chest radiograph (a) showed a patchy opacity located in the right hilum, the thickened markings in the bilateral lungs, and scattered miliary nodules in the bilateral lungs, especially in the peripheric lungs and at the base. CT scans (b–f) demonstrated the consolidation of the dorsal segment of right lower lobe surrounded by ground-glass-like patchy opacities, diffuse miliary nodules in the bilateral lungs, especially at the subpleural area and bilateral lower lobe near diaphragmatic surface. HRCT scan revealed diffuse small nodules of different size as well as centrilobular emphysema in the bilateral lungs. CT scans (h, i) showed the consolidation of the dorsal segment of right lower lobe, and the enlarged lymph nodes beside the trachea and at the inferior knob. After 2 weeks, chest radiograph showed the fields of both lungs were clearer than before, the small miliary nodules were significantly absorbed in the bilateral lungs and the lesions in the inferior lobe of right lung were better improved than before (j).

12.2 Imaging features

The pulmonary infections caused by multiple pathogens in AIDS patients are commonly characterized by dissemination, complexity and multiplicity of the lesions. Imaging performance are overlapped, predominantly one sign (i.e. ground-glass opacity, cavity, milliary nodules, multiple alveolar consolidations, diffuse interstitial lung disease or diffuse alveolar damage) combined with other signs, which attribute to the difficulty in the differential imaging diagnoses.

Editors: Bihua Chen, Wanshan Chen, Chibiao Yin, Qingxin Gan

13 Imaging findings of AIDS-related Lymphoma

13.1 Introduction

After infected with human immunodeficiency virus (HIV), the incidence of lymphoma is as high as 4%–10%, secondary to of Kaposi sarcoma. In terms of the incidence, Non-hodgkin's lymphoma (NHL) is obviously higher than Hodgkin's lymphoma in HIV-infected group, 60 times than which in normal people group.

Lymphoma is divided into two categories (color fig. 13.0): Hodgkin's disease (HD) and Non-Hodgkin's lymphoma (NHL).

Hodgkin's disease is classified as nodular lymphocyte predominance, lymphocyte predominance type, lymphocyte depletion type, nodular sclerosis type and mixed cellularity.

Non-hodgkin's lymphoma include two main types: B cell lymphoma and T/NK cell lymphoma. The subtypes are listed as below in Table 13.1.

Table 13.1: Types of non-Hodgkin's lymphoma

B cell lymphoma	T/NK cell lymphoma
– Precursor B cell lymphoid neoplasms: B lymphoblastic leukemia/lymphoma	– Precursor T cell lymphoid neoplasms: T lymphoblastic leukemia/lymphoma
– Mature B cell lymphoma	– Mature T-cell lymphoma
– B chronic lymphocytic leukaemia/lymphoma	– T cell prolymphocytic leukaemia
– B prolymphocytic lymphocytic leukaemia	– T cell large granular lymphocytic leukaemia
– Lymphoplasmacytic lymphoma	– Aggressive NK cell leukaemia
– Splenic B cell marginal zone lymphoma	– Adult T cell leukaemia/lymphoma
– Hairy cell leukaemia	– Extranodal NK/T cell lymphoma, nasal type
– Plasma cell myeloma/Plasmacytoma	– Enteropathy-associated T cell lymphoma
– Extranodal marginal zone lymphoma of mucosa-associated lymphoid tissue (MALT lymphoma)	– Hepatosplenic T cell lymphoma
	– Subcutaneous panniculitis-like T cell lymphoma
– Nodal marginal zone lymphoma	– Mycosis fungoides/Sézary syndrome
– Follicular lymphoma	– Anaplastic large cell lymphoma: T/null cell, primary cutaneous type
– Mantle cell lymphoma	– Peripheral T cell lymphoma, NOS
– Diffuse large B cell lymphoma	– Angioimmunoblastic T cell lymphoma
– Burkitt lymphoma	– Anaplastic large cell lymphoma: T/null cell, primary systemic type

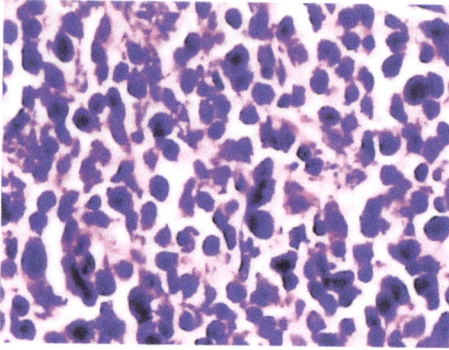

Fig. 13.0: Non-Hodgkin's lymphoma (large B cell type, HE stain, ×100)

In most cases, AIDS-related lymphoma (ARL) includes diffuse large cell type, small uncleaved cell Burkitt type and large immunoblast type. HIV-associated NHL predominantly involves B lymphocyte in spite of HIV attacking T cell. Although it is unidentified in terms of etiological factors and mechanism, ARL is assumed to have possible relationships with reactivation of Epstein-Barr virus (EBv).

Most of ARL belong to NHL, which occurs in advanced stage of HIV infection when the CD4+ lymphocytes in peripheral blood are less than 200/µl. It always leads to a poor prognosis because of its high malignancy as well as its extensive involvement in lymph nodes and extranodal organs in early stage.

13.2 Radiologic findings

Case 13.1 (Fig. 13.1 a–l)

A 30-year-old male patient complained of bellyache for more than ten days, fever and vomiting for 12 hours. Body temperature at admission was 39.8 °C. In the right groin, an enlarged lymph node sized 2.0 cm × 3.0 cm was palpated, tenacious and painless. The right anterior superior iliac spine was palpable tender and the liver was palpable 2 cm below the costal margin, soft and painless and the spleen was not palpable. There were some bean-curd-like substances on the surface of tongue, mild ingestion of pharynx, and rough rales in the bilateral lungs. CD4+ cell count was 35/µl. The biopsy of the right iliac mass identified Non-Hodgkin's lymphoma and giant B cell lymphoma. Blood and bone marrow cultures were PM positive. The patient was diagnosed with AIDS (C3)-related lymphoma combined with pulmonary infection (disseminated PM). Sadly, the patient died of shock and circulatory collapse after 19 days hospitalization.

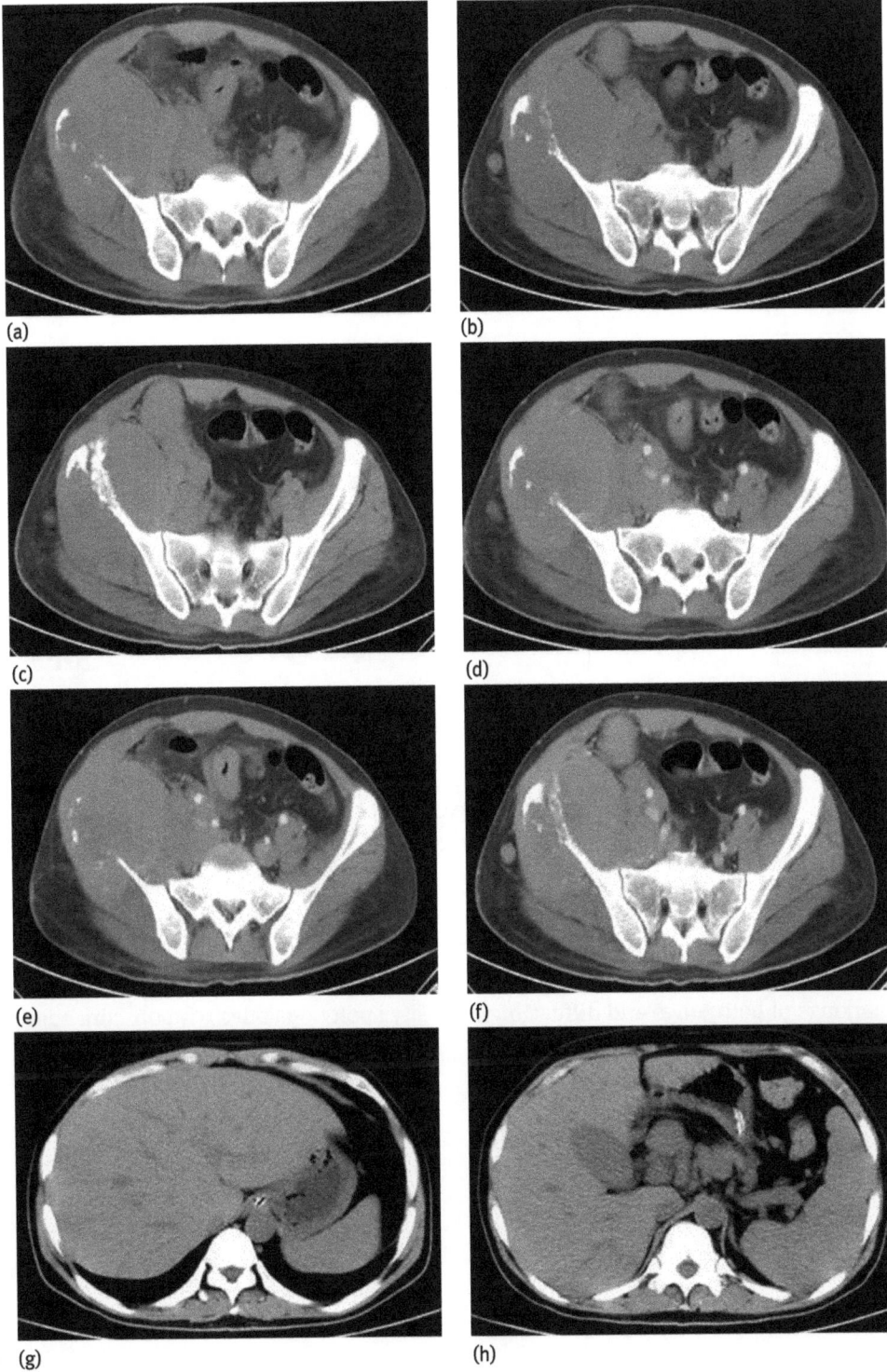

Fig. 13.1 a–k: AIDS-related lymphoma combined with pulmonary infection (Disseminated PM).

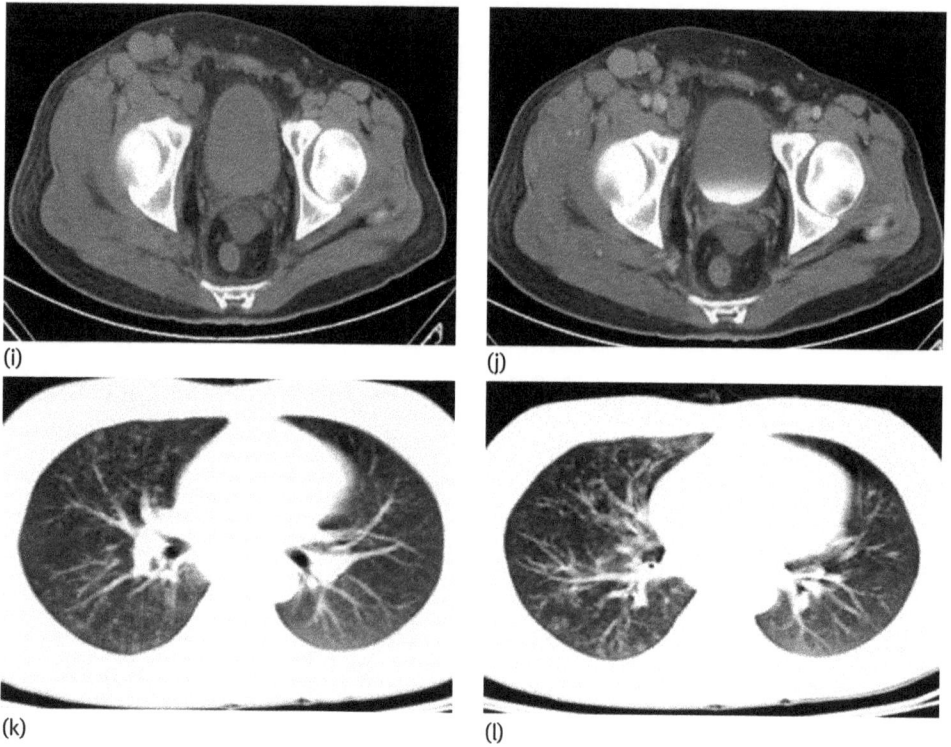

(i)

(j)

(k)

(l)

Fig. 13.1: (continuing)

Plain CT scans (a–c) showed a wide range of osteolytic bone destruction in the right ilium surrounded by blurry-edged soft tissue density masses, accompanied with adjacent muscles swelling obviously. Enhanced CT scans (d–f) showed mildly enhanced swelling soft tissues (d–f), hepatosplenomegaly (g, h). CT scans (i) showed enlarged lymph nodes in the right groin, which manifest with enhancement in contrast-enhancement scan (j). Thoracic CT scans (k, l) showed multiple blurry-edged thickened markings of both lungs and diffuse high-density spotty opacities with obscure edge, presenting a sign of "tree-in-bud".

Case 13.2 (Fig. 13.2 a–h)

A 36-year-old male patient presented recurrent epigastric pain for 16 months and subaxillary mass for 9 months. Body temperature at admission was 36.8 °C. Examination: A mass sized 10 cm × 15 cm at the left armpit was palpable, hard, smooth on surface and painless. There were some red papules with clear edge on his forearms. The abdomen was flat and soft and the right upper abdomen was tender. The liver was palpable 2 cm below the right costa and 6cm beneath the xiphoid process, hard, blunt in the edge, smooth on the surface and no tender. The spleen was palpable 2 cm below the left costa, moderate in nature, blunt at the edge, smooth on the surface and

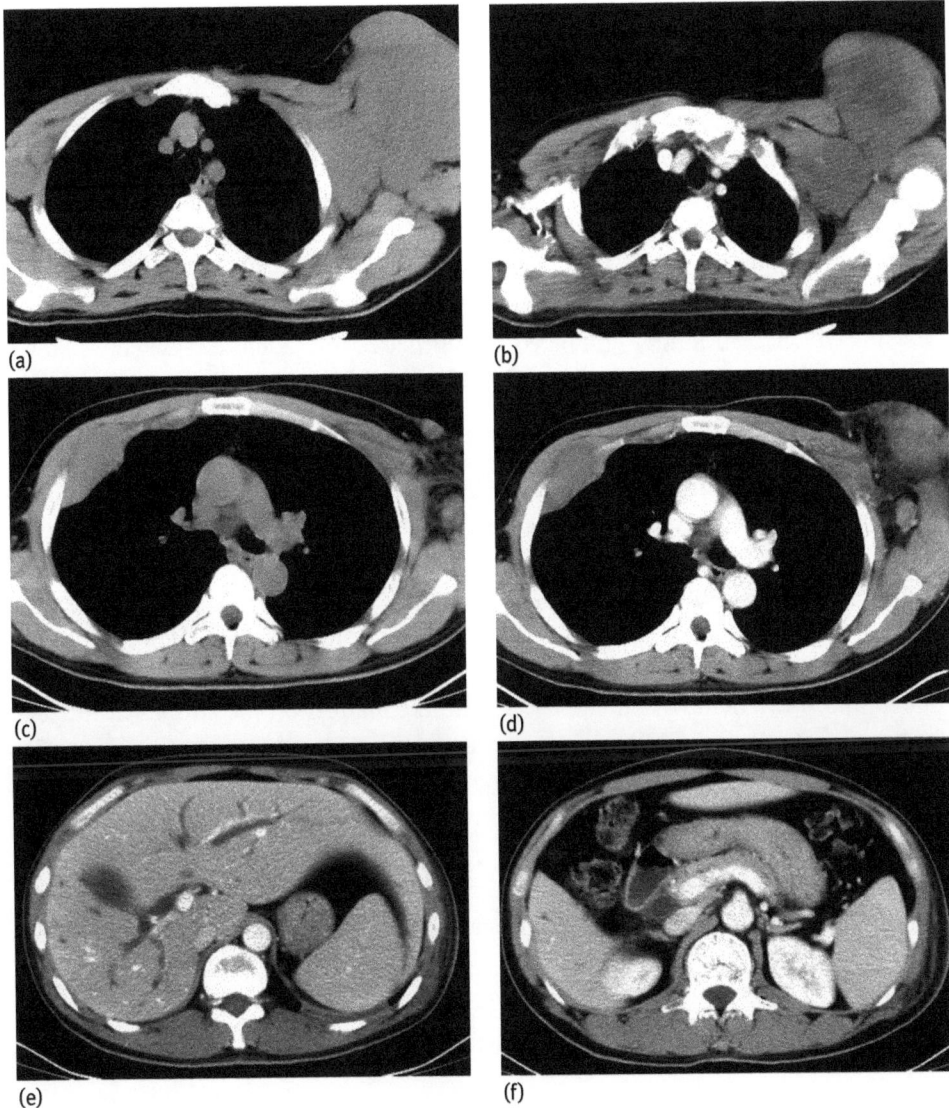

(a)   (b)

(c)   (d)

(e)   (f)

Fig. 13.2 a–h: AIDS-related lymphoma.

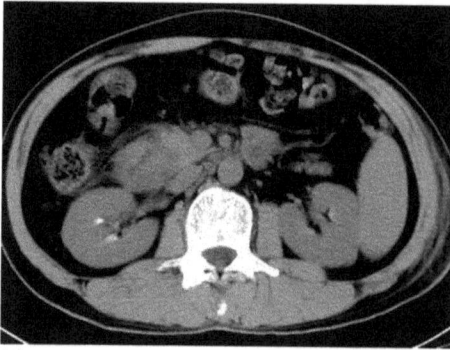
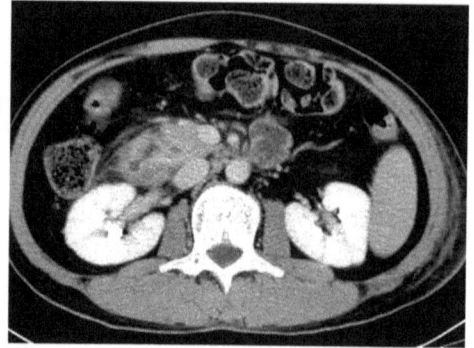

(g) (h)

Fig. 13.2: (continuing)

no tender. Murphy' sign was positive. The breath sounds of bilateral lungs were clear, without dry or moist rales. CD4+ cell count was 73/µl. The biopsy from the axillary nodes identified diffuse B cell non-Hodgkin's lymphoma. The patient was diagnosed with AIDS (C3)-related lymphoma.

Plain CT scans (a) showed multiple enlarged bilateral axillary lymph nodes of various sizes, obviously in the left side, and some of the nodes were fusing. Enhanced CT scans (b) showed mildly enhanced lymph nodes and some low-density patchy necrotic zones in the central giant lymph nodes. CT (c) showed relatively low density masses of soft tissues in the right intercostal space, which aren't enhanced by enhanced scanning (d). The plain scans (e–g) showed dilated intra and extra-hepatic bile ducts and irregularly thickened nodular wall of descending segment of duodenum, which present unevenly enhancements by enhanced scanning (h).

Case 13.3 (Fig. 13.3 a–j)

A 56-year-old male patient, complained of right blepharoptosis for 2 months, accompanied with blurred vision, ghost images and nausea. Body temperature at admission was 36.5 °C. There were some bean-curd-like matters on the surface of tongue. The breath sounds of the bilateral lungs were clear, without dry or moist rales. The abdomen was palpated flat and no tenderness. The liver and spleen were not palpable below the costa. There were mild edemas in both lower extremities. Systemic superficial lymph nodes were not palpable. CD4+ cell count was 115/µl. The biopsy of duodenal tumor obtained from gastroscopy indentified non-Hodgkin's lymphoma, diffuse large B cells type. The patient was diagnosed with AIDS (C3)-related lymphoma.

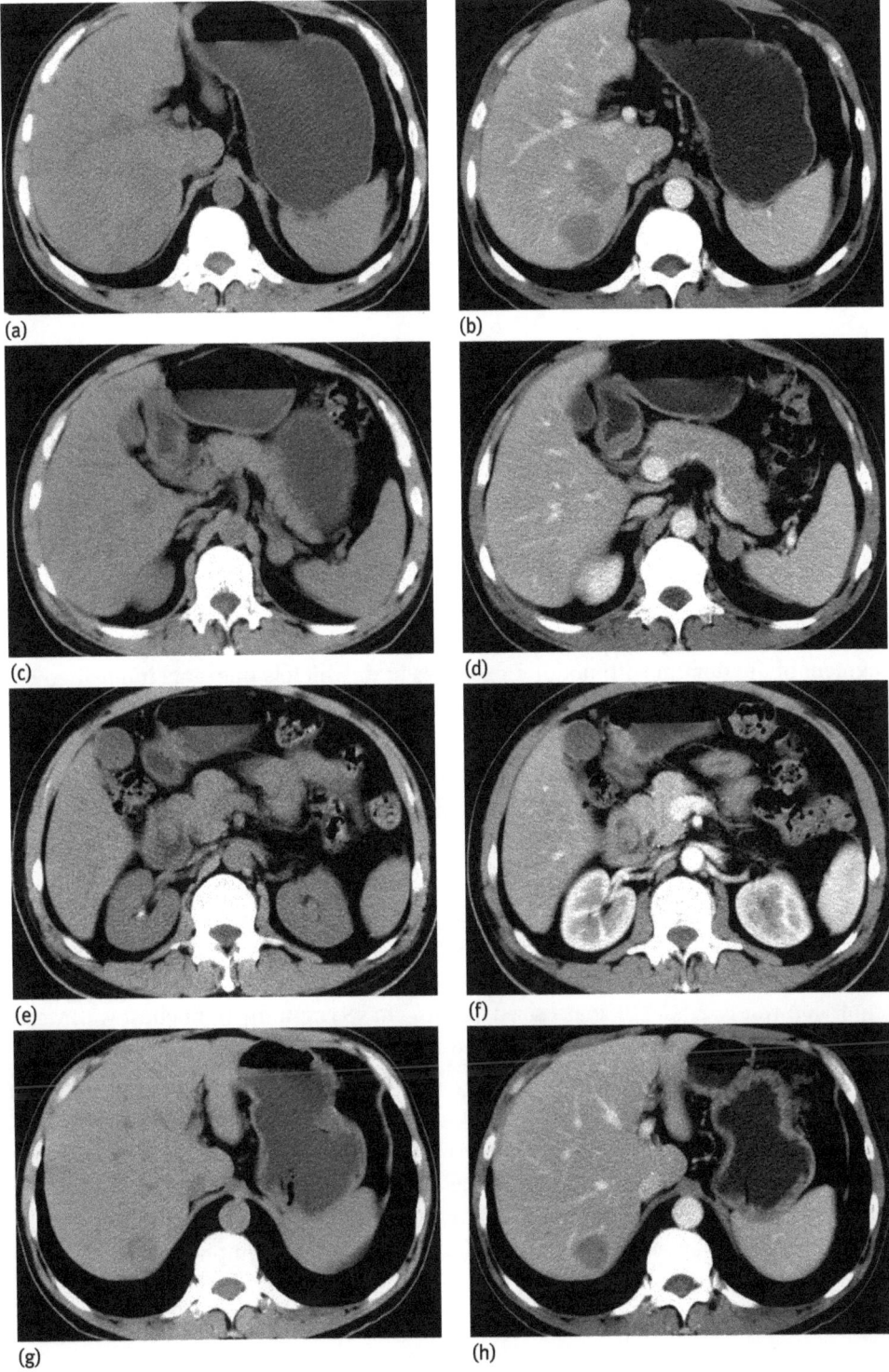

Fig. 13.3 a–j: AIDS-related lymphoma.

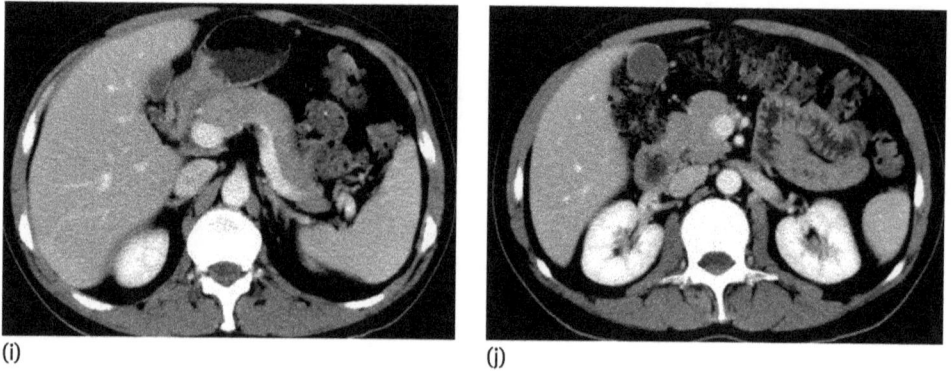

(i)   (j)

Fig. 13.3: (continuing)

Plain CT scans (a) showed a low-density blurry-edged nodular lesion in the right posterior lobe of liver. Enhanced CT scans (b) demonstrated insignificant enhancement
on the lesion and relatively low-density sharp-edged lesion in portal venous phase.
CT scans (c) showed a small nodular lesion in left adrenal gland, which is mildly
intensified by the enhanced scanning and presents relatively low density in the portal
venous phase (d). Plain CT scans (e) showed irregularly thickened wall of descending
segment of duodenum with nodular opacities in it, which is unevenly intensified by
enhanced scanning (f). After 3 weeks chemotherapy, CT scans showed the low-density
nodule in the posterior lobe of right liver obviously shrank (g, h), the small nodular
lesions disappeared in the left adrenal gland (i), the wall of descending segment of
duodenum recovered to normal and the nodules in the lesion disappeared (j).

Case 13.4 (Fig. 13.4 a–l)

A 62-year-old male patient complained of a mass in the right chest, without pain or
fever 2 months before hospitalization, the mass progressively grew and spread into
the right armpit,accompanied with occasional touched tender. Body temperature at
admission was 36.5 °C. The mass sized about 7 cm × 9 cm in the right chest wall were
palpable, and the one sized about 5 cm × 6 cm in the right armpit were connected to
the former. The latter was uneven on the surface, palpable no tender and inactive
with adhesion. There were some bean-curd-like matters on the surface of tongue but
no hairy leukoplakia on the lingual side. The breath sounds of bilateral lungs were
clear, without dry or moist rales. CD4+ cell count was 262/μl. The biopsy from the
right chest wall identified pathologically non-Hodgkin's lymphoma, diffuse large B
cells type. The patient was diagnosed with AIDS (B3)-related lymphoma.

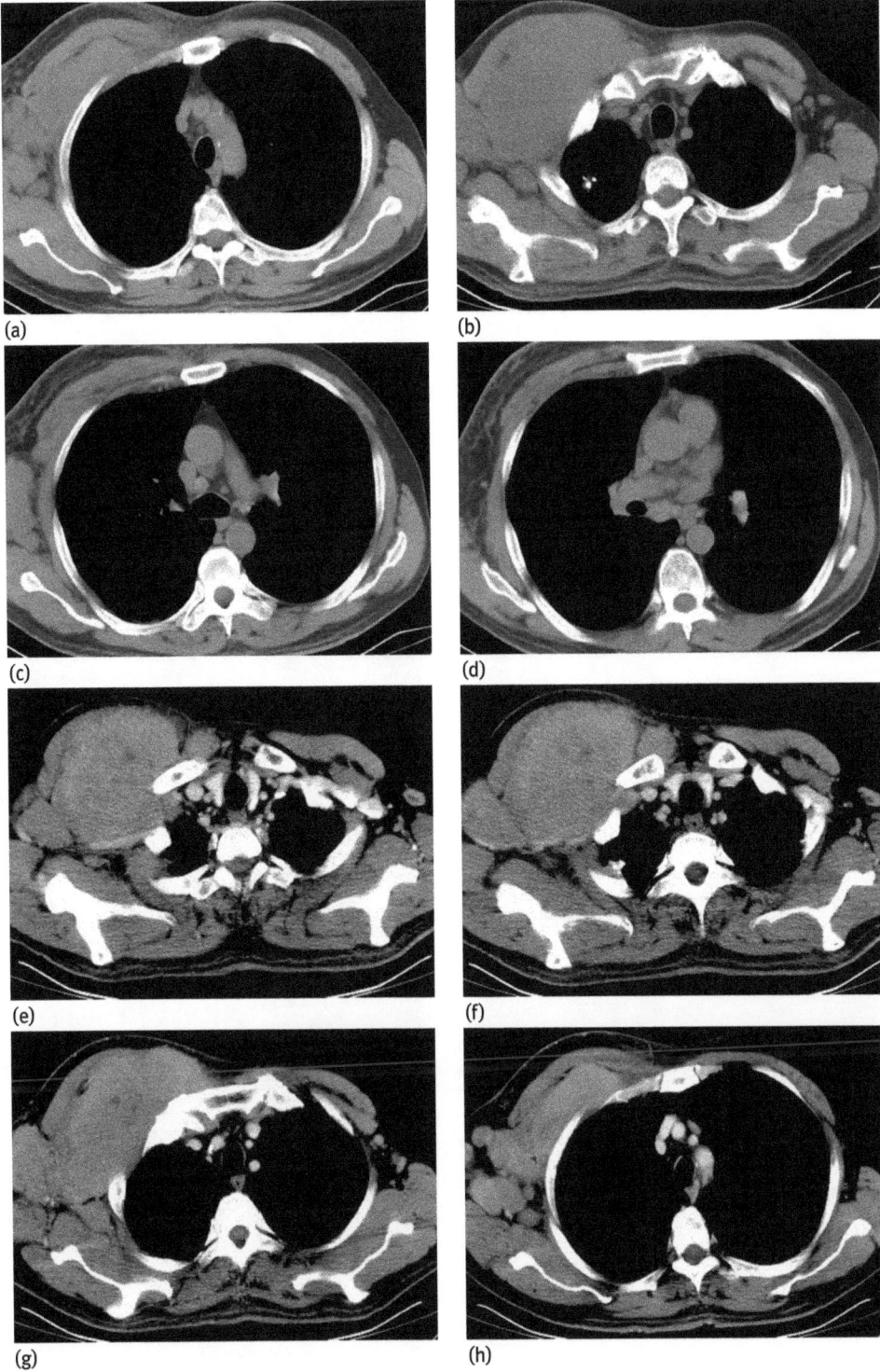

Fig. 13.4 a–l: AIDS-related lymphoma.

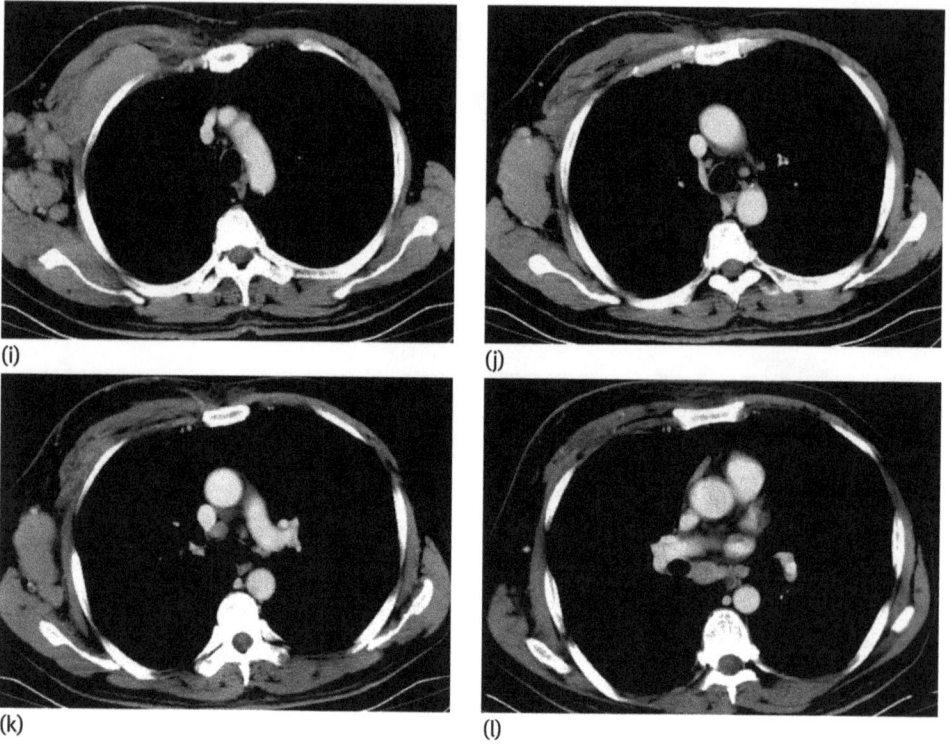

(i)

(j)

(k)

(l)

Fig. 13.4: (continuing)

Plain CT scans showed enlarged multiple lymph nodes in the right armpit, infracla-vicular region and mediastinum, mainly located in axilla (a–d). Enhanced CT scans showed mild enhancement of the enlarged lymph nodes, little patchy low-density necrosis can be seen in the center of right axillary giant lymph nodes, and some of the enlarged lymph nodes fused with each other (e–l).

13.3 Imaging features

The AIDS-related lymphoma is characterized by the following imaging manifestations:

1. Enlargement of systemic lymph nodes: especially of the superficial lymph nodes, and partially of the mediastinal and abdominal lymph nodes.
2. Involvement in the extranodal organs including chest, abdomen, brain, muscles and bones.
   a) The chest imaging manifestations include lung nodules, pulmonary exudative lesions, pleural effusion, seldom-seen tumors on chest walls and occasionally-found osteolytic destructions.
   b) The abdominal imaging manifestations include involvements mainly in the stomach and small intestine, presenting irregular thickening in mucosa and nodular lesions, combined with penetrating ulcers and stenosis of bowel, enlargements of the liver, spleen and kidney and focal lesions.
   c) The brain imaging manifestations include focal low density lesions, frequently combined with edema.
   d) The imaging manifestations of bone, joint and soft tissue include osteolytic destructions to bones mainly of lower limbs, cranial bone, spine and pelvis, and involvements in psoas major muscles and lower extremity muscles.

Editors: Songfeng Jiang, Chunliang Lei, Xiaoping Tang,Deyang Huang

14 Abdominal CT findings in AIDS

14.1 Introduction

Because the account of CD4+ cells decreases significantly, AIDS patients often concomitant with opportunistic infections and AIDS-associated malignant tumor, the abdominal tissues and organs are frequently involved, which is a major cause of multiple organ failure and mortality.

14.1.1 Liver and spleen

1. Non-specific changes: CT findings include hepatosplenomegaly, the reduction of the liver density caused by hepatic steatosis, liver cirrhosis and so on. According to Trojan etc. analyzed 227 cases retrospectively, except 29 (13%) cases without any change, most of the patients have different kinds of liver lesions, and the liver weight increases generally, hepatic steatosis were occurred in 77 cases (34%), which is the most frequent change in non-specific changes. Liver cirrhosis has main etiological factors such as hepatitis and alcohol addiction in common globally, and viral hepatitis, e. g., type B or C hepatitis, most commonly in China.
2. Opportunistic infections in the liver and spleen: CT scan shows low density nodules and masses in the liver and spleen, liver abscess, hepatomegaly, the reduction of liver density, heterogenous enhancement of the liver parenchyma. There is a variety of pathogens. Trojan analyzed 227 cases, liver with opportunistic infections were found in 50 patients (22%), CMV infections account for 19 (8%), mycobacterium infections account for 16 (7%), and toxoplasma infections account for 11 (5%), other rare pathogens include leishmania, cryptococcus neoformans, pneumocystis. The incidence of infection in liver is higher than that of spleen infection.
   a) fungal infection: in south China and Southeast Asia, the warm and humid weather allows the AIDS patients with susceptibility to fungal infections by PM. Blood and spiral marrow culturing make a definite diagnosis. Lung, liver, spleen, lymph node, intestines, which are in rich in macrophage are often involved. So CT examinations could observe above-mentioned organs involved at the same time. Other common fungi include *Candida albicans*, cryptococcus neoformans and coccidioides immitis etc.
   b) *Mycobacterium tuberculosis* (MTB) infection: according to WTO, the patients with HIV/MTB double infection increases about 7 folds in 1990's in Asia. China is one of the most severely MTB-hit regions. Some signs of abdominal CT should draw our attention, such like the low-density nodules in liver and spleen, calcification occasionally, and some perform as miliary tuberculosis in liver and spleen.

c) *Mycobacterium avium*-intracellulare complex (MAC) infection: a common opportunistic infection in AIDS patients in developing countries, often occurs in AIDS advanced stage, incidence of MAC infection will increase accordingly, when the infections caused by other pathogens are under control. In imageology, the abdominal CT findings are similar to those MTB infection.

d) bacterial liver abscess: it is highly epidemic among AIDS patient with bacterial septicemia as well as the drug addicts. As for the imaging, the CT findings are similar to those liver abscess in non-AIDS people.

e) bacillary peliosis hepatitis (BPH): CT scans show hepatomegaly and no abnormal focal lesions or capsular foci in liver. The enhancement scanning may show blood vessel-like intra-capsular enhancement. Specifically, the diagnosis of the disease is based on histological examination of liver and spleen, the pathogen is Bartonella Rochalimaea henselae.

f) CMV infection: CT may present multiple low density lesions in liver, the accurate diagnosis is based on biopsy.

3. AIDS-associated malignant tumor in liver and spleen:

a) lymphoma: most are NHL, include Burkitt lymphoma, often invades extranodal tissues, the frequency of organ involvement is gastrointestinal tract, CT scans display multiple localized low density nodules in liver and spleen, often accompany with retroperitoneal and mesentery lymphadenectasis.

b) Kaposi sarcoma (KS): also known as multiple idiopathic hemorrhagic sarcoma. In China, the incidence of AIDS-associated Kaposi sarcoma is lower than in Europe and America so that the lesions in liver and spleen are rarely reported except with skin lesions in most cases.

14.1.2 Biliary system

AIDS with gallbladder and bile duct lesion is also seen, CT scan shows cholecystitis, dilation of intra- and extra- hepatic duct, duodenal papilla edema, transendoscopic biopsy of duodenal papilla and common bile duct, we can see mucous chronic inflammation, pathogens may be able to be found, such as CMV, cryptozoite etc.

14.1.3 Retroperitoneal and mesentery lymph nodes

CT exams display mesentery, hepatic hilar region, hepatoduodenal ligament region and para-aortic soft tissue nodes, mesentery sandwich sign could be seen in severe cases, display lymphadenectasis of the anterior and posterior part of mesentery, mesentery vessels could be seen in the centre. CT contrast enhancement shows ring like enhancement, most occurs in opportunistic infections, the predilection infections are fungals and tubercle bacillus.

14.1.4 Kidney and adrenal glands

AIDS patients involve with kidney is rare, is a localized disseminated infection, CT scans show unclear margin in kidney, high density in perirenal adipose capsule, the perfusion of renal parenchyma decreases inhomogeneously in contrast enhancement, the involvement in adrenal glands in CT show unilateral or bilateral lesions. It is difficult to differential from space occupying lesion in adrenal glands, most are CMV infection, and the lesions will disappear after systemic infection under control. According to research reports, CMV has a predilection of adrenal glands. Klatt reports 164 cases about HIV, 81 cases is CMV infection, 75% of adrenal glands is with CMV lesions.

14.1.5 Digestive tract

Intestine wall thickening complicated with digestive tract obstruction, seen in cryptozoite which result in chronic diarrhea. Penicilliosis marneffei also lead to intestine wall thickening, the main infection organ are duodenum and jejunum. Ileocecal junction wall thickening and luminal stenosis also seen in TB infection. AIDS-associated lymphoma also lead to intestine wall thickening, that is rare in Kaposi sarcoma.

14.1.6 Pelvic cavity and abdominal

The prediction of pelvic infection is female, CT examination shows pelvic abscess, bacterial septicemia lead to psoas abscess; the imaging finding is similar to general people.

14.1.7 Peritonitis and ascites

Great fluid in peritoneal cavity or with peritoneal thickening, the cause is complicated. All kinds of chronic liver disease that lead to hypoproteinemia, various kinds of opportunistic infections that lead to peritonitis and AIDS-associated tumors will result in ascites. If that is bacterial peritonitis, the CT scan shows encapsulated effusion.

In conclusion, AIDS often involves all organs and tissues in abdomen, accompanying with opportunistic infections, and the abdominal CT findings is non-specific. The definite diagnosis needs biopsy and germiculture, fungus cultivation. Because abdominal biopsy is difficult, the finding of the lesions depends on image examination. The abdominal CT mainly displays lesion involvement, and evaluates the size of the lesion. The radiologist should link clinical and epidemiology closely to make the diagnosis and differential diagnosis.

This chapter will mainly discuss the abdominal CT manifestations of PM and TB infection in AIDS patients.

14.2 Abdominal CT findings of PM infection in AIDS

14.2.1 Introduction

PM infection has become one of the most common opportunistic infections in Southeast Asia and has been regarded as an indicator of AIDS. In affecting human, enicilliosis marneffei (Color figure 14.0) often invades mononuclear phagocyte system, forming the granulomatous, suppurative, unresponsive and necrotic lesions and bringing about lesions in organ and tissues rich in mononuclear phagocytes. For example, the abdominal organs such as liver, spleen and lymph nodes are vulnerable to the affection.

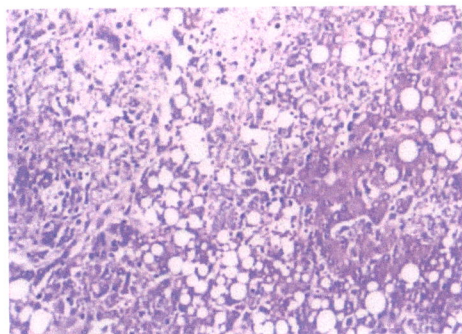

Fig. 14.0: PM in liver tissue (HE stain, ×100).

The cadaveric liver biopsies by microscopy showed multifocal lytic necrosis in liver parenchyma as well as a large number of penicillium spores in necrotic lesions, sinus hepaticus and periportal area: some looking like sausage and others having diaphragm. Besides, the autopsies may show effusive hepatic steatosis.

14.2.2 Radiologic findings

Case 14.1 (Fig. 14.1 a–f)
A 35-year-old male patient complained of recurrent fever for 3 months, and aggregated with bellyache for 5 days before hospitalization. There were erythematous maculopapular rashes on the body trunk and face. CD4+ cell count was 18/μl, with CD4+/CD8+: 0.25. Blood and spiral marrow cultures were PM positive. The patient was diagnosed AIDS (C3) and disseminated PSM. These symptoms were improved after 1 month treatment.

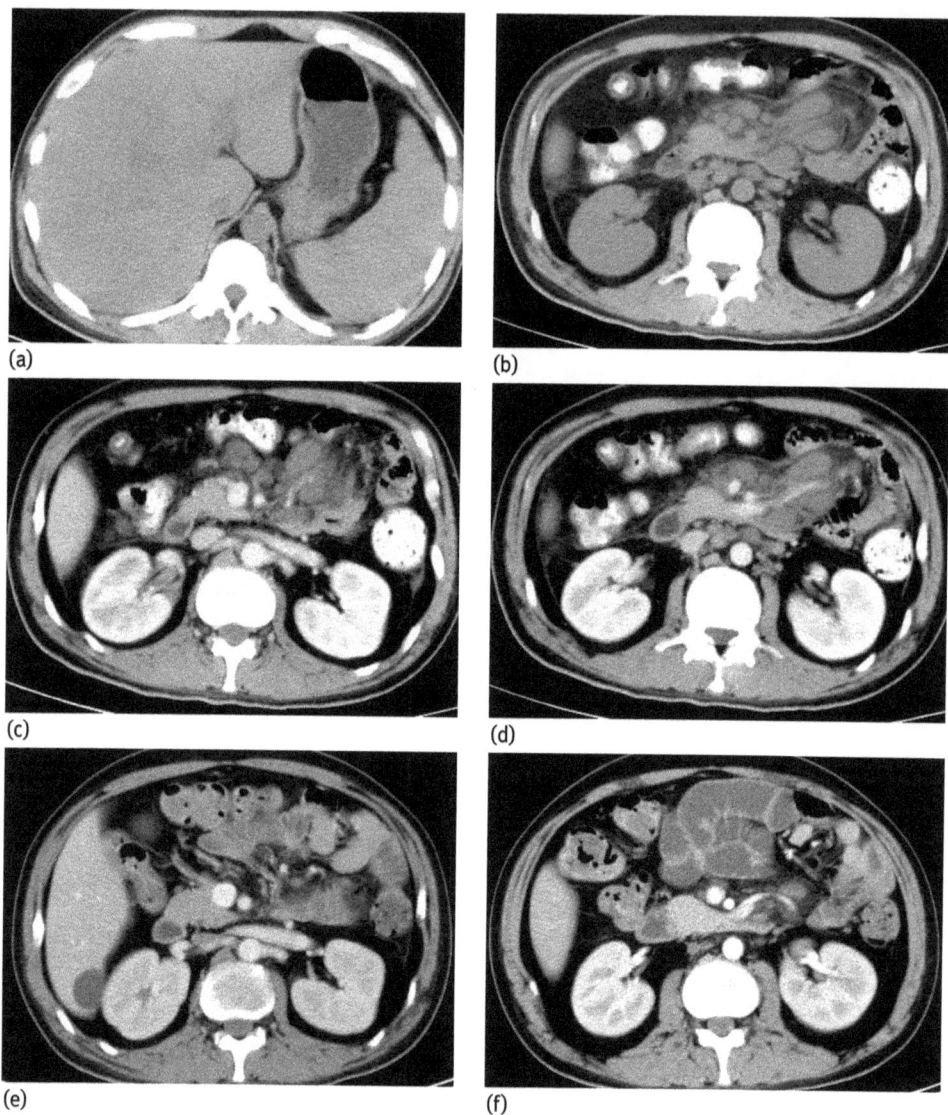

Fig. 14.1 a–f: Disseminated Penicilliosis marneffei disease.

The upper abdominal plain CT scans showed hepatosplenomegaly (a) and enlarged mesenteric and para-aortic lymph nodes of different sizes mainly located in the mesentery (b). Enhanced scans showed mildly and homogeneously enhanced lymph nodes and a sandwich on the mesentery (c, d). After 4 weeks of anti-fungal therapy, the enlarged mesenteric and para-aortic lymph nodes obviously shrunken (e, f).

Case 14.2 (Fig. 14.1 a–l)

A 33-year-old male patient was admitted into a local hospital for cervical mass, fever for more than 3 months, skin rashes for more than 2 months, the biopsy suggesting tuberculous lymphadenitis. The anti-tuberculosis treatment for 2 weeks was ineffective in improving the symptoms. CD4+ cell count was 1/μl, CD4+/CD8+: 0.002. Bone marrow culture was PM positive. The patient was diagnosed with AIDS (C3) combined with disseminated PSM.

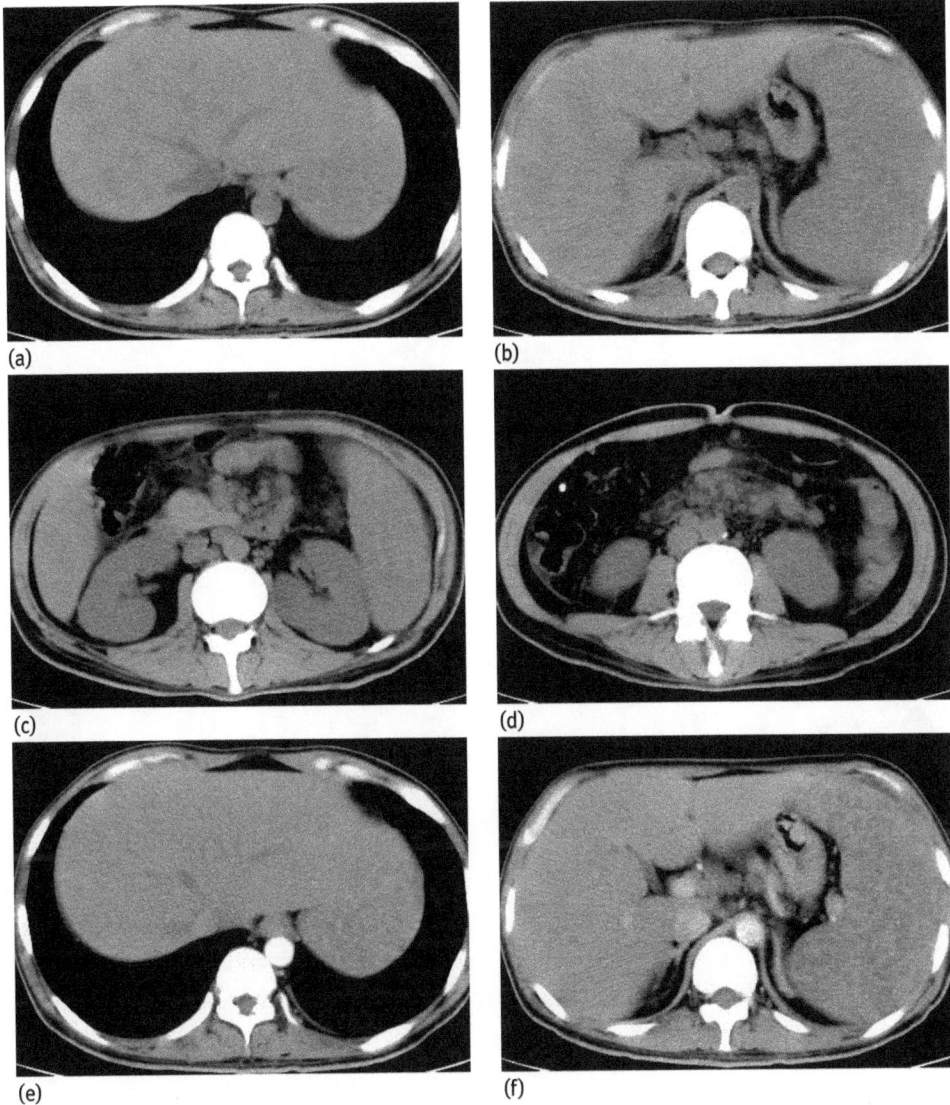

(a)　　(b)
(c)　　(d)
(e)　　(f)

Fig. 14.2 a–l: Disseminated PSM.

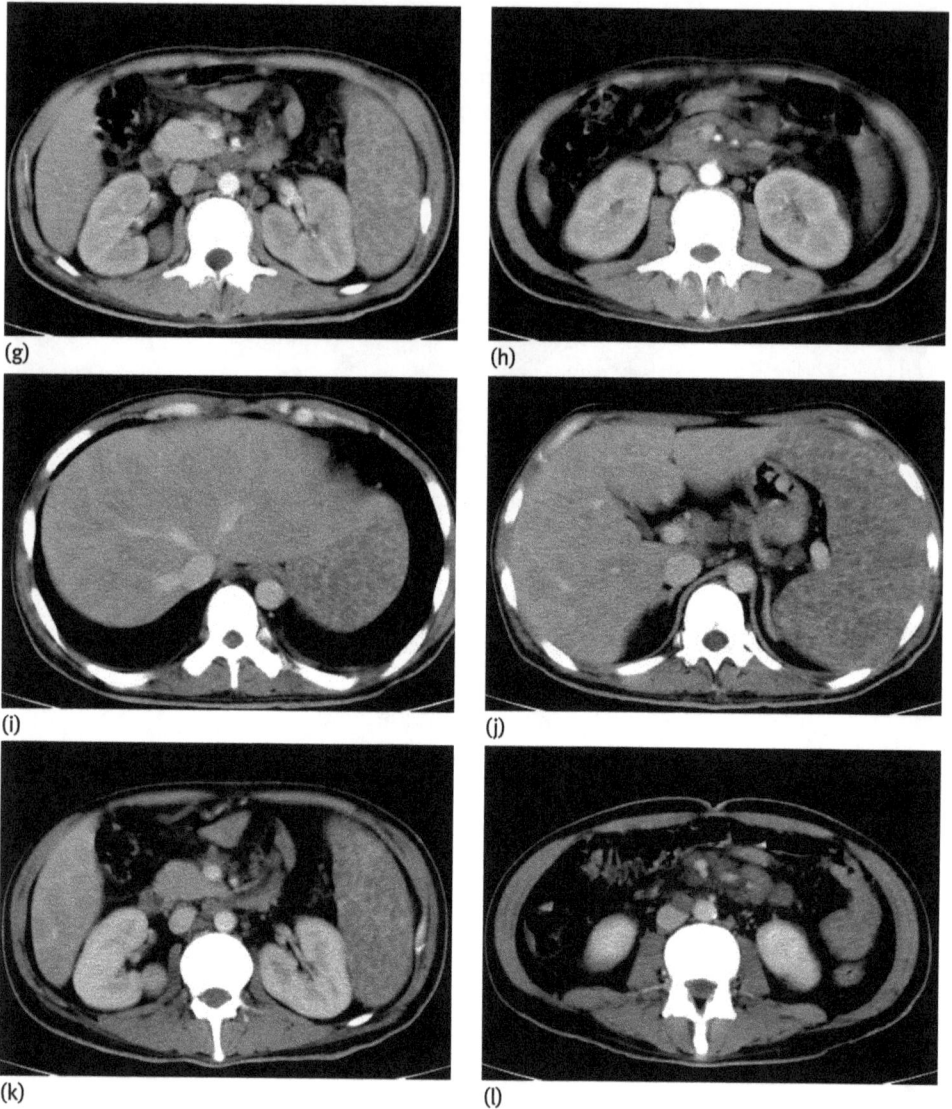

Fig. 14.2: (continuing)

Plain CT scans showed multiple low-density round lesions in liver (a–c) and the enhanced CT scans show the low-density lesions still in the liver, low-density lesions around the small branch of the portal vein in portal venous phase, central high-density shadow on the portal vein (e–g, i–k). The plain scans showed evident enlargement of spleen and low-density miliary lesions in spleen and the enhanced scans show unevenly enhanced hollow-like spleen in portal venous phase (i–k). The plain scans showed enlarged lymph nodes in mesentery, hepatic hilar region and abdominal aorta, most evidently in mesentery, which present soft tissue nodular opacities of various sizes and the enhanced scans show slightly homogeneous enhancement on the lesions (b–d, f–h, j–l).

Case 14.3 (Fig.14.3 a–l)

A 27-year-old male patient presented with skin rash and abdominal swelling and pain for 10 days, when maculopapules covered the face, some looking like hilar depression and there were systemic enlargement of superficial lymph nodes. The abdominal B ultrasonography suggested hepatomegaly with coarse liver echoes. CD4+ cell count was 35/μl, CD4+/CD8+: 0.11. Blood and bone marrow cultures were PM positive. The patient was diagnosed with AIDS (C3) combined with disseminated PSM.

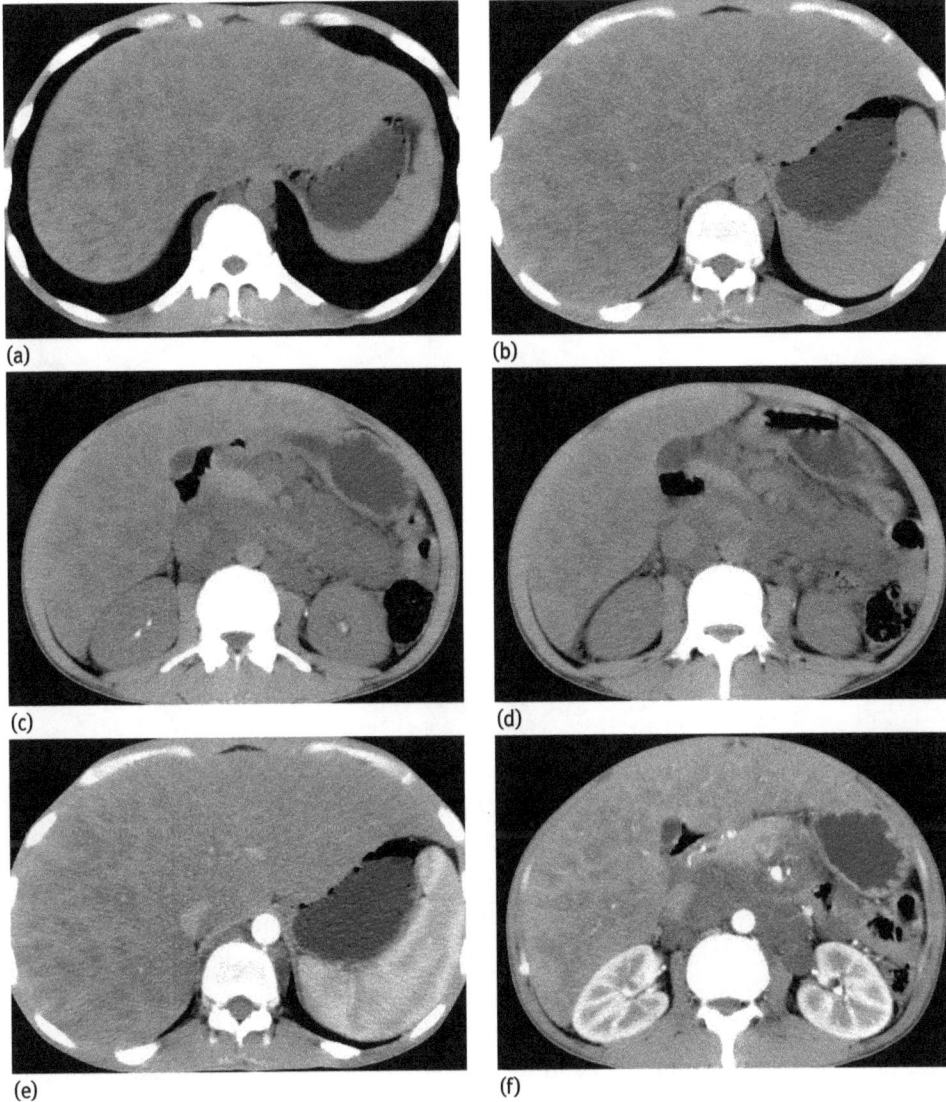

Fig. 14.3 a–l: Disseminated PSM.

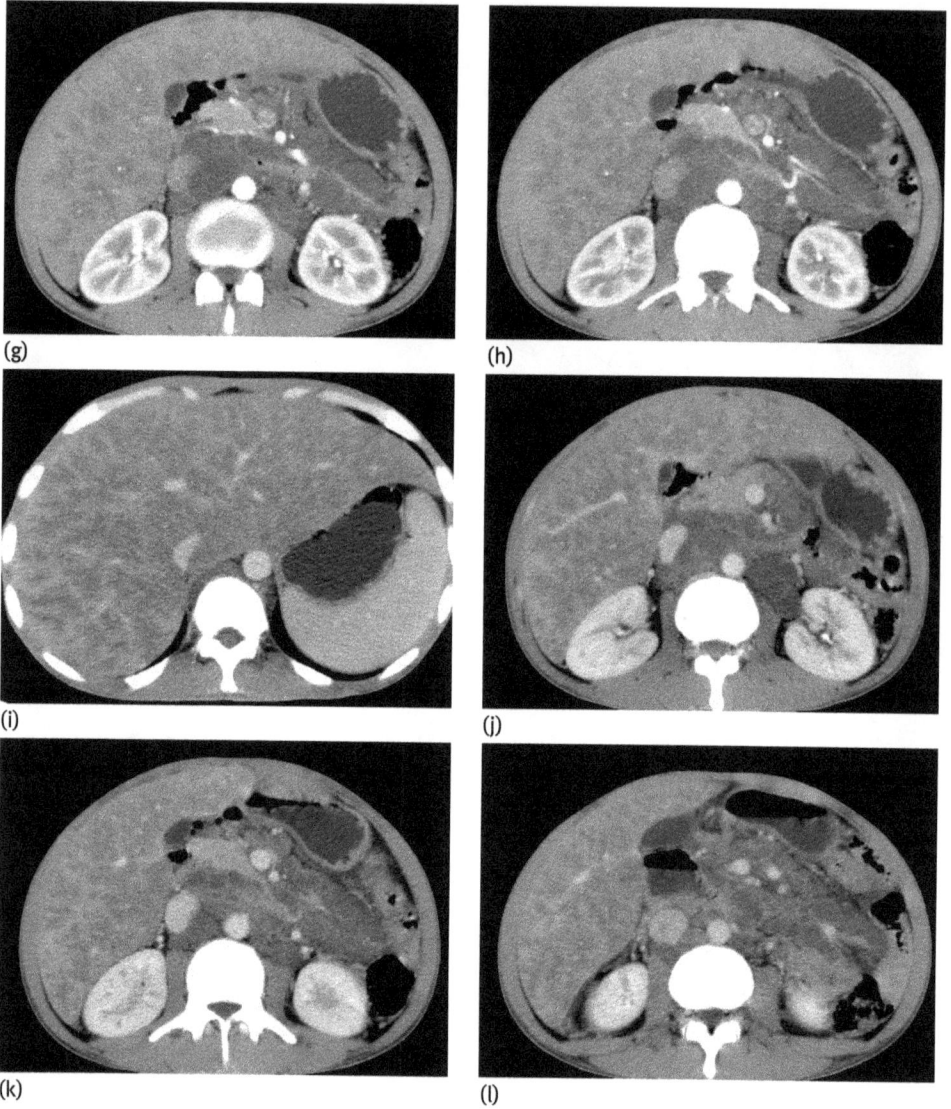

(g)

(h)

(i)

(j)

(k)

(l)

Fig. 14.3: (continuing)

The upper abdominal plain CT scans (a, b) showed hepatomegaly and liver parenchyma with irregularly decreased density. The enhanced scans showed (e–l) diffuse
low-density opacities around the portal area and 'hollow' liver parenchyma with
funicular or plate enhancement in arterial phase and portal venous phase (e–l), and
extensively enlarged lymph nodes in the abdominal cavity (c–d) with partial fusion
of the nodes mainly in the mesentery, indicating a sandwich sign and presenting with
rim enhancement (f–h, j–l).

Case 14.4 (Fig. 14.4 a–l)

A 38-year-old male presenting with lassitude, lack of appetite, and fever for 2 months at admission. CD4+ cell count was 4/µl, with CD4+/CD8+: 0.02. Blood and bone marrow cultures were PM positive. The patient was diagnosed with AIDS (C3) combined with disseminated PSM.

The upper abdominal plain CT scans show hepatosplenomegaly and liver parenchyma with irregularly decreased density (a, b), a small quantity of pleural effusions in both sides (A) and mildly enlarged mesenteric lymph nodes (c, d). The enhanced scans

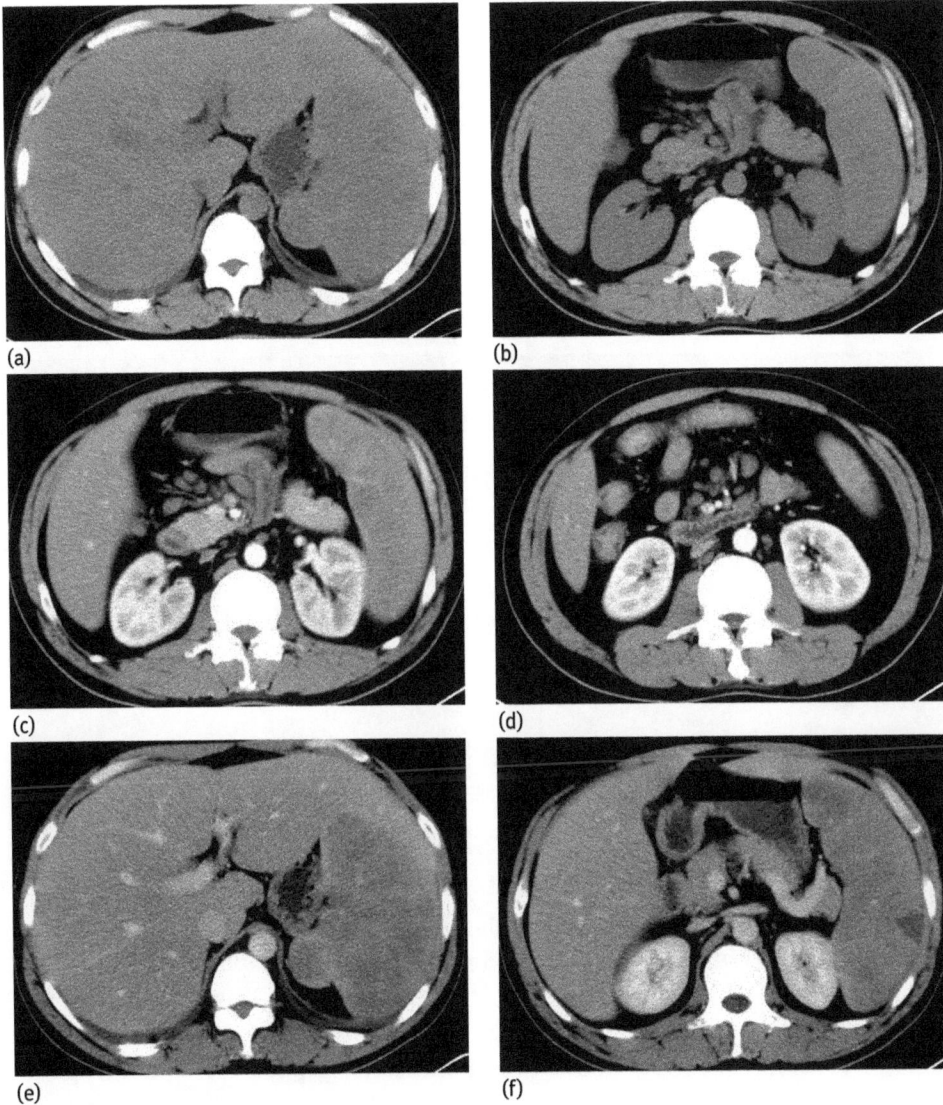

(a) (b) (c) (d) (e) (f)

Fig. 14.4 a–l: Disseminated PSM.

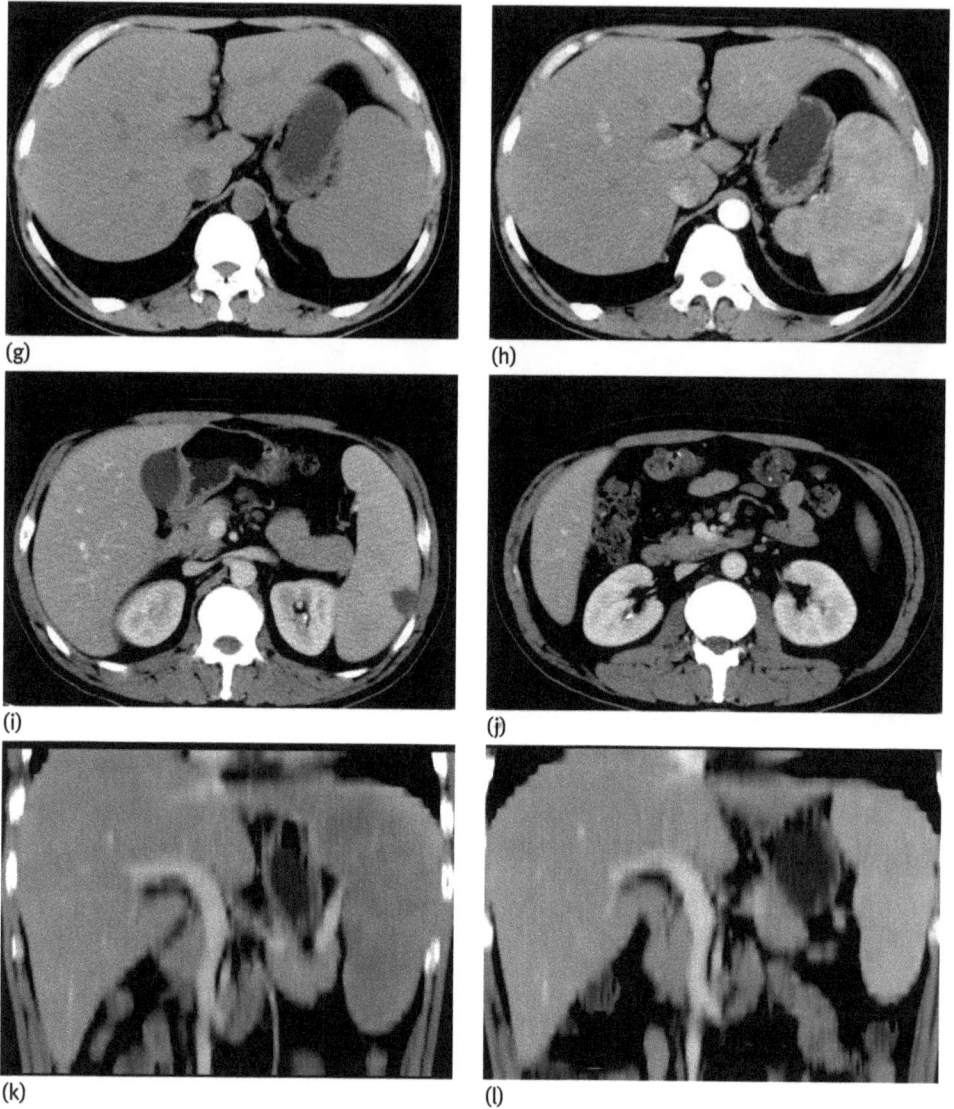

(g)

(h)

(i)

(j)

(k)

(l)

Fig. 14.4: (continuing)

at portal venous phase show irregularly enhanced spleen with uneven low-density patchy opacities and a local wedge-shaped infarct in the outer edge of inferior pole of the spleen (e, f). After 9 days treatment, the liver and spleen shrank, their paren-chyma resumed to normal and the remaining infract in the inferior pole of the spleen, as showed on the CT scans (g–i). By enhanced scanning, the liver and spleen were both irregularly enhanced and the mesenteric lymph nodes shrank as showed on the scans (h–j). MPR scans shows the significant differences in the liver and the spleen between pre-treatment and post-treatment (k before treatment, l after treatment).

Case 14.5 (Fig. 14.5 a–l)
A 37-year-old male patient, presenting with fever for 3 months for no specific reasons, his temperature peaking at 39 °C. He complained about cough with less sputum 3 days ago, dyspnea and 5 kg weight loss within a year. CD4+ cell count was 7/µl, with CD4+/CD8+: 0.05. Blood and bone marrow cultures were PM positive. The patient was diagnosed with AIDS (C3) combined with disseminated PSM.

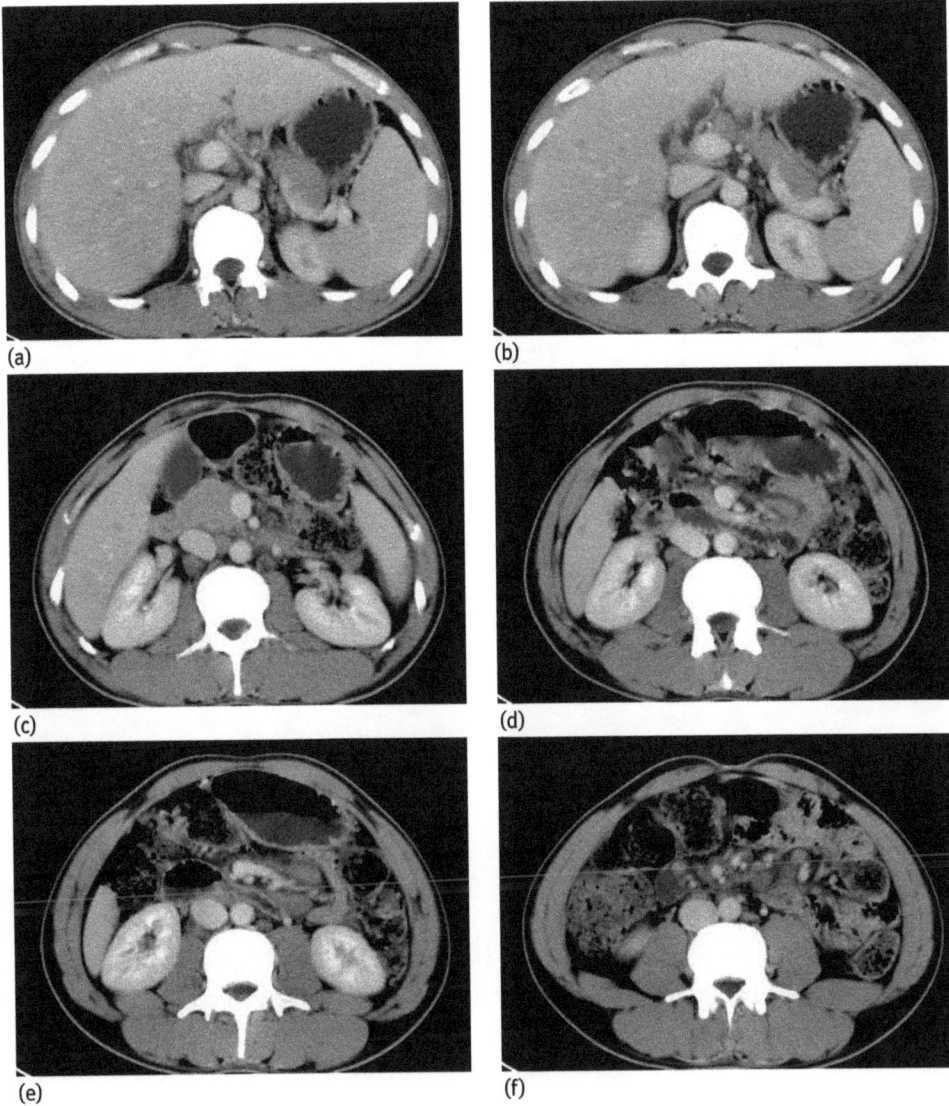

Fig. 14.5 a–l: Disseminated PSM.

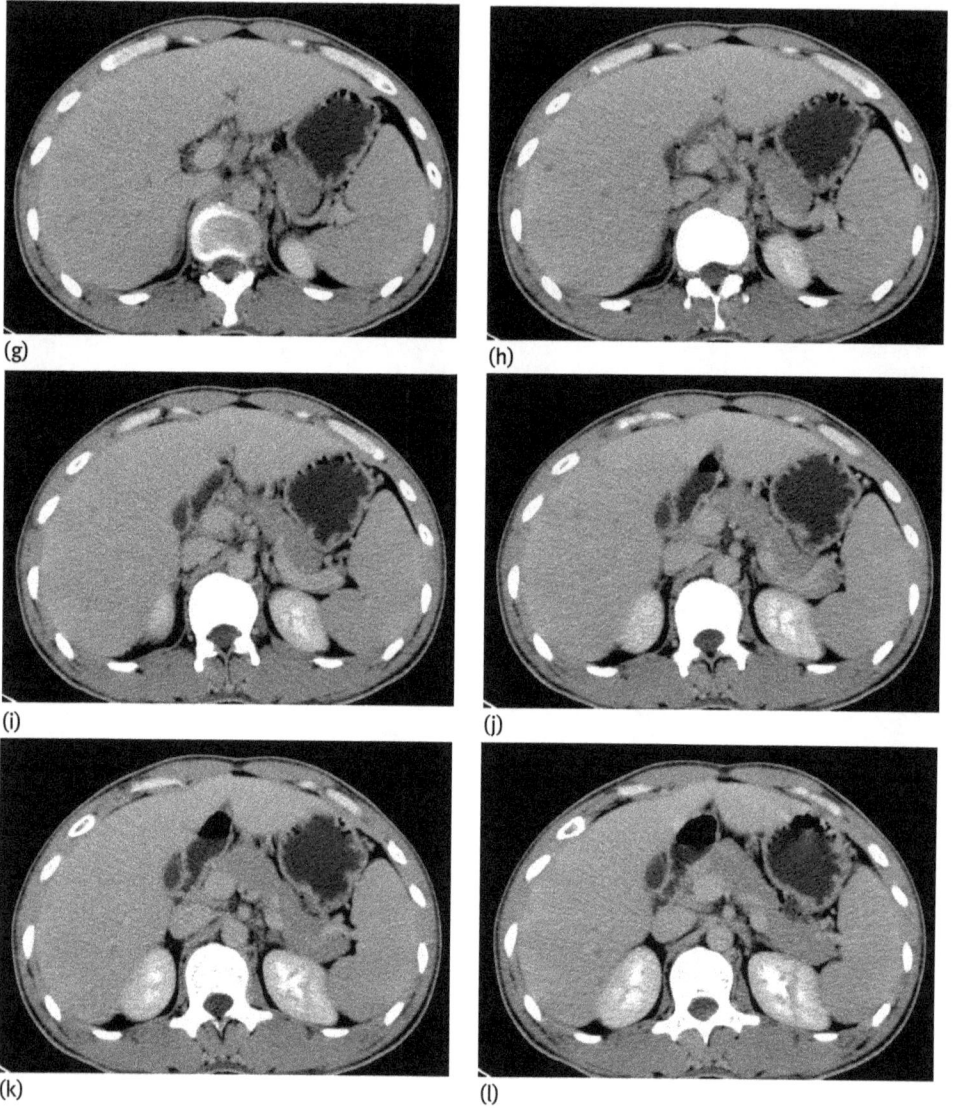

Fig. 14.5: (continuing)

The upper abdominal enhanced CT scans show multiple low-density miliary nodules in the liver parenchyma in portal venous phase (a–d), enlarged mesenteric and para-aorta lymph nodes as well as enlarged lymph nodes in the hepatic hilar region (d–f), and hepatosplenomegaly (g). The thin-layer chromatographic scanning shows clear lesions (g–l).

Case 14.6 (Fig. 14.6 a–l)

A 40-year-old male patient had a history of going for whores. He was confirmed HIV positive for 8 months and complained about dysphagia, asthenia, nausea and occasional coughs with white mucal sputum, for 20 days ago. The gastroscopy suggested mycotic esophagitis. CD4+ cell counting was 9/μl, with CD4+/CD8+: 0.07 Blood and bone marrow cultures were PM positive. The patient was diagnosed with AIDS (C3) together with disseminated PSM.

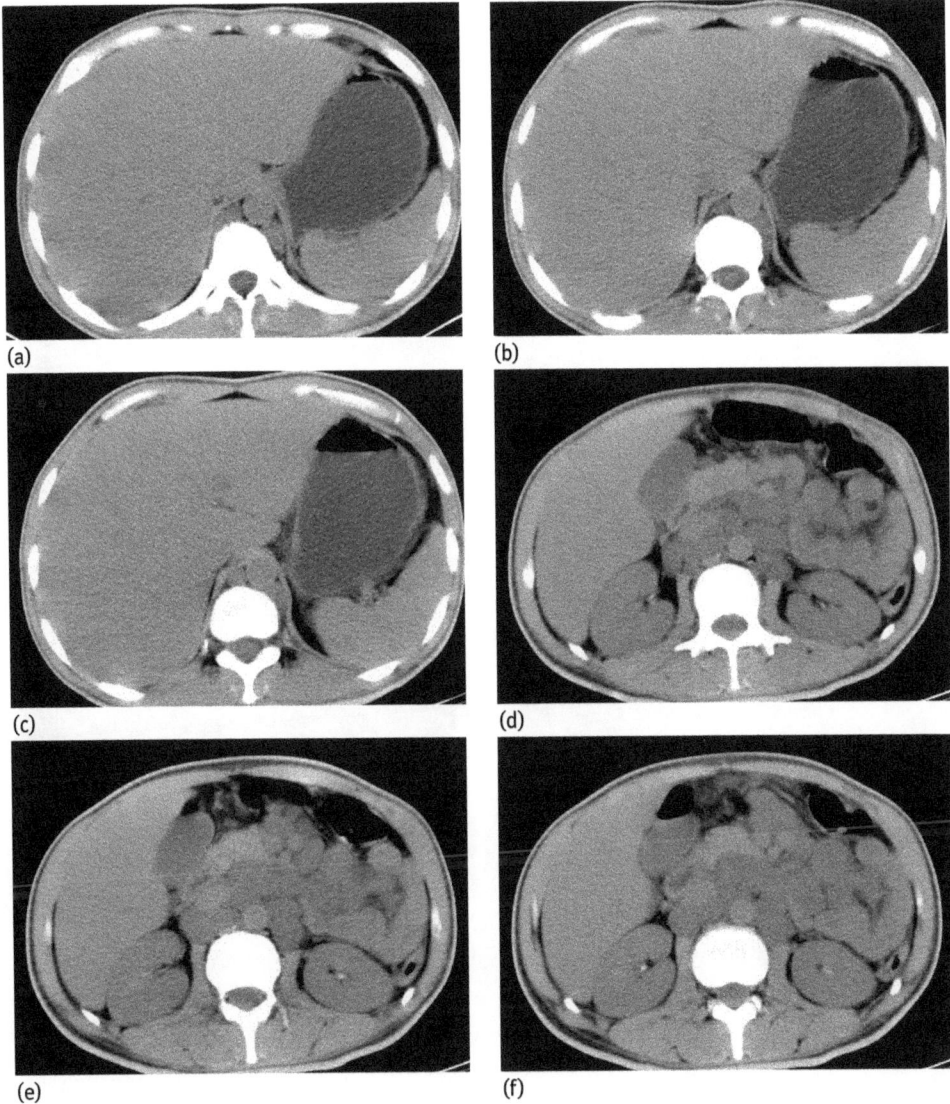

(a) (b) (c) (d) (e) (f)

Fig. 14.6 a–l: Disseminated PSM.

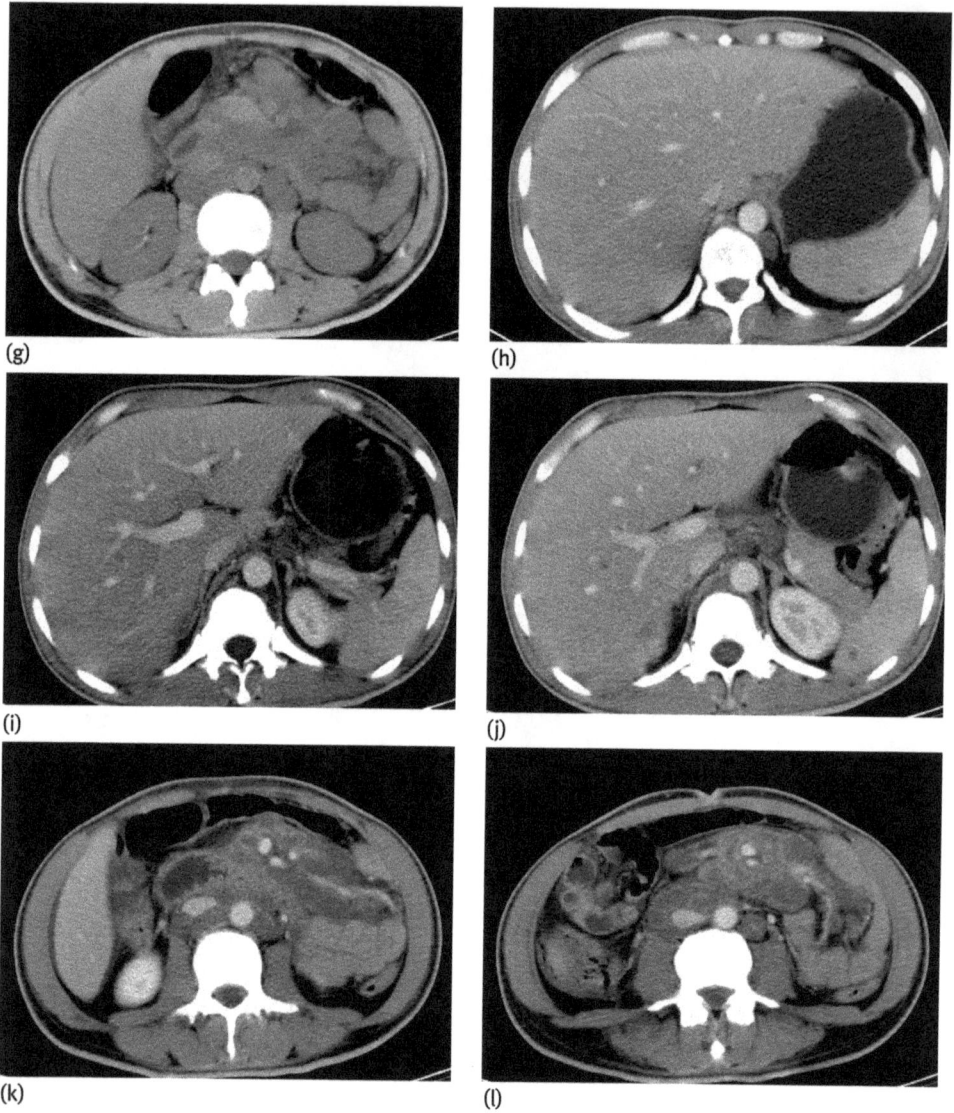

(g)

(h)

(i)

(j)

(k)

(l)

Fig. 14.6: (continuing)

The upper abdominal plain CT scans show hepatomegaly and the liver and spleen with decreased density (a–c), multiple low-density lesions in them in the portal venous phase (h–j) and enlarged mesenteric and retroperotoneal lymph nodes as well as enlarged lymph nodes in the hepatic hilar region but mainly located in the mesentery, indicating a sandwich sign and presenting a rim enhancement (d–g, j–l).

Case 14.7 (Figure 14.7 a–l)

A 38-year-old male, presenting with recurrent hypogastralgia for half a year which was aggravated with fever for 1 week. CD4+ cell count was 17/μl, CD4+/CD8+: 0.03. Blood and bone marrow cultures were PM positive. The patient was diagnosed with AIDS (C3) together with disseminated PSM.

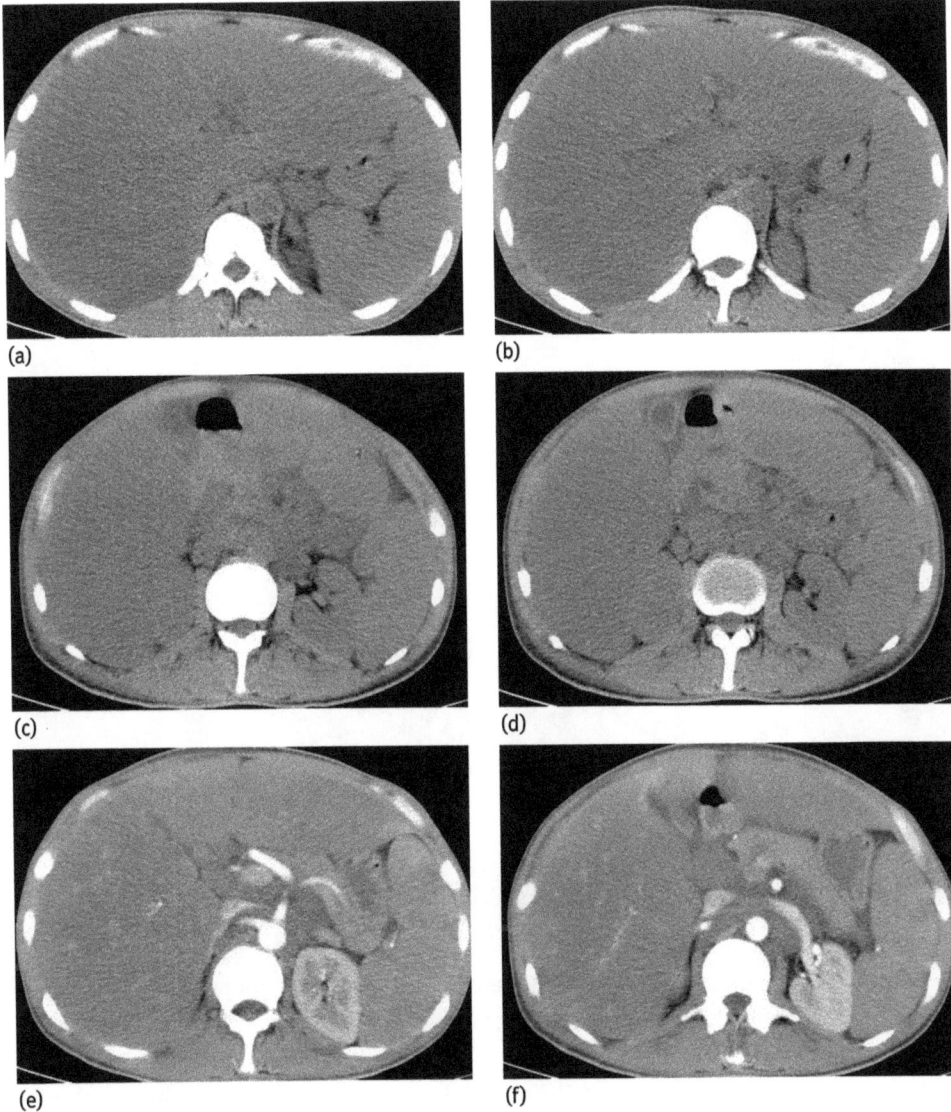

Fig. 14.7 a–l: Disseminated PSM.

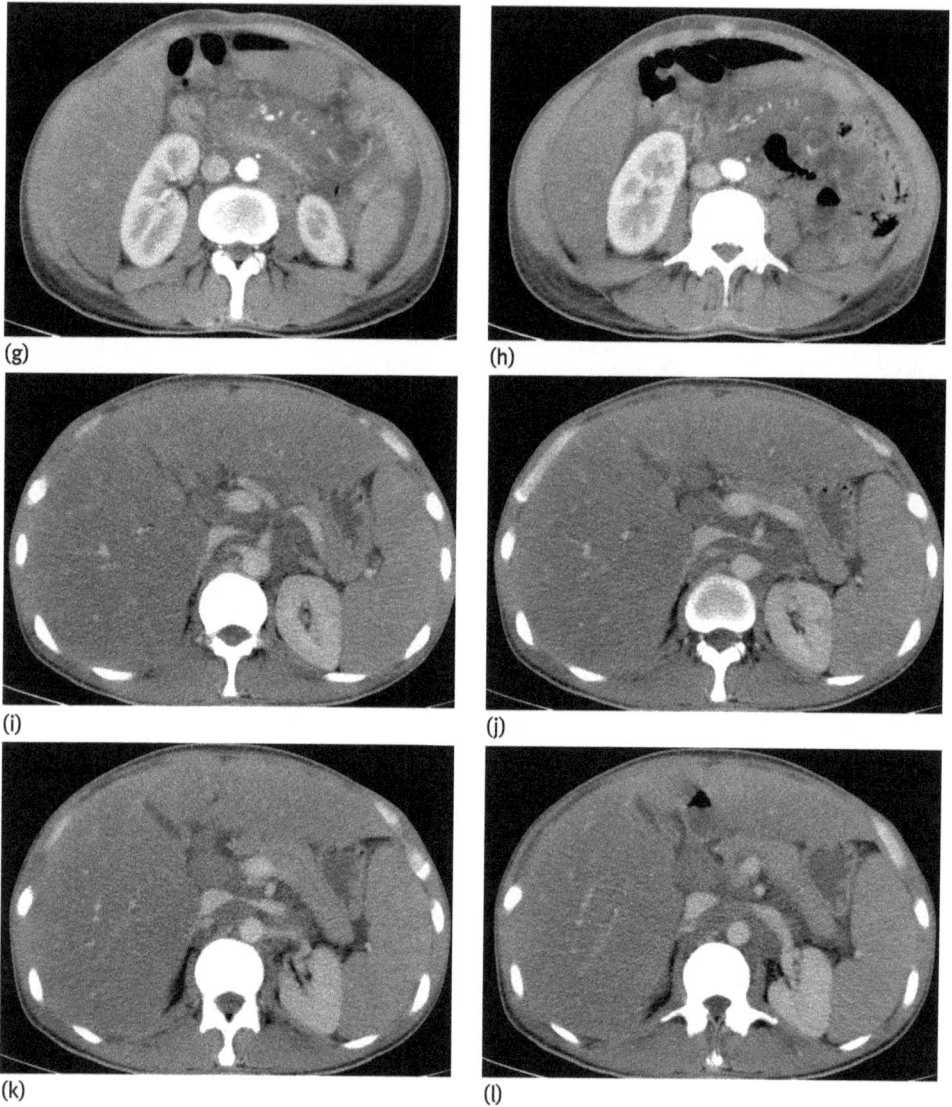

(g)

(h)

(i)

(j)

(k)

(l)

Fig. 14.7: (continuing)

The plain CT scans show hepatosplenomegaly, the liver and spleen with decreased density (a–d), extensively enlarged mesenteric and retroperotoneal lymph nodes as well as enlarged lymph nodes in the hepatic hilar region with partial fusion of the nodes, and the lesion-surrounded Celiac trunk, mesentery vessels, main portal vein and renal veins (e–l).

Case 14.8 (Fig. 14.8 a–l)

A 35-year-old male patient, presenting with fever for 2 months and epigastric pain for 1 month. CD4+ cell count was 27/μl, CD4+/CD8+: 0.08. Blood and ascites cultures were PM positive. The patient was diagnosed with AIDS (C3) together with disseminated PSM. Sadly the patient died for multiple organ failure (MOF). The biopsy of liver indicated: liver steatosis, slight increase of portal area, less lymphocyte infiltration, lytic necroses in liver parenchyma and hepatic sinusoid with spore pathogens in the lesions.

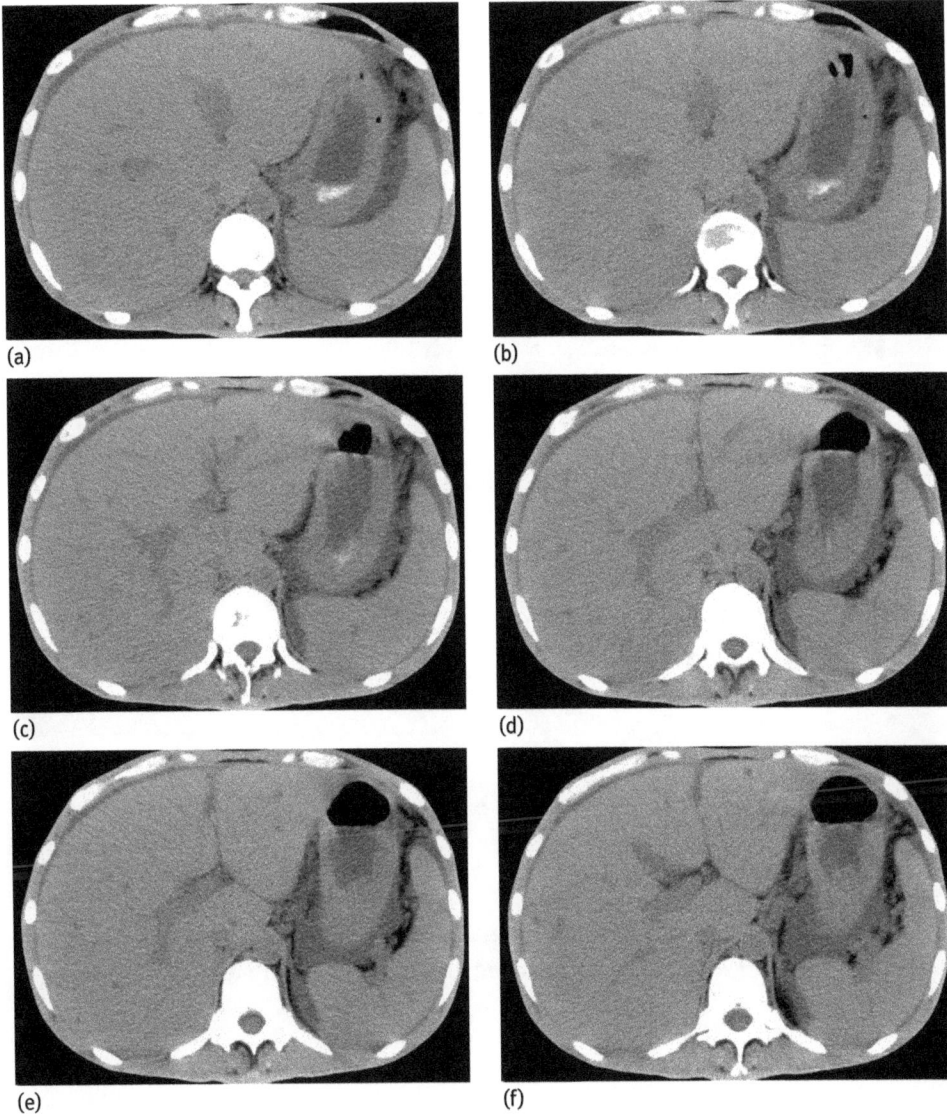

Fig. 14.8 a–l: Disseminated PSM.

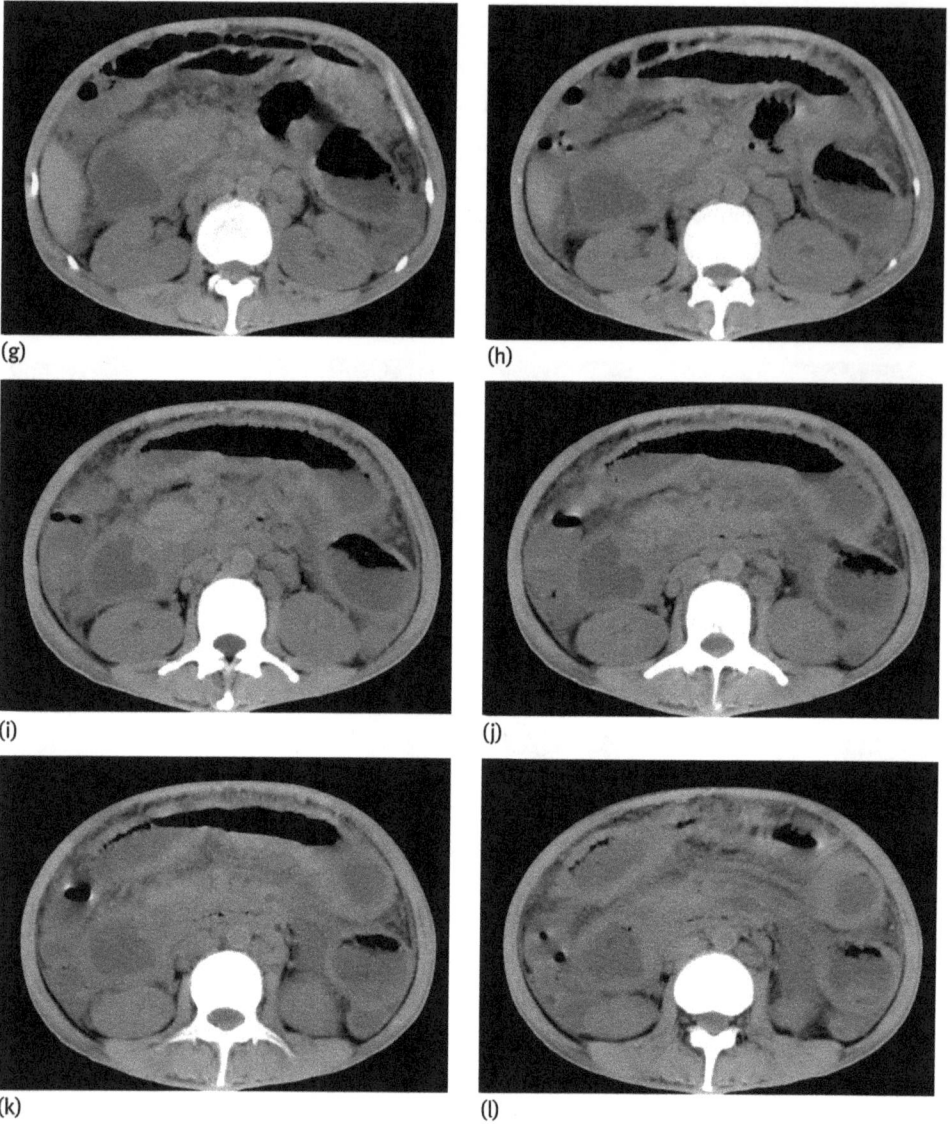

Fig. 14.8: (continuing)

The plain CT scans show hepatosplenomegaly, a small amount of free ascites in the peritoneal cavity (a–f), thickened duodenal and intestinal walls, dilated intestinal canals (g–l) and density-increased thickened great omentum with fuzzy structure (g–l).

Case 14.9 (Fig. 14.9 a–l)

A 33-year-old male patient, presented with recurrent fever for more than 3 months. 3 days after admission, he complained of abdominal pain, and was diagnosed with acute pancreatitis, which was improved after symptomatic treatment. CD4+ cell count was 32/μl, CD4+/CD8+: 0.03. Bone marrow culture was PM positive. The patient was diagnosed with AIDS (C3) with disseminated PSM.

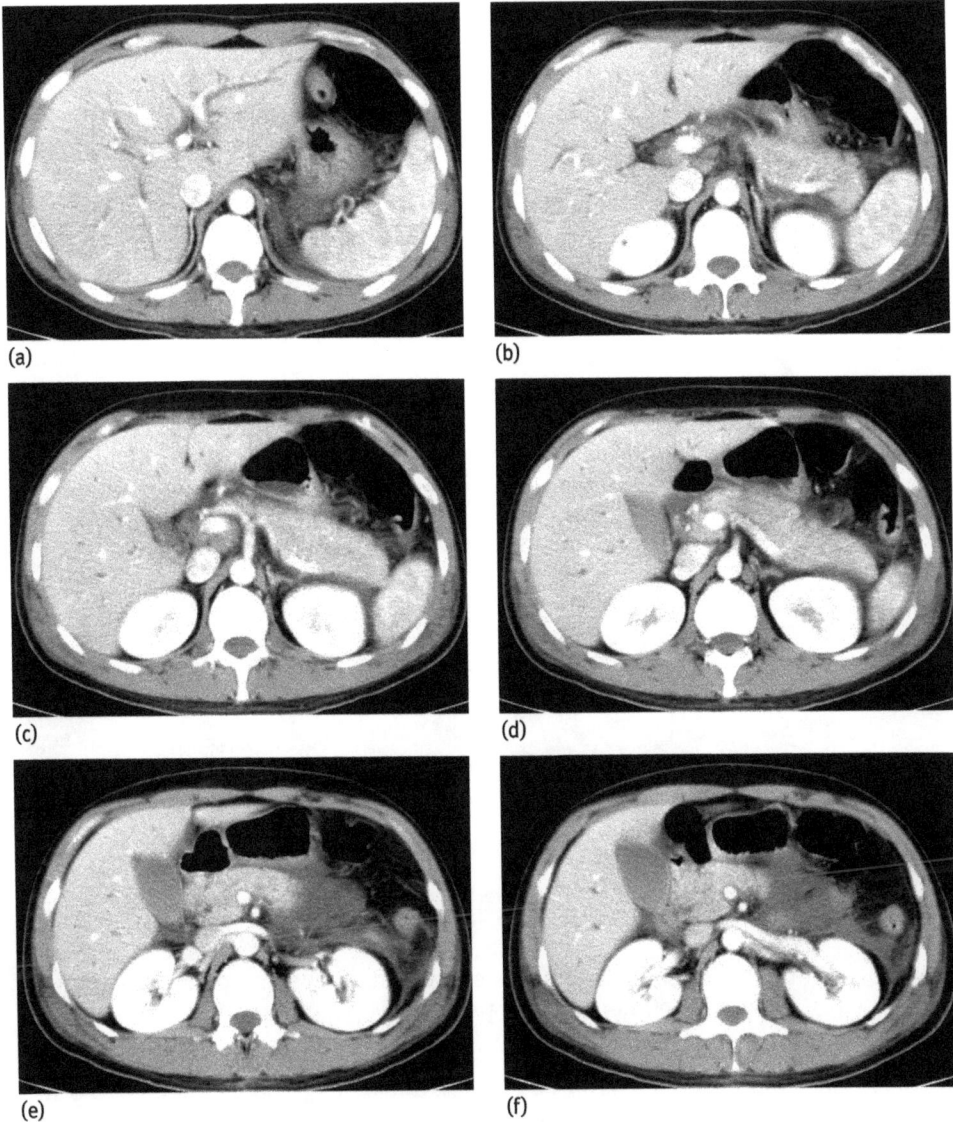

(a)

(b)

(c)

(d)

(e)

(f)

Fig. 14.9 a–l: Disseminated PSM combined with acute pancreatitis.

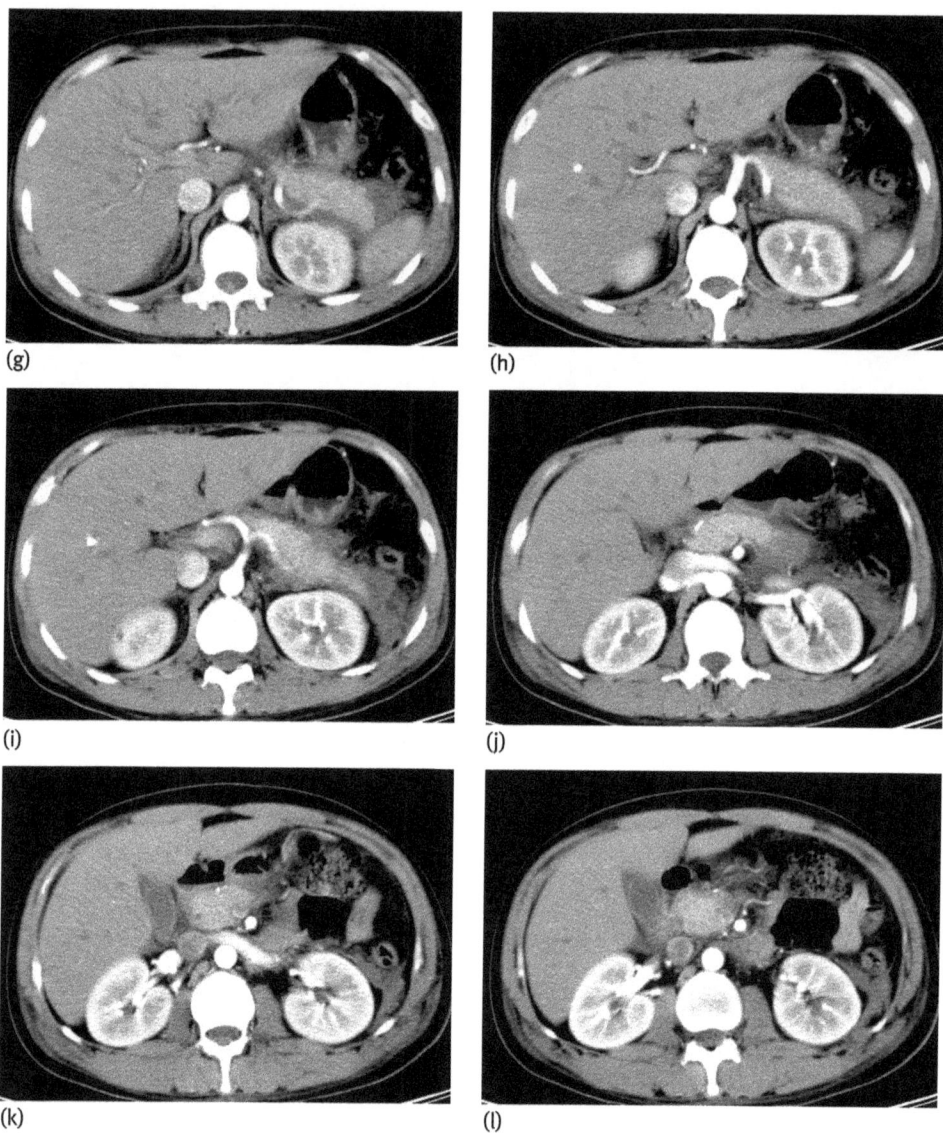

(g)

(h)

(i)

(j)

(k)

(l)

Fig. 14.9: (continuing)

The upper abdominal enhanced CT scans show diffuse swelling pancreas, peripancreatic edema and hydrops, obviously thickened fascia in the left anterior kidney and mildly dilated intrahepatic bile ducts in the later arterial phase (a–f). After 3 weeks treatment, the swelling pancreas shrank in size, alleviated peripancreatic edema and previously-thickened fascia in the left anterior kidney, and evidently improved dilation of intrahepatic bile ducts in the later arterial phase (g–l).

Case 14.10 (Fig. 14.10 a–f)

A 30-year-old male presented with fever with chill but no algor for indefinite reasons 1 month ago. The temperature once went up to 38.9 °C. He began to get abdominal distension, abdominal pain. CT scan showed abdominal mass, multiple lymphadenectasis and loss weight more than 5 kg. CD4+ cell count was 12/μl, CD4+/CD8+: 0.12. Blood and bone marrow cultures were PM positive. The patient was diagnosed with AIDS (C3) and disseminated PSM.

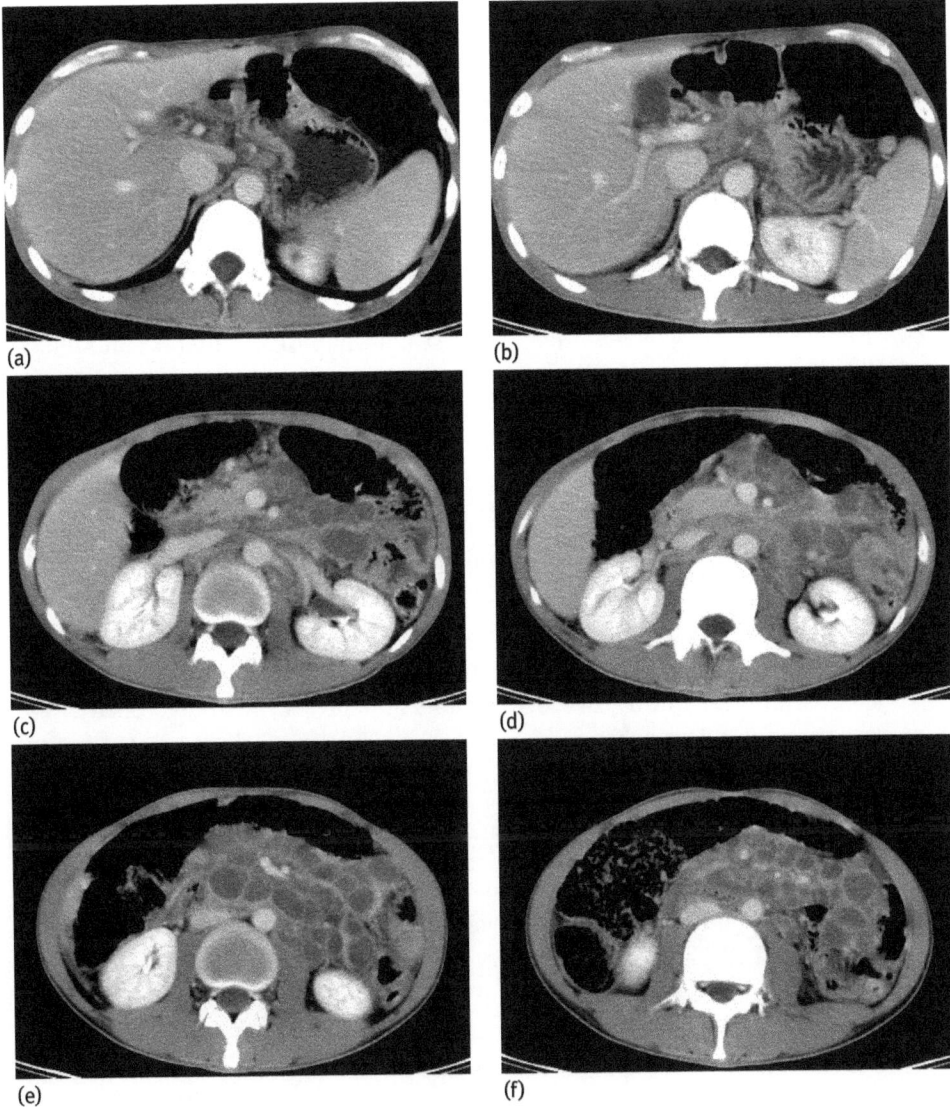

Fig. 14.10 a–f: Disseminated PSM.

The enhanced abdominal CT scans show evident extensive enlargement of mesenteric and retroperitoneal lymph nodes and in the hepatic hilar region in the portal venous phase (a–f), with rim-enhancements of different sizes which are more evident in the mesentery and present a sandwich sign (e, f).

14.2.3 Imaging features

1. The abdominal CT findings of disseminated PM infection in AIDS patients (C3)
   a) For retroperitoneal and mesentery lymphadenectases induced by PM, the CT scans may show multiple soft tissue density nodules in mesentery, hepatic hilar region, hepatoduodenal ligament region and abdominal para-aorta, with a sign of sandwich because of lymphadenectases of the anterior and posterior part of mesenterium clamping the central blood vessels. The enhanced CT scanning confirms the sign by showing an enhanced ring. After effective antifungal treatment, the retroperitoneal and mesentery lyphadenectases shrank obviously by CT examination.
   b) Hepatosplenomegaly is evident on CT scans when AIDS patients contract PM infection.
   c) The PM infection in AIDS patients may invade liver and spleen, leading to focal lesions. In this case, the imaging scans firstly may show low density nodules in the liver with low density opacities by plain scanning, and scattered or effusive nodules of different sizes less than 1.5 cm in diameter by enhancement scanning. Secondly, the scanning may show low density nodules in the spleen which are similar to those in the liver in terms of the appearance and size and they may coexist with lesions in the liver. Some lesions are showed to be ill-edged miliary nodules by plain scanning and to be hollow by enhancement scanning. Thirdly, the focal lesions may present with decreased effuse density of the liver and unevenly-enhanced liver parenchyma. Some lesions are hollow, which is much evident by enhancement scanning, especially in portal venous phase. For other cases, the plain scanning may display the low density lesions around portal vein and portal area and the enhancement scanning still present low density lesions and the portal veins in the center.
   d) When gastrointestinal tract is involved, the imaging may show thickened intestinal walls, especially thickened duodenum and jejunum, combined with digestive tract obstruction.
   e) Besides, few cases may affect acute pancreatitis, peritonitis, and ascites.
2. The abdominal imaging manifestations and pathological diagnoses of disseminated PM infection in AIDS (C3) patients
   a) Retroperitoneal and mesentery lymphadenectases: When AIDS patients are affected by PM, the imaging scans show retroperitoneal and mesentery lymphadenectases with a rim enhancement on the image. The CT images of more

than half of the cases present hilar and mediastinal lymphadenectases, which are part of systemic lymphadenectases with an incidence up to 77 %. Pathologically, blood and spiral marrow cultures indicate the invasion of PM in systemic mononuclear phagocyte system.

b) Hepatosplenomegaly and focal or diffuse lesions in liver and spleen: The CT scans for the AIDS patients with PM infection may identify hepatolienal nodular lesions with effuse abnormal density and abnormal enhancement. In contrast, the biopsies of cadaveric liver tissues suggest hepatic steatosis, multiple lytic necroses with allantospore (PM) in them, and enlarged portal area with allantospores in it as well. The necroses by pathological detection are in accordance with nodular lesions by imaging, while the steatoses and necroses match the images of density-decreased lesions.

c) The hollow lesions in liver and spleen: The 'hollow' sign is more evident when CT scanning is done in portal venous phase, the imaging features including extensive low density lesions, blurry edges and non-eminence of liver and spleen in appearance. The hollow lesions are related with effuse lytic necroses of liver and spleen parenchyma and the areas with normal density and enhancement are the remaining liver and spleen.

d) Diffuse low-density lesions around portal vein: It is believed in our minds to have relations with a predilection of PM to blood vessels. In the study by Peiqing Ma etc. (2006), moruloid, rhagoid mycelium and spores were identified around vessel wall in liver of AIDS patients with PM infection. Interestingly, Guangzhou No. 8 People's Hospital also identified a large number of allantospores in portal area using needle biopsy of liver.

e) Other involved organs: One example is thickened intestinal wall. Peiqing Ma et al. (2006) reported one biopsy of duodenal mucosa, finding PM spores in inflammatory mucosa and between glands. Peritonitis and ascites were seen in some cases and cultivation of ascites also pointed to PM, indicating the possible relations with PM or with hypoproteinemia. A few cases manifest as possibly non-specific acute pancreatitis, and the heteropathy is effective.

14.3 Abdominal CT findings of abdominal tuberculosis in AIDS

14.3.1 Introduction

Pyrenomycetes usually leads to pulmonary tuberculosis when it invades population with normal immunity, but seldom to extra-pulmonary tuberculosis. For AIDS patients, however, the opportunistic extra-pulmonary infections by Pyrenomycetes are of high possibility due to immunocompromise, and involve abdomen narrowly less frequently than lung. In the advanced stage of HIV infection, the immunologic function is seriously impaired, giving rise to the higher TB incidence of tuberculosis, so that the abdominal organs, intestinal tract, lymph node and peritoneum are easy to be involved. Succeeding

Pathologically, the immune response of HIV patients at early stage or TB patients with following HIV infection is pale. Therefore, TB develops into tuberculous granuloma which is typically evident by microscopy. As showed in Color figure 14-I a), the cheesy necroses are smaller, MTB is fewer in number and many CD4 lymphocytes, epithelioid cell, Langerhans cells are around the lesions, helping them localized and repaired. In the medium-term of HIV infection when the immune suppression is weaken, the cheesy necroses expand in size, CD4 lymphocytes, epithelioid cells and Langerhans cells decreases in number and MTB increases in number. In case of TB in advanced stage of HIV, the severely-impaired cellular immunity produces no immune response to MTB. As a result, the lesions are deprived mostly of epithelioid cells and Langerhans cells, nearly giant cells and lymphocytes so that uppurative and coagulative necrosis takes the place of granuloma formation and MTB bloom (Color figure 14-I a and b), as identified by biopsy and autopsy indicative of disseminated miliary TB and unresponsive TB.

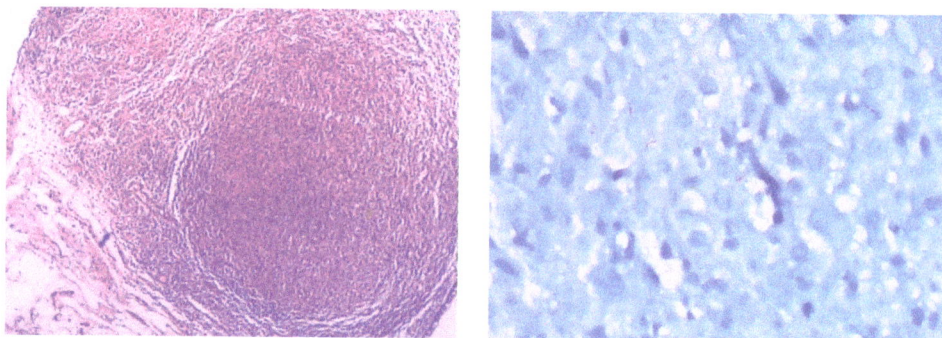

Color Fig.14-I a–b: Intestinal tuberculosis granuloma, HE stain, ×100 (A) Intestinal acid-fast bacilli, acid-fast staining, ×400 (B).

14.3.2 Radiologic findings

Case 14.11 (Fig. 14.11 A–f)

A 34-year-old male, presenting with cervical mass for 1 month. He had a history of intravenous drug addiction. At visit, multiple masses were palpable in bilateral neck, right axillary and left inguen, the largest sized about 6 cm × 7 cm, most fused, poor in activity, sharp in edge, tender, fluctuating, high in skin temperature and some red. CD4+ cell count was 9/μl, with CD4+/CD8+: 0.04. The smear and cultures of sputamentum and abscess of neck were MTB positive and the fungal smear was MTB negative. Tuberculosis antibody was TB-IgM negative and TB-IgG positive. The patient was diagnosed with AIDS (C3) and disseminated tuberculosis.

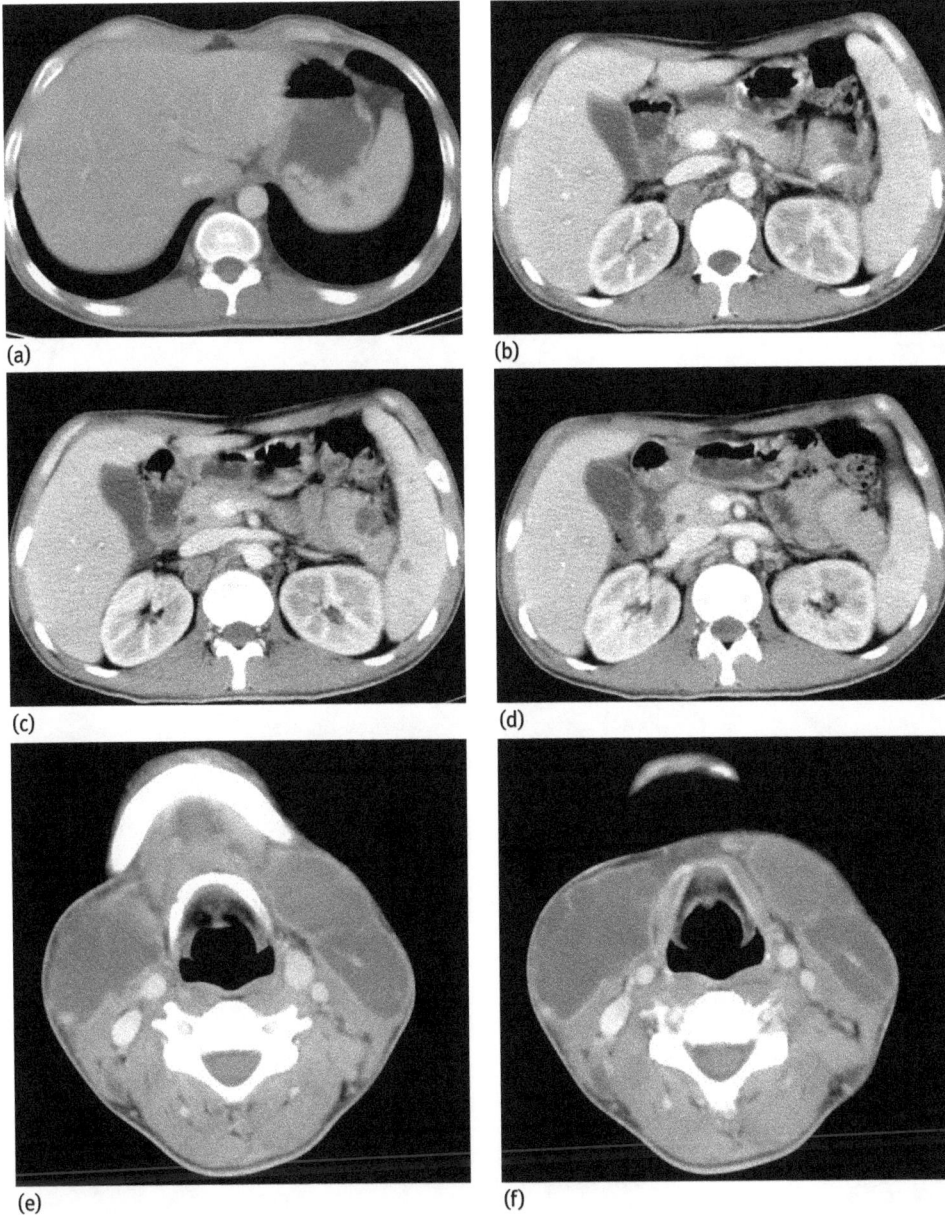

Fig. 14.11 a–f: Disseminated tuberculosis in abdominal tract and neck.

The plain CT scans show multiple low-density nodules in the spleen (a–d), enlarged lymph nodes in the splenic hilum and retroperitoneum with rim enhancement by enhanced scanning (b, c), and obviously enlarged even-density lymph nodes in the bilateral necks, with complete liquidation in the interior nodes and rim enhancements of the thin wall (e, f).

Case 14.12 (Fig. 14.12 a–l)

A 39-year-old female presented dyspnea, recurrent fever and cough for half a year. CD4+ cell count was 7/μl, CD4+/CD8+: 0.02. The bronchoalveolar lavage fluid smear and culture identified MTP positive. The patient was diagnosed with AIDS (C3) and disseminated tuberculosis (in lung, pericardium, liver and abdominal cavity).

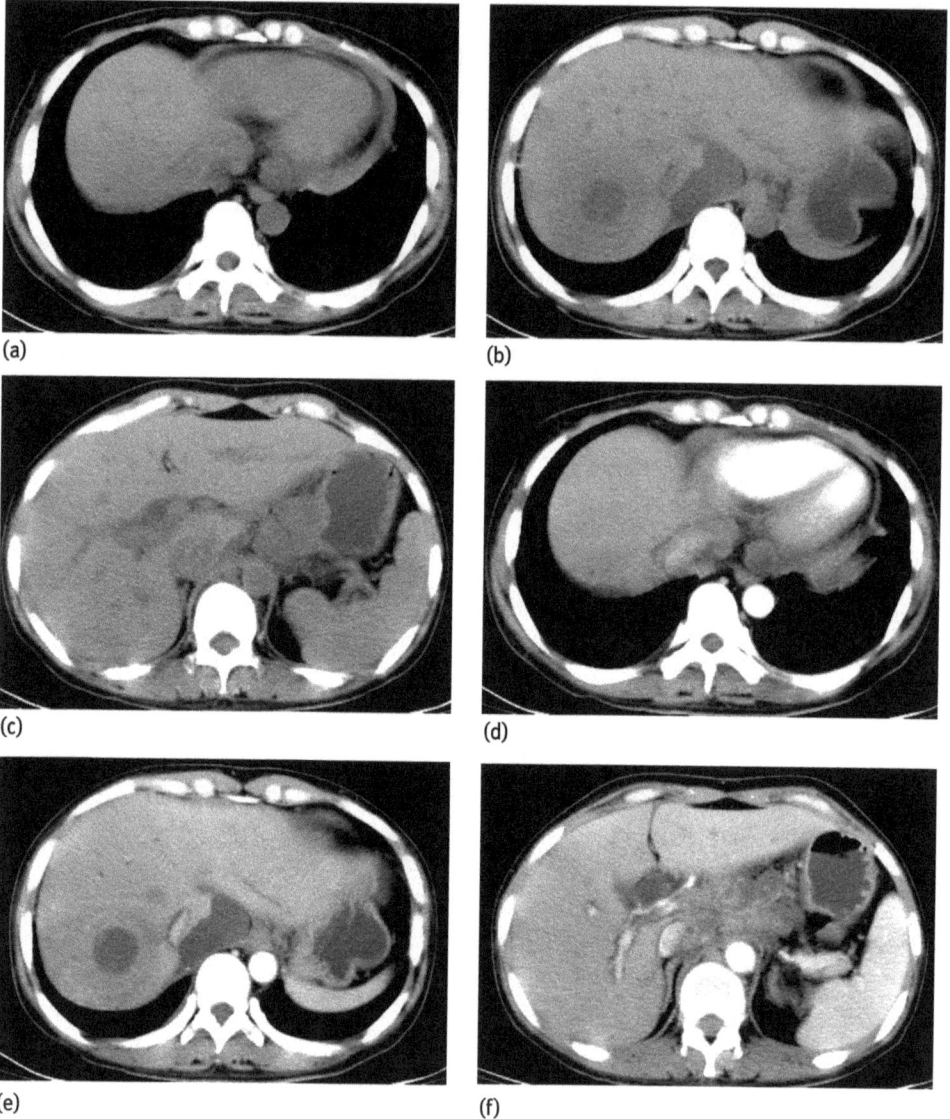

Fig. 14.12 a–l: Abdominal tuberculosis.

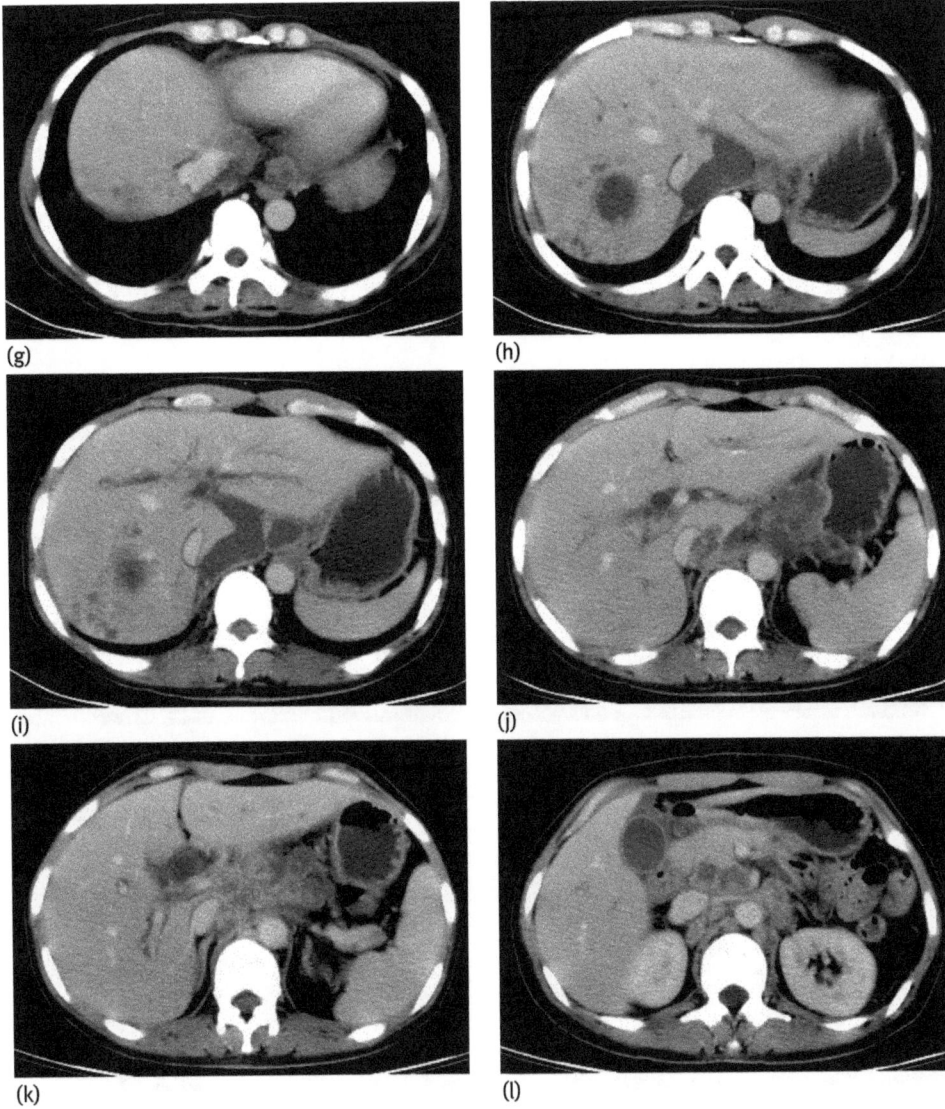

Fig. 14.12: (continuing)

The plain CT scans show a low-density round lesion (tuberculous abscess) in the right lobe of the liver, with a mildly high-density ring-like opacity around it and peripheral patchy liver parenchyma with unevenly decreased density. The enhanced scans show mild rim-enhancement of the low density lesion, and unevenly-enhanced liver parenchyma around it and multiple low-density lesions in it (b, e, h, i). The CT scans show multiple enlarged lymph nodes with rim enhancement in the hepatogastric ligament region, hepatic hilar region retroperitoneum and around the esophageal hiatus (a, c, d, f, g, j–l), dropsy in the superior omental recess of fissure in ligamentum venosum (b, h, i) and pericardial effusion (a).

Case 14.13 (Fig. 14.13 a–l)

A 30-year-old male patient presented with recurrent fever for more than 2 months. At physical examination, a lymph node about 1cm in diameter in the left supraclavieular and bilateral axillary was palpable. The right lymph node grew larger in size and liquefied gradually one month after admission. The body temperature was high at night, up to 39.5 °C. CD4+ cell counting was 185/μl, CD4+/CD8+: 0.35. The smear and culture of right neck abscess were MTB positive. The tests with tuberculosis antibody showed TB-IgM negative and TB-IgG positive. The patient was diagnosed with of AIDS (C3) and tuberculous lymphadenitis.

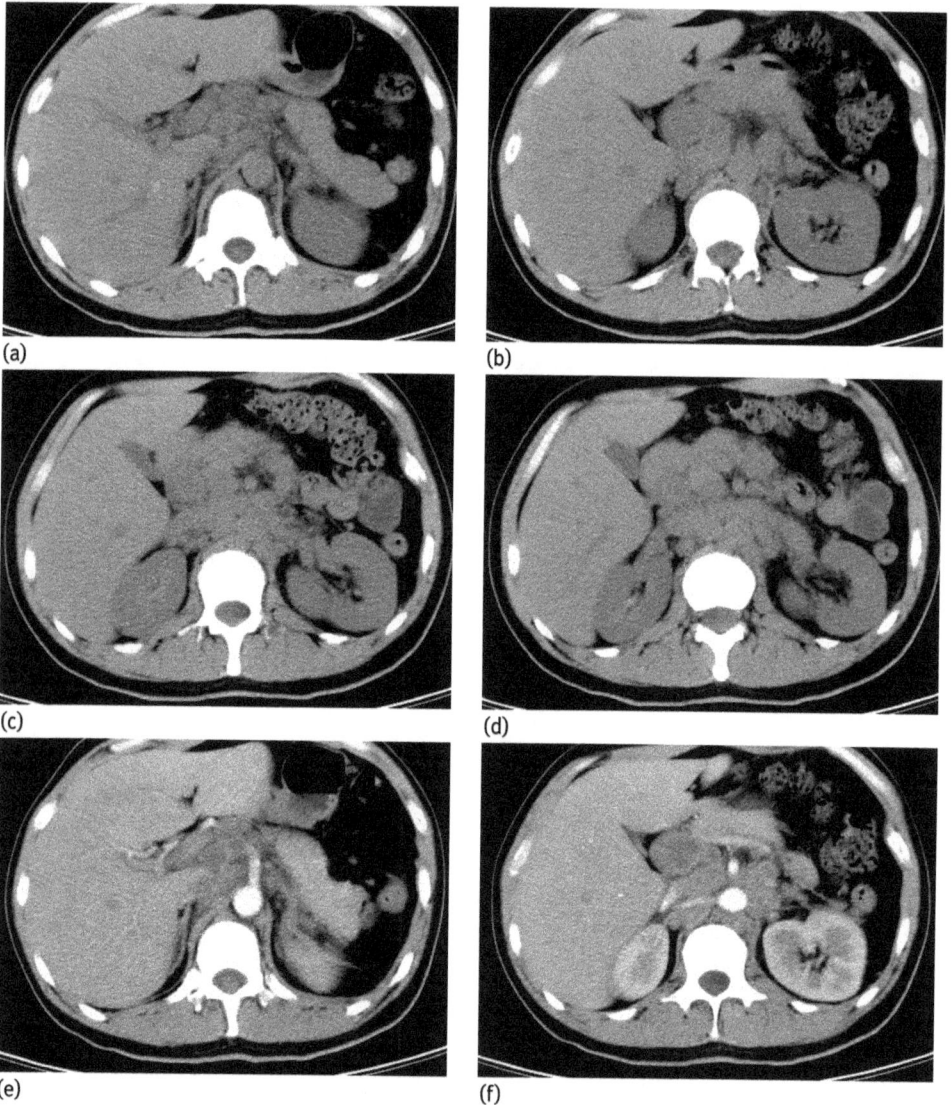

Fig. 14.13 a–l: Tuberculous lymphadenitis.

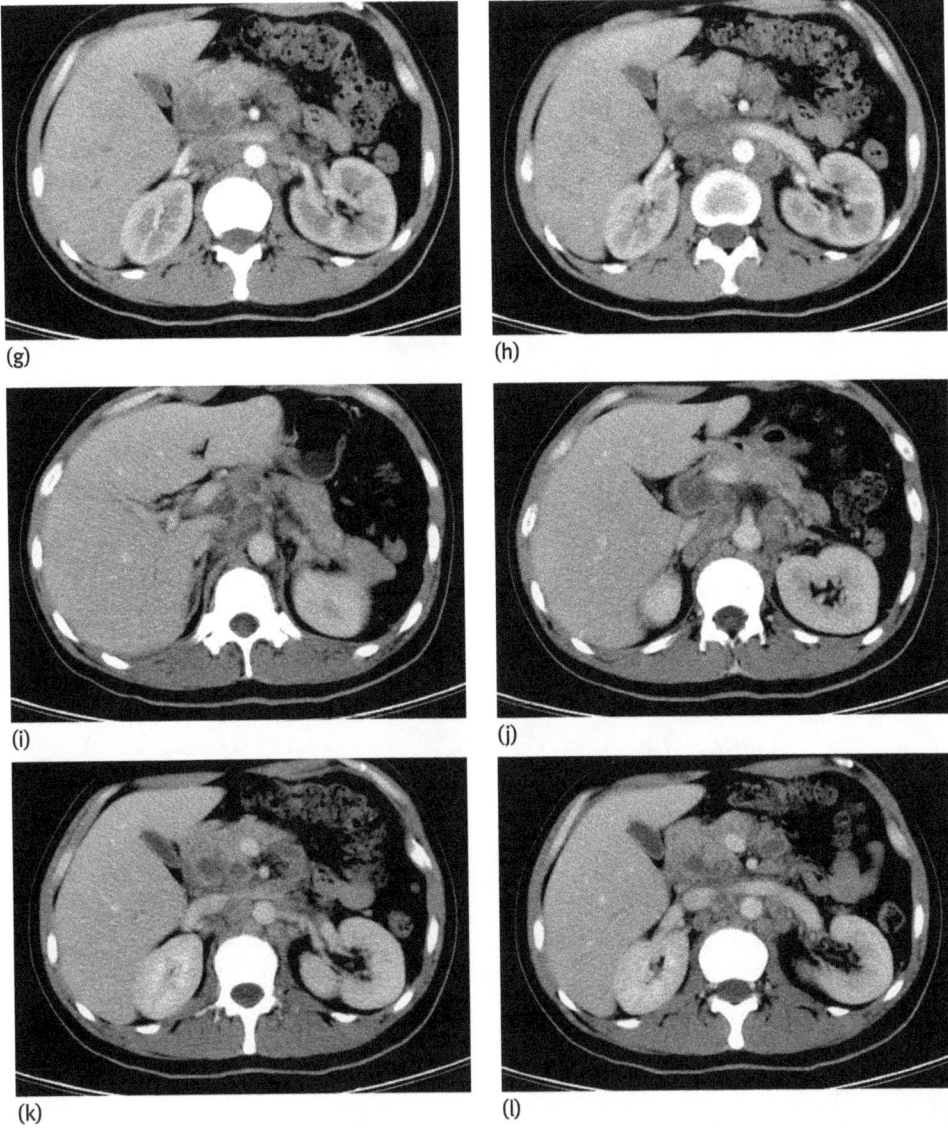

Fig. 14.13: (continuing)

The CT scans show lymph nodular enlargements of different sizes in the mesentery, retroperitoneum, hepatic hilar region, most evident in the retroperitoneum and the hepatic hilar region, together with rim enhancement (a–d: on plain scans; e, f: at arterial phase; g–l: at portal vein phase).

Case 14.14 (Fig. 14.14 a–l)

A 43-year-old male patient presented with recurrent lower abdomen pain for 1 month and a fever for a week. He had a history of drug addiction. CD4+ cell count was 30/μl, CD4+/CD8+: 0.12. Then the enteroscopic biopsy identified (terminal ileum, cecum) caseous tubercle. The patient was diagnosed with AIDS (C3) together with intestinal tuberculosis and peritoneal tuberculosis.

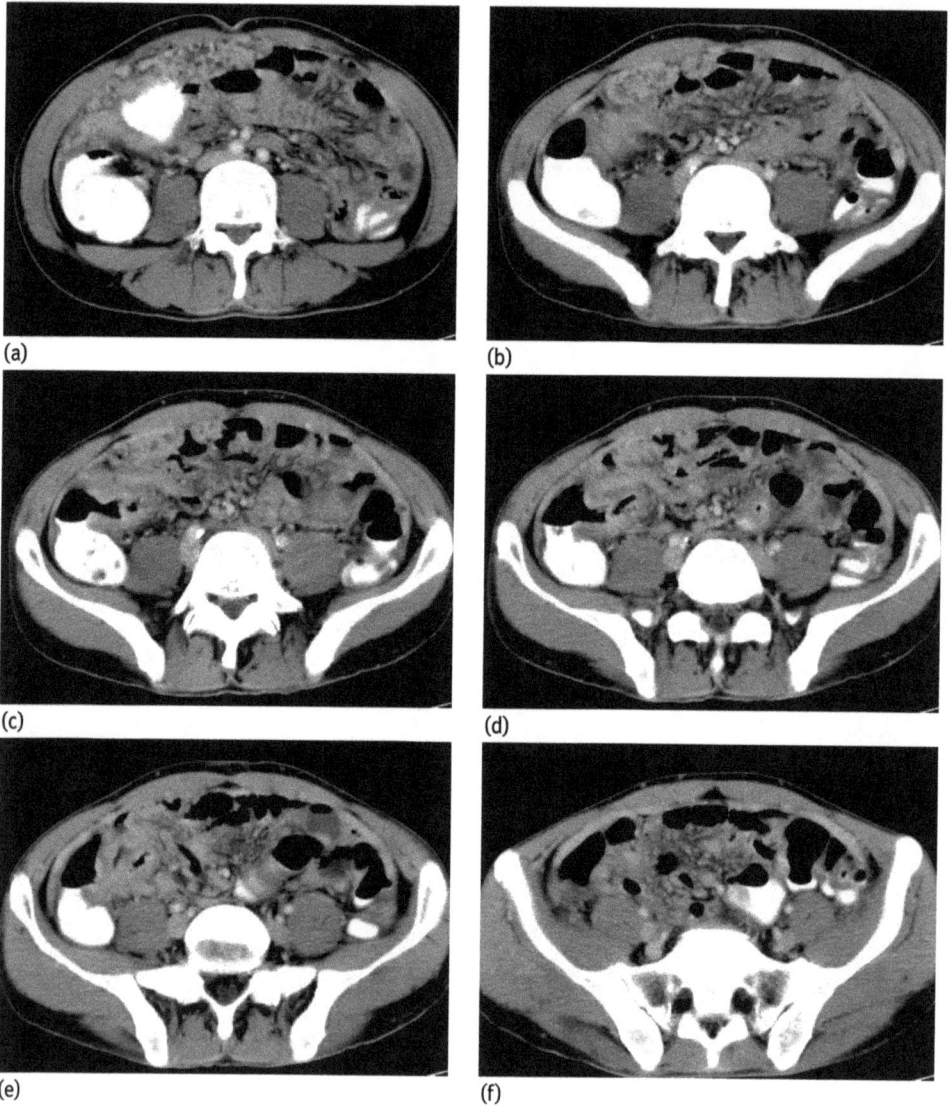

(a) (b)

(c) (d)

(e) (f)

Fig. 14.14 a–l: Intestinal tuberculosis and peritoneal tuberculosis.

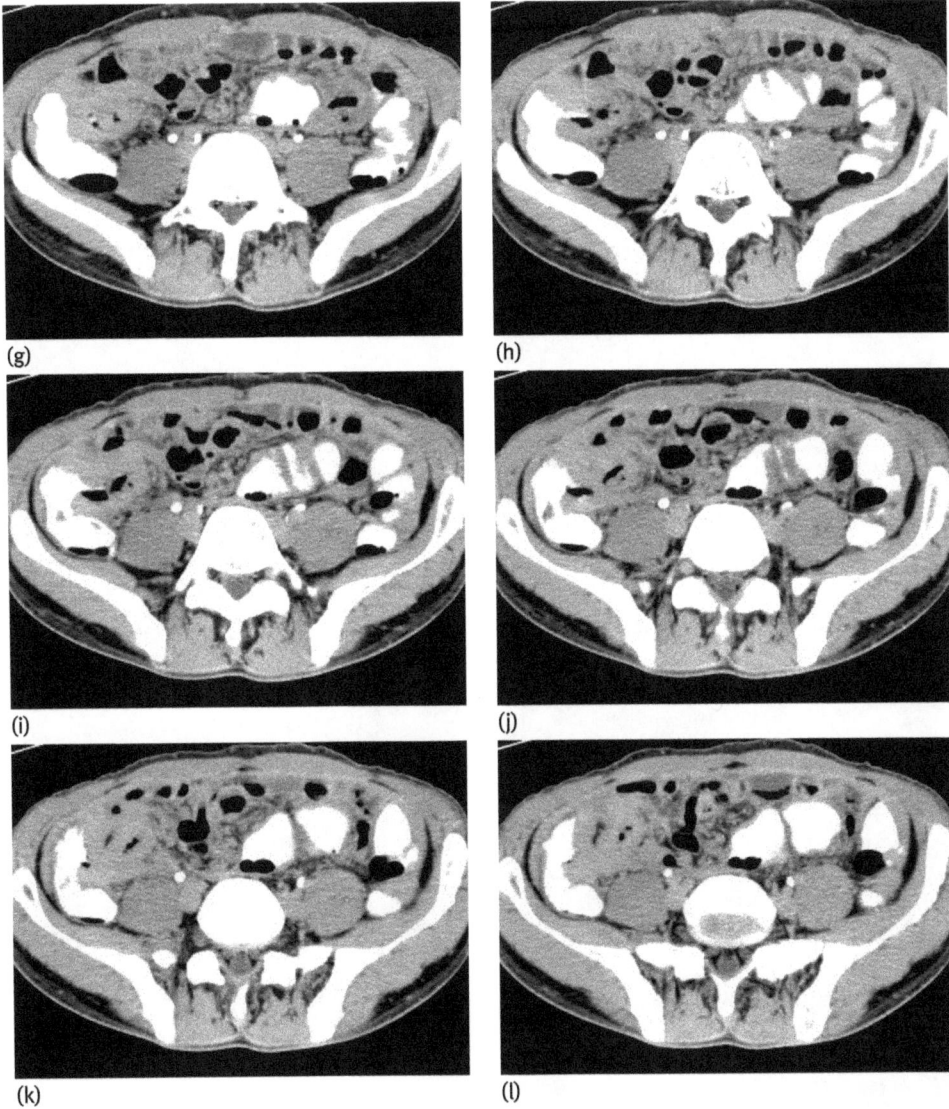

Fig. 14.14: (continuing)

The plain CT scans show thickened pie-like greater omentum with increased density, thickened peritoneum which is unevenly enhanced by the enhanced scanning, evidently irregularly thickened walls of the terminal ileum, cecum and adjacent ascending colon, density-increased mesentery with increased dense small lymph nodes (a–l) (a–f: enhanced scans in venous phase at a slice thickness of 6.5 mm on supine position; g–l: enhanced scans in delayed phase at a slice thickness of 3.2 mm on prone position)

Case 14.15 (Fig. 14.15 a–l)

A 37 year-old female patient presented recurrent fever, cough for 6 months, lack of appetite for 4 months and mental problems for a week. CD4+ cell count was 9/μl, CD4+/CD8+: 0.06. After anti-tuberculosis treatment, her general symptoms were greatly improved. She was diagnosed with AIDS (C3) and disseminated phthisis.

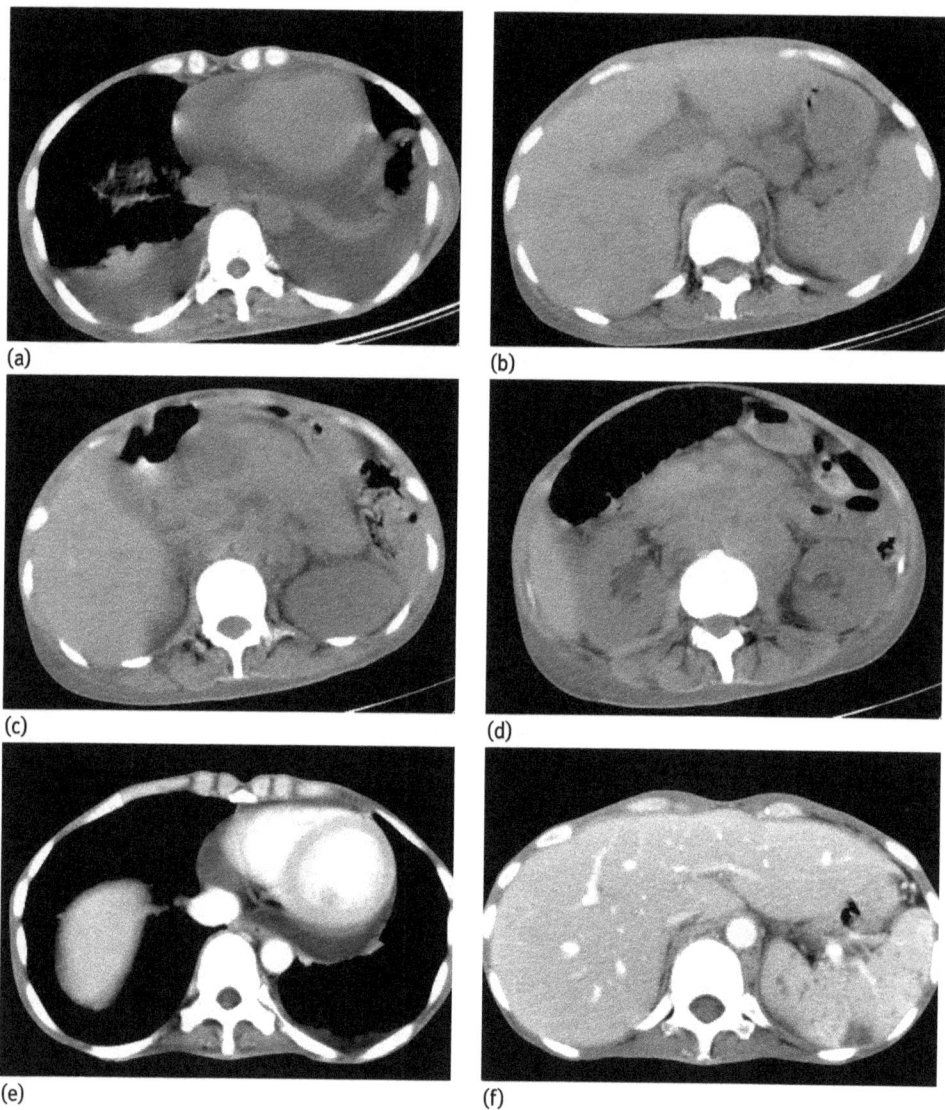

(a)

(b)

(c)

(d)

(e)

(f)

Fig. 14.15 a–l: Abdominal tuberculosis.

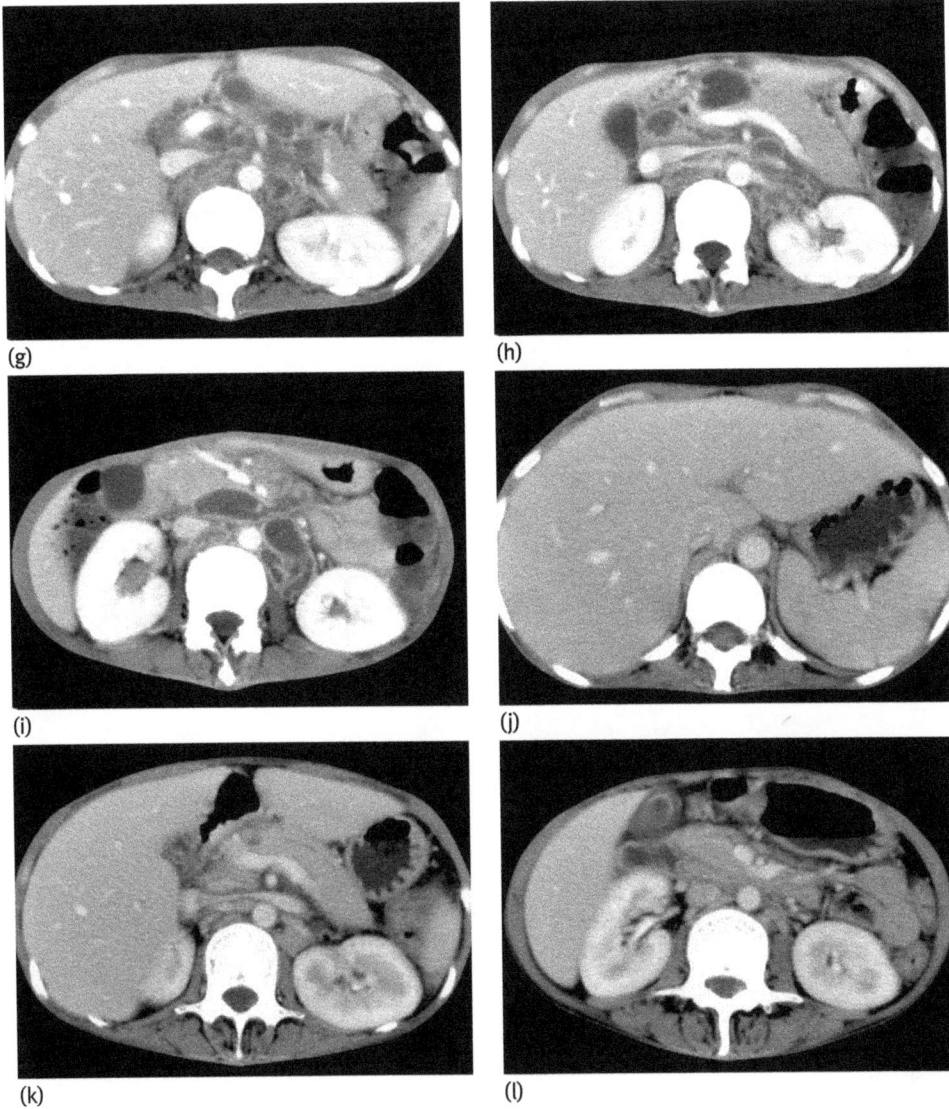

Fig. 14.15: (continuing)

Before treatment: The plain CT scans show pericardial effusions and bilateral pleural effusions (a), enlarged lymph nodes with decreased central density in the hepatic hilar region and retroperitoneum which are most evident at superior head of pancreas with aquatic density inside them, relatively mildly enlarged mesenteric lymph nodes (b–d), and the spleen with uneven density (b).

2 weeks after anti-tuberculosis treatment: The enhanced CT scans show evidently absorbed and decreased pericardial effusions and bilateral pleural effusions (e), the evidently reduced enlargements of lymph nodes in the hepatic hilar region and retroperitoneum and evidently decreased central density, similar to cholecystic density

inside them, the shrinking lesions at superior head of pancreas, relatively improved enlargement of mesenteric lymph nodes even with rim enhancement (g–i), the spleen with irregular density and low-density small diffuse miliary lesions in it, presenting no evident enhancement by the enhanced scanning (f).

5 months after anti-tuberculosis treatment: The contrast-enhancement CT scans show significant shrinking of the enlarged lymph nodes in the hepatic hilar region, retroperitoneum and superior pancreas, no more enlargement of mesenteric lymph nodes, significant shrinking of the swelling lymph nodes in superior pancreas, the spleen with regular density and complete absorption of the low-density military lesions (j–l).

Case 14.16 (Fig. 14.16 a–l)

A 57 year-old female patient presented fever, chill but no algor for infinite reasons for 4 month. The temperature peaked at 41 °C, accompanied with mild cough with white sputamentum but no hemoptysis. The temperature fell after treatment. The weight loss was about 15kg over the past four months. CD4+ cell count was 114/μl, CD4+/CD8+: 0.37. The bronchofiberscope biopsy identified infiltrative tuberculosis. The patient was diagnosed with AIDS (C3) and disseminated tuberculosis (lung, liver, spleen and lymph nodes).

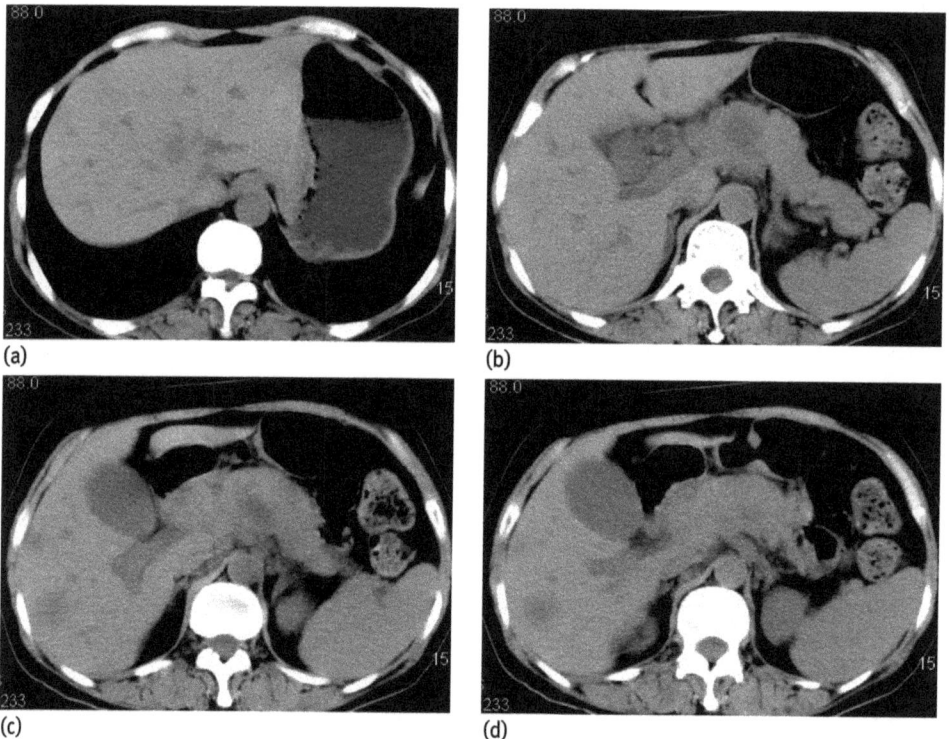

(a)

(b)

(c)

(d)

Fig. 14.16 a–l: Abdominal tuberculosis in liver, spleen and lymph nodes.

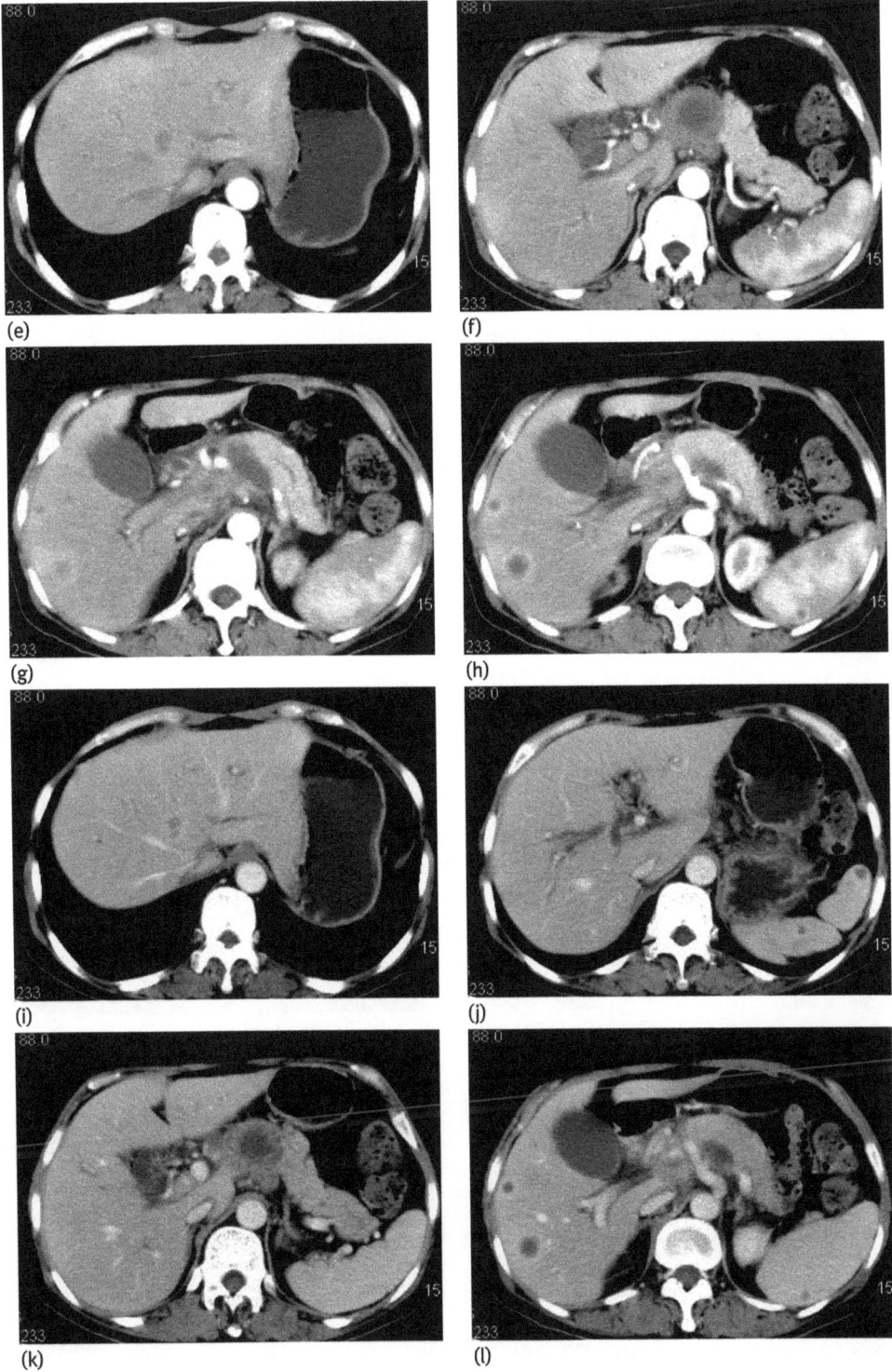

Fig. 14.16: (continuing)

The upper abdominal plain CT scans show multiple low-density round nodules of different sizes in liver parenchyma with relatively low central density and enlarged lymph nodes in the hepatic hilar region which are more evident in the superior pancreatic head with evenly-liquidized central density (a–d). The enhanced scans show low-density lesions with rim enhancement in the liver, enlarged lymph nodes with mild enhancement in the right coeliac trunk with lower density than that of pancreas, pressed common bile duct, mildly dilated intraheptic bile duct, superior spleen head with rim enhancement and internal regular liquid density and multiple small low-density nodules in the spleen with mild rim enhancement by the enhanced scanning (e–h: at arterial phase; i–l: at portal vein phase).

Case 14.17 (Fig. 14.17 a–l)

A 26-year-old male patient presented recurrent fever, temperature fluctuated at 38–39 °C, highest at night and combined with chill and mild headache, occasional cough with a little white sputamentum and spontaneous perspiration at night. CD4+ cell counting was 23/μl, CD4+/CD8+: 0.06. The radiograph showed diffuse miliary lesions, which were absorbed after 1 month's anti-tuberculosis treatment. The bronchoalveolar lavage smear and culture were MTB positive. The patient was diagnosed with AIDS (C3) and disseminated tuberculosis (lung, abdominal and lymph nodes).

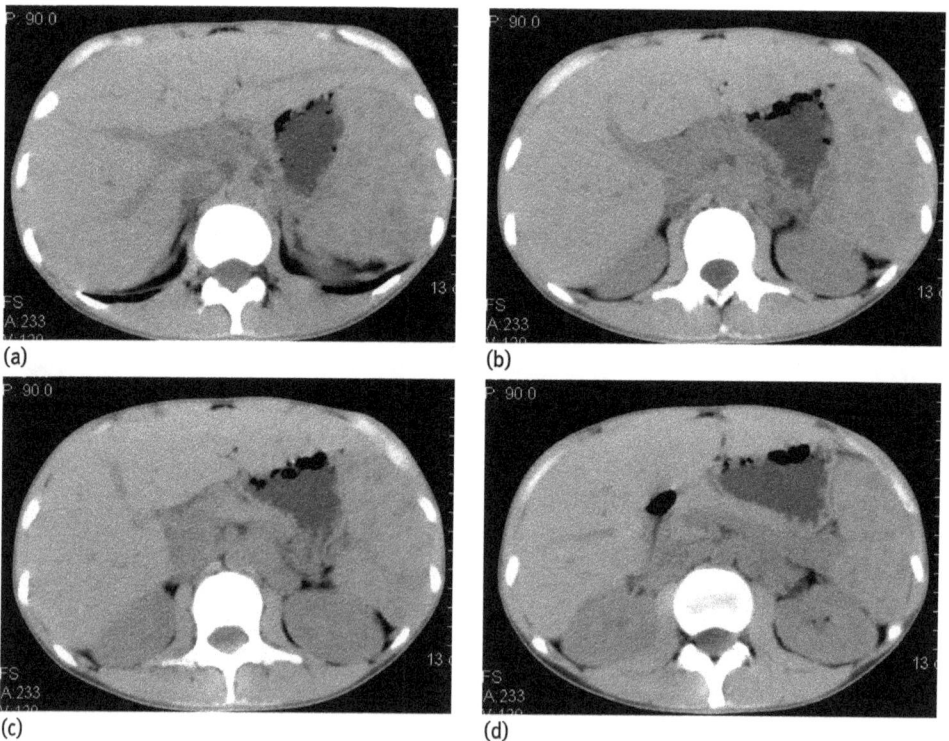

Fig. 14.17 a–l: Abdominal tuberculosis in spleen and lymph nodes.

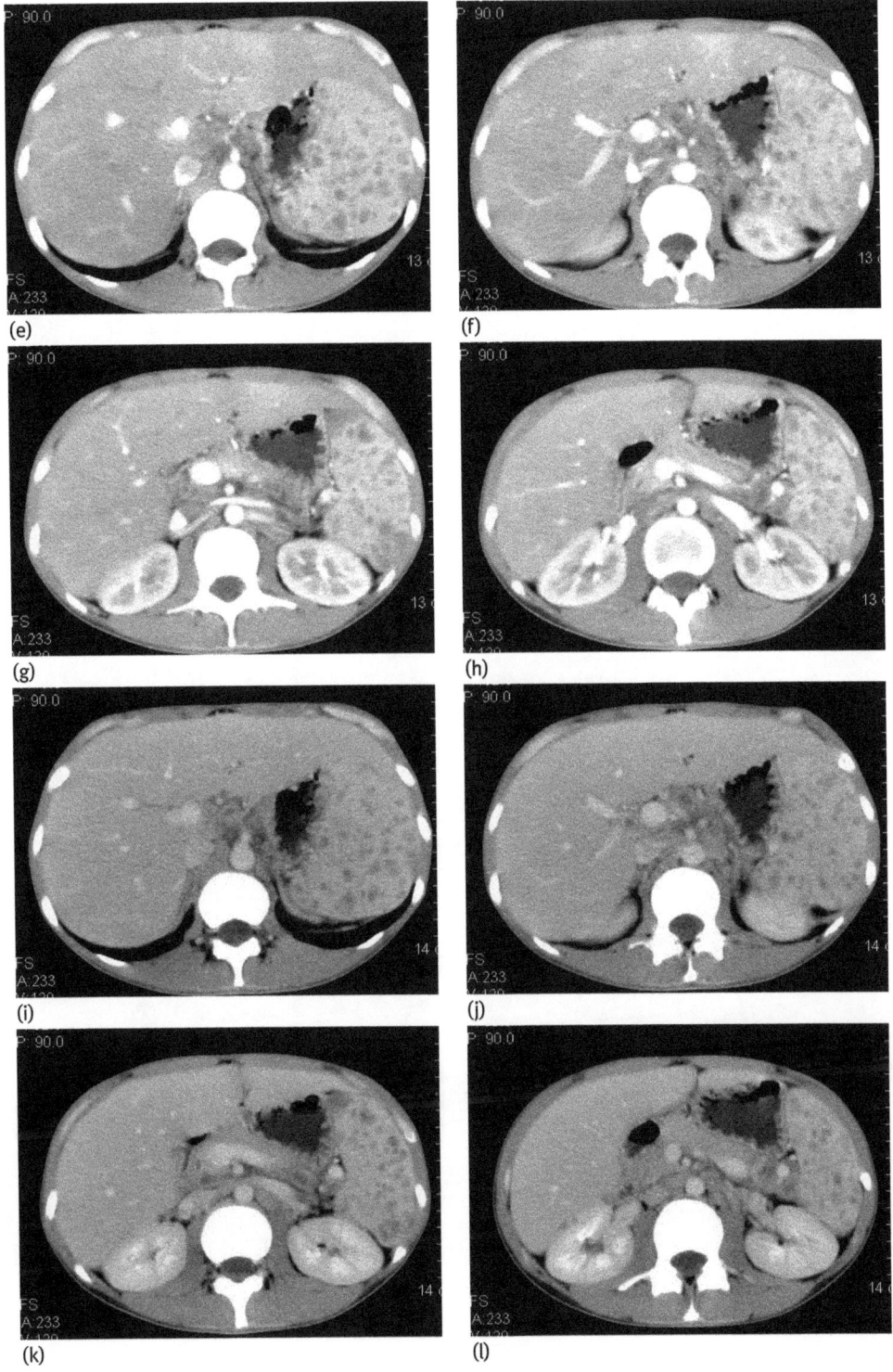

(e)

(f)

(g)

(h)

(i)

(j)

(k)

(l)

Fig. 14.17: (continuing)

The upper abdominal plain CT scans show splenomegaly, blurry-edged diffuse low-density miliary nodules in the spleen and enlarged lymph nodes in the hepatic hilar region and retroperitoneum (a–d). The enhanced scans show sharp-edged and not evidently enhanced low-density miliary nodules in the spleen and blurry-edged enlarged lymph nodes in the hepatic hilar region and retroperitoneum, some presenting rim enhancements by the enhanced scanning (e–h: at arterial phase; i–l: at portal vein phase).

Case 14.18 (Fig. 14.18 a–l)

A 34 year-old male patient presented recurrent fever and bellyache for more than 1 month before hospitalization. CD4+ cell count was 29/μl, CD4+/CD8+: 0.06. After 1 month's anti-tuberculosis treatment, the general symptoms were improved. The patient was diagnosed with AIDS (C3) combined with tuberculous peritonitis.

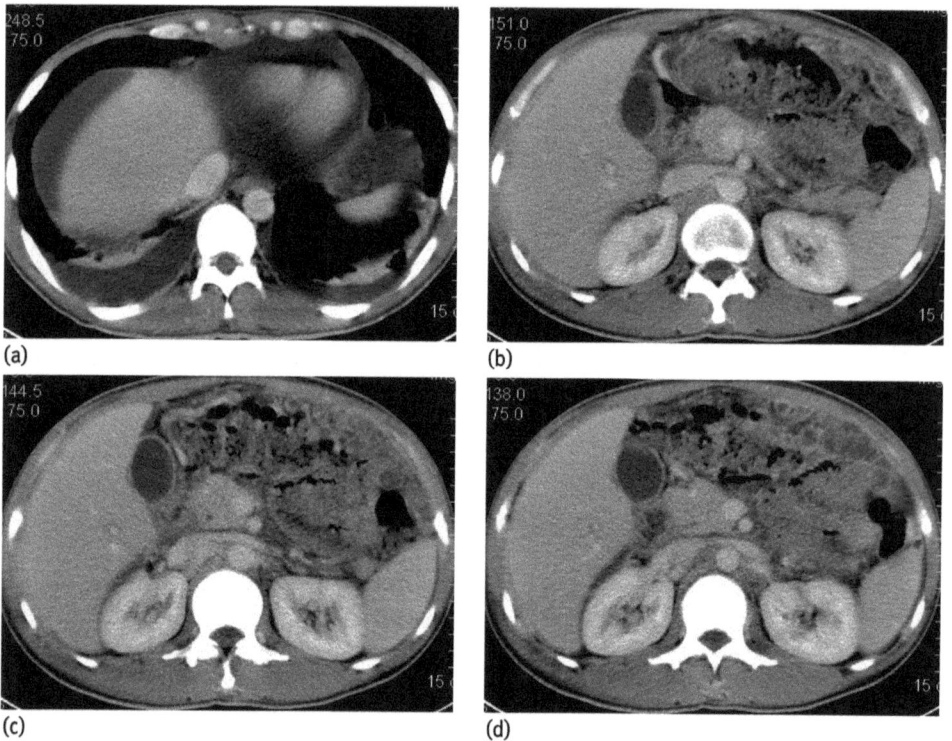

(a)

(b)

(c)

(d)

Fig. 14.18 a–l: Tuberculous peritonitis.

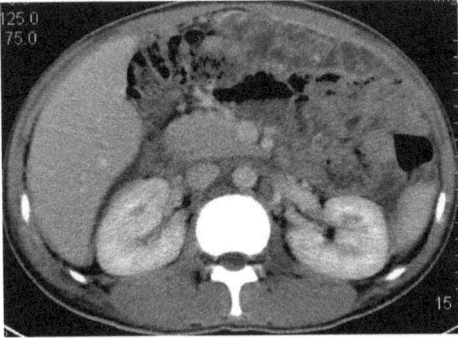

(e)

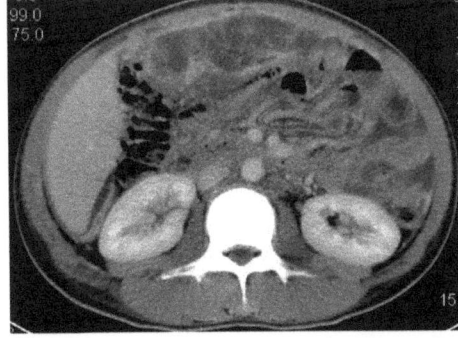

(f)

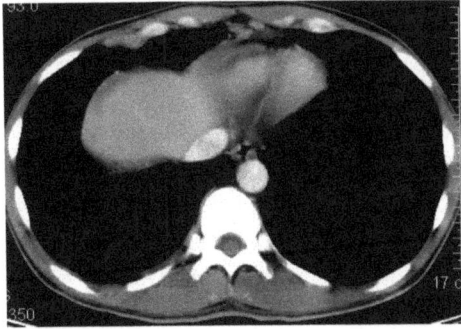

(g)

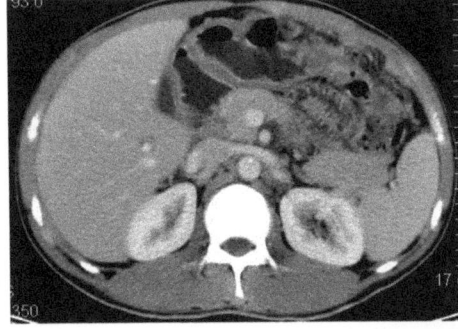

(h)

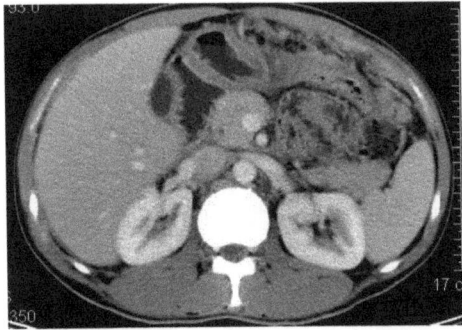

(i)

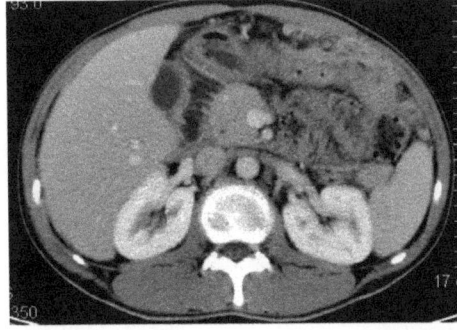

(j)

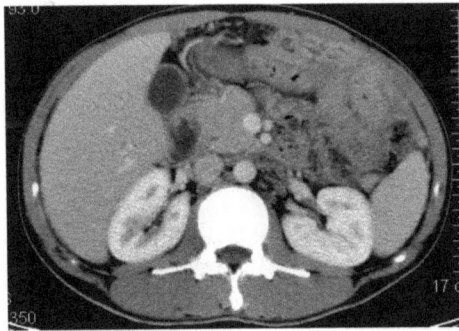

(k)

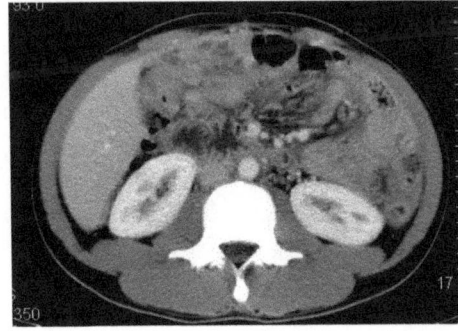

(l)

Fig. 14.18: (continuing)

The abdominal enhanced CT scan shows seroperitoneum, bilateral pleural effusions, pericardial effusions in the portal venous phase (a), extensively thickened perito- neum, evidently thickened pie-like great omentum with coarsened internal omental vessels with multiple rim enhanced nodular lesions and blurry edge between the under-part and the intestinal canal and thickened fuzzy mesentery (b–f). At the recheck 4 weeks after treatment, the ascites bilateral pleural effusions and pericardial effusion evidently were decreased (g), the lesions in the great omentum were obvi- ously reduced, the abdominal intestinal canal was clearer and thickened peritoneum and mesentery were significantly alleviated (h–l).

Case 14.19 (Fig. 14.19 a–f)
A 35-year-old male patient. He was admitted for hospitalization because of fever and chest pain for 2 months and palpable tumors in the right neck for 5 days. Multiple enlarged lymph nodes at the size of a bean were palpable in the bilateral necks, sub- maxilla, subaxil and inguen. Besides, a sized of 2 cm × 3 cm lymph node in the right neck was palpated hard, poor in activity, clear in boundary and without haphalgesia. The right upper quadrant of the abdomen was mildly tender. The CD4+ cell count was 8/µl, CD4+/CD8+: 0.01. Blood and bone marrow cultures were MTB negative, but the smear and culture of bronchoalveolar lavage identified MTB. He was eventually diagnosed with AIDS (C3) together with disseminated phthisis (lung, abdominal and lymph nodes).

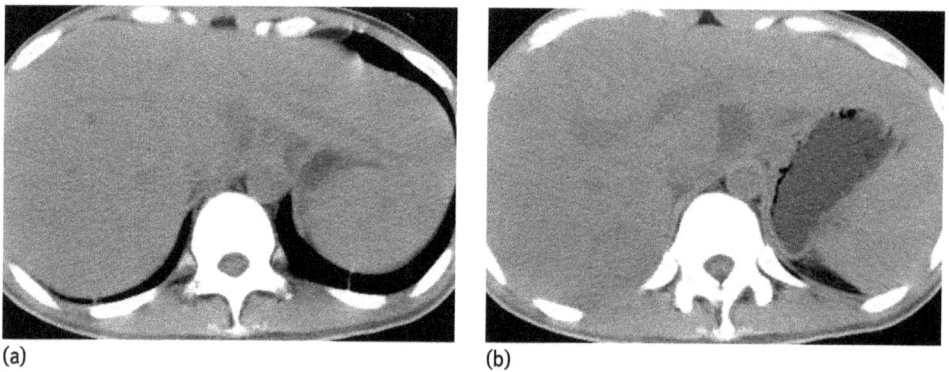

(a)   (b)

Fig. 14.19 a–f: Abdominal tuberculosis in liver, spleen and lymph nodes.

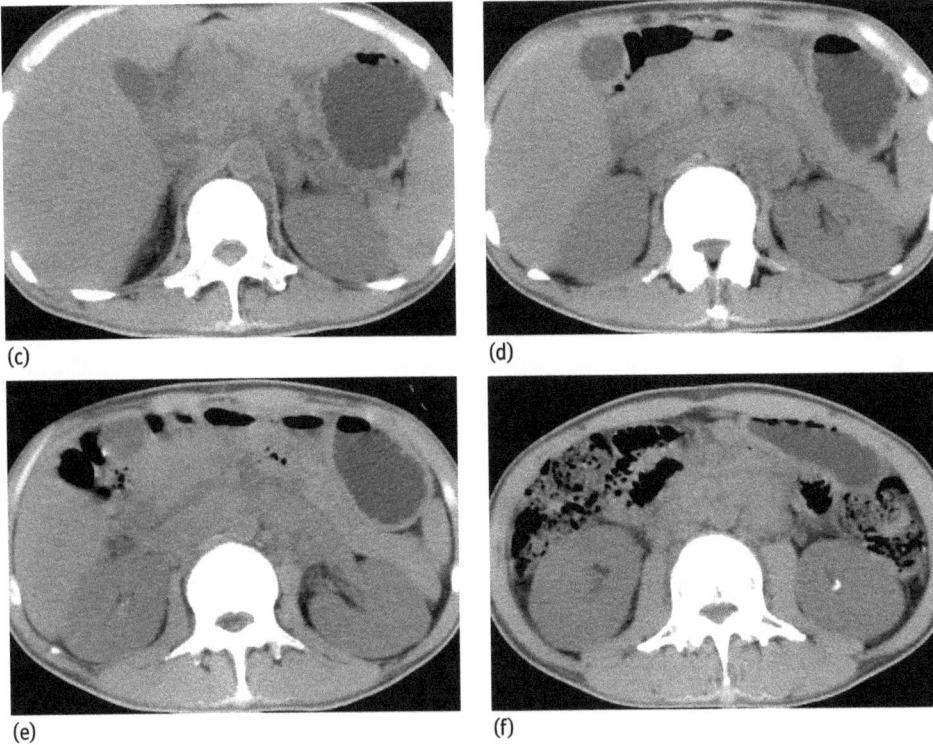

Fig. 14.19: (continuing)

The plain CT scans show a small low-density nodule in both upper and lower poles of the spleen (a–d), multiple small low-density miliary nodules in the liver (a–c) and widely enlarged blurry-edged lymph nodes in the hepatic hilar region and retroperitoneum, mainly located in the retroperitoneum (a–f).

14.3.3 Imaging features

When the abdominal TB combined with AIDS involves multiple abdominal organs and tissues, the main CT findings are summarized as follows:

1. Low-density nodular lesions in the liver and spleen: More often they are miliary, which can be evident more by the contrast-enhanced imaging than by plain scanning.

2. TB abscesses in liver and spleen: It occurs more often in the liver, showing similarities to bacterial liver abscess on CT scans and specificity due to the frequent complications of lesions in lung, abdominal cavity lymph nodes or intestines.

3. Abdominal lymphadenectasis: TB leads to lymphadenectasis even involving mesentery and retroperitoneal lymph nodes, which manifests as rim enhancement on the contrast-enhanced scans.

4. Intestinal TB: It is most commonly found in terminal ileum, cecum and adjacent ascending colon. The CT findings show irregularly-thickened wall or tumor formation.
5. Peritoneal TB: The images show extensively thickened peritoneum, especially the thickened great omentum. It takes the shape of pie, with multiple nodular lesions in the peritoneum and rim-enhanced shadow on them.

When AIDS patients are affected by TB, the images may show pulmonary TB lesions or systemic lymphoid TB lesions. Compared with the TB patients with normal immunity, they are prone to tuberculosis abscesses, with more extensive and complete central liquefaction necrosis of the swelled lymph nodes.

Editors: Lieguang Zhang, Xiejie Chen, Weiping Cai,Yan Ding

15 Thoracic and abdominal imaging features of pediatric AIDS

15.1 Introduction

Children contract HIV mainly via vertical transmission, blood transfusion and use of blood products. HIV infection progresses rapidly to onset of AIDS in children with a remarkably short course, only because of their immature immune barrier as well as the developmental disorder and malnutrition from HIV infection. As a result, children may expose to more opportunistic infections than adults.

The common manifestations in AIDS children clinically include recurrent fever of undetermined origin (over a month), growth retardation (especially in infants), recurrent respiratory tract infection, persistent interstitial pneumonia, oral ulcer and thrush, protracted diarrhea, enlargement of the liver, spleen and superficial lymph nodes, enlargement of the parotid gland of undetermined origin, significant weight drop (more than 10 % of the baseline in 3 months) and tuberculosis infection and other opportunistic infections.

The pediatric AIDS is characterized by the following findings:

1. The incubation period of HIV is shorter, followed by acute onset and rapid progress to AIDS;
2. The growth retardation causes evident developmental deviation from the normal growth curve and the younger they are, the earlier and the more severely the AIDS sets on.
3. The AIDS children are susceptible bacterial infections, especially the infection by polysaccharide capsule bacteria.
4. They are prone to contract encephalopathic syndrome, which is earlier at onset, rapid in progress and poor in prognosis.

15.2 Radiologic findings

Case 15.1 (Fig. 15.1 a–g)

A 11-year-old boy who was admitted to hospital because of recurrent fever for more than 1 month. Some enlarged nodes in the left supraclavicular and cervical region were palpated smooth, without adhesion and tender. CD4+ cell count was 21/μl, with CD4+/CD8+: 0.05. Bone marrow culture was *Penicillium marneffei* positive. The patient was clinically diagnosed as AIDS (C3) combined with disseminated penicilliosis marneffei and interstitial pneumonia.

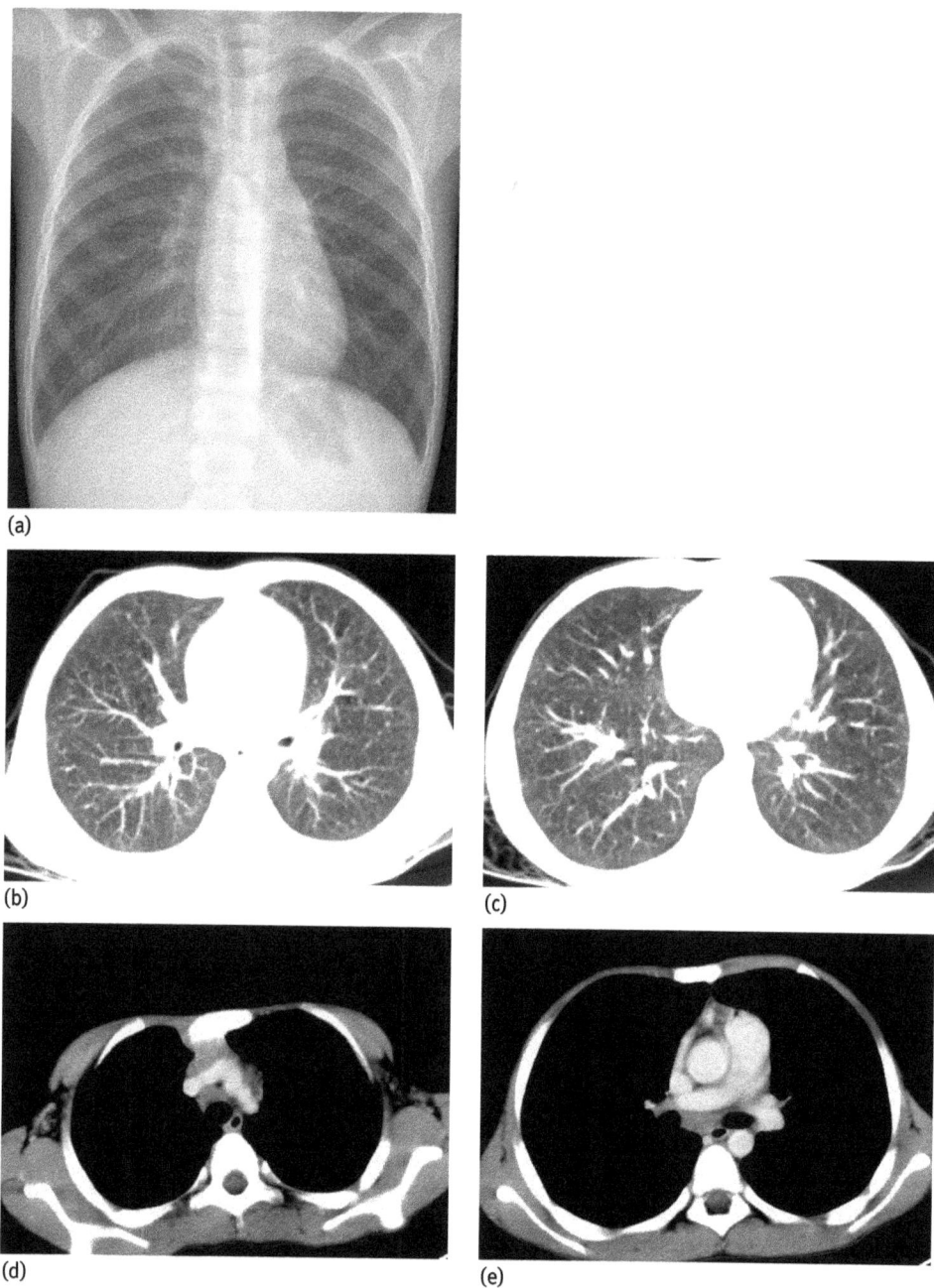

Fig. 15.1 a–g: Penicilliosis marneffei septicemia and interstitial pneumonia.

Chest radiograph showed coarsened lung markings and broadened right upper mediastinum (a). CT scans with lung windows showed scattered miliary nodules with a diameter less than 3 mm, mainly centrilobular nodules in the bilateral lungs, indicating tree-in-bud sign (b, c). CT scans with mediastinal windows showed enlargements

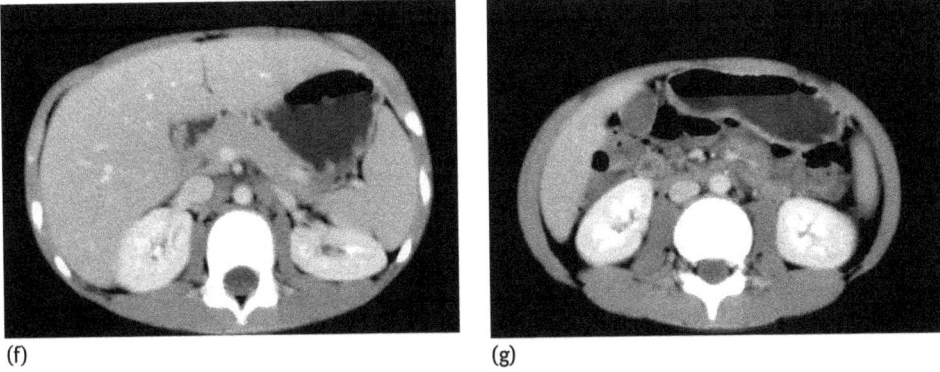

(f)　　　　　　　　　　　　　　　　　(g)

Fig. 15.1: (continuing)

in mediastinal lymph nodes (d, e). Enhanced abdominal CT scans showed enlarged mesenteric lymph nodes, indicating a "sandwich" sign (f, g).

Case 15.2 (Fig. 15.2 a–l)

A 5-year-old boy was admitted to hospital because of recurrent fever and bellyache for more than 2 months. He was relatively thin, for his weight was 15 kg. The superficial lymph nodes in the neck, armpit and groin were palpated to be enlarged, moderate in nature, movable and little tender. The patient had abdominal distention, with tenderness in his whole abdomen but no rebound tenderness. CD4+ cell count was 17/μl, CD4+/CD8+: 0.04. Blood culture was *Penicillium marneffei* positive. The patient was diagnosed with AIDS (C3) combined with disseminated penicilliosis marneffei. The patient's conditions got better after anti-infection treatment for 1 month.

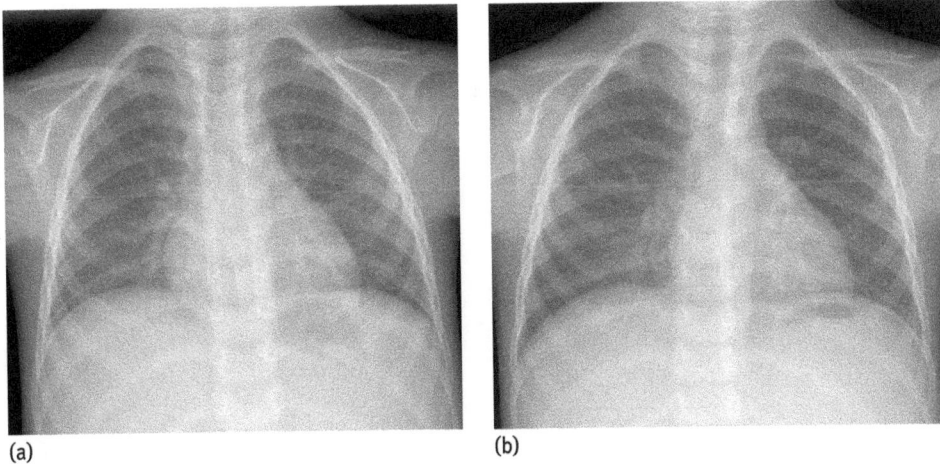

(a)　　　　　　　　　　　　　　　　　(b)

Fig. 15.2 a–l: Disseminated penicilliosis marneffei.

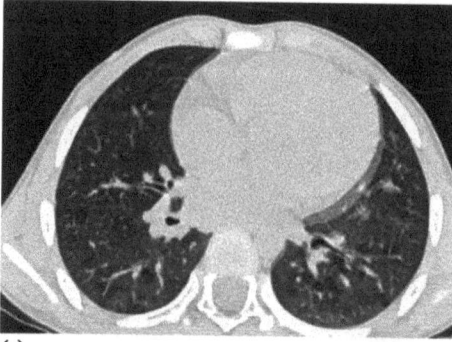
(c)

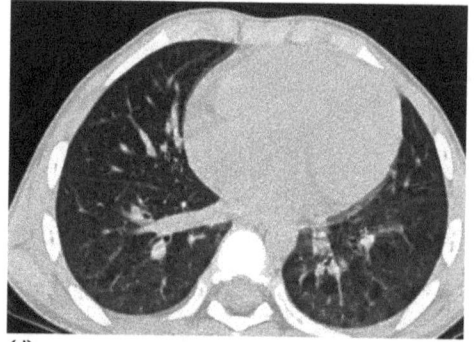
(d)

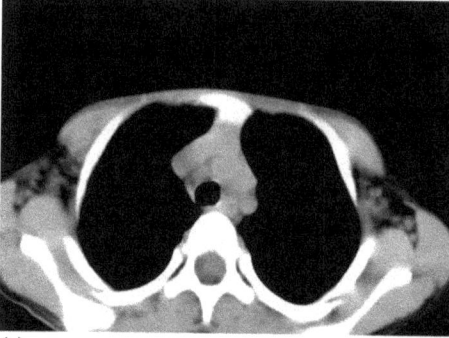
(e)

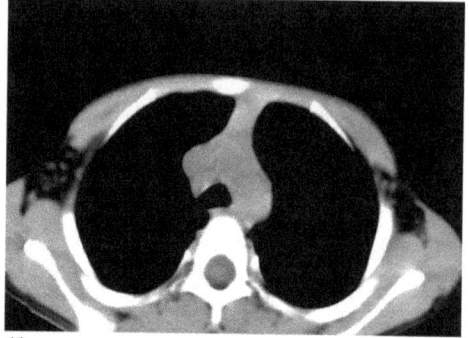
(f)

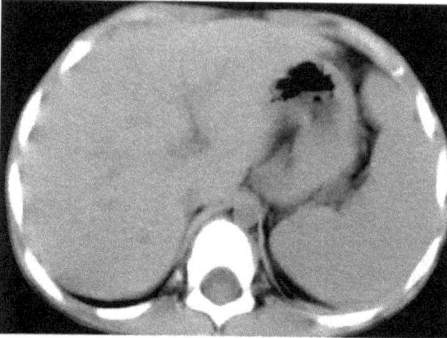
(g)

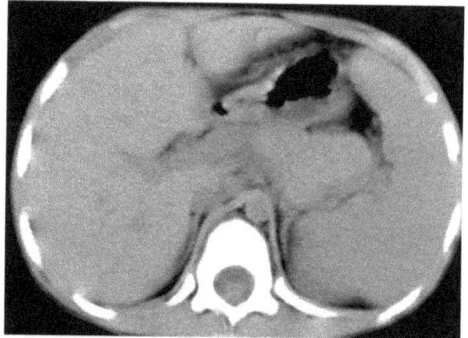
(h)

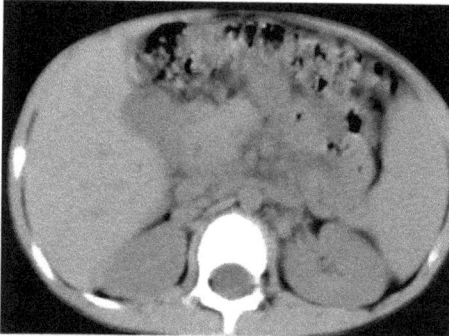
(i)

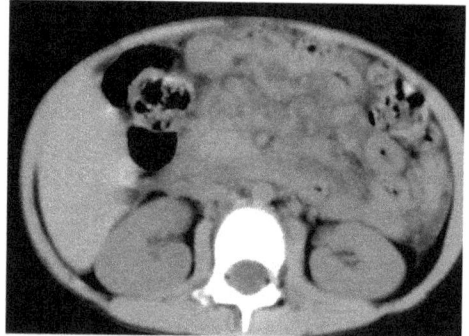
(j)

Fig. 15.2: (continuing)

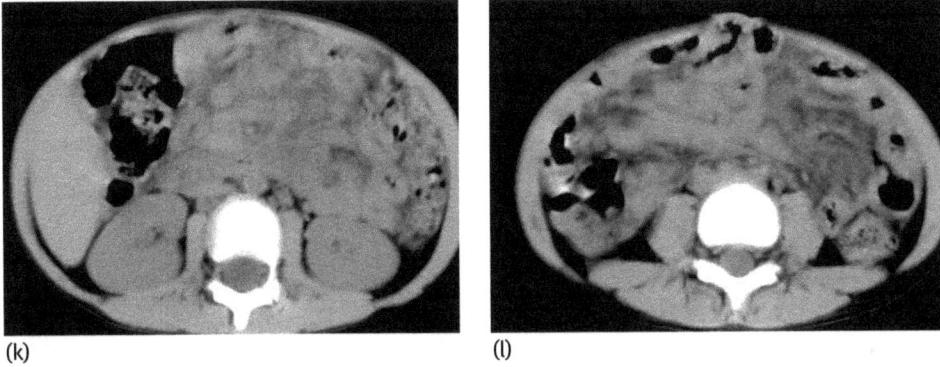

(k) (l)

Fig. 15.2: (continuing)

Chest radiograph showed thickened lung markings (a), and a little improvement after 6 weeks compared with the previous film (b). HRCT scans showed interlobular septal thickening in the bilateral lung and local centrilobular emphysema in lower lobes of the bilateral lung (c, d). CT scans with mediastinal window showed enlarged paratracheal lymph nodes (e, f). The plain abdominal CT scans showed hepatosplenomegaly, the increased-density thickened fuzzy mesentery and the mildly thickened intestinal wall (g–l)

Case 15.3 (Fig. 15.3 a–i)

A 9-year-old boy was admitted to hospital with fever and cough for 1 month. He was poorly grew with a wasting body type. Multiple lymph nodes in the patient's neck, supraclavicular area and groins were palpable. The patient's breathing sounds were rough with a lot of dry and moist rales, especially in the right lung. CD4+ cell count was 34/μl, CD4+/CD8+: 0.03. Sputum direct smear examination was acid-fast bacilli negative but Gram's positive bacteria positive. Hemolysis staphylococci were found in bone marrows cultivation. Bone marrow culture was *Penicillium marneffei* positive. The patient was diagnosed with AIDS (C3) combined with pulmonary infection (PCP, bacteria), sepsis (*Penicillium marneffei*, hemolysis staphylococcus) and HIV wasting syndrome. After 1 month of treatment, the patient's conditions improved.

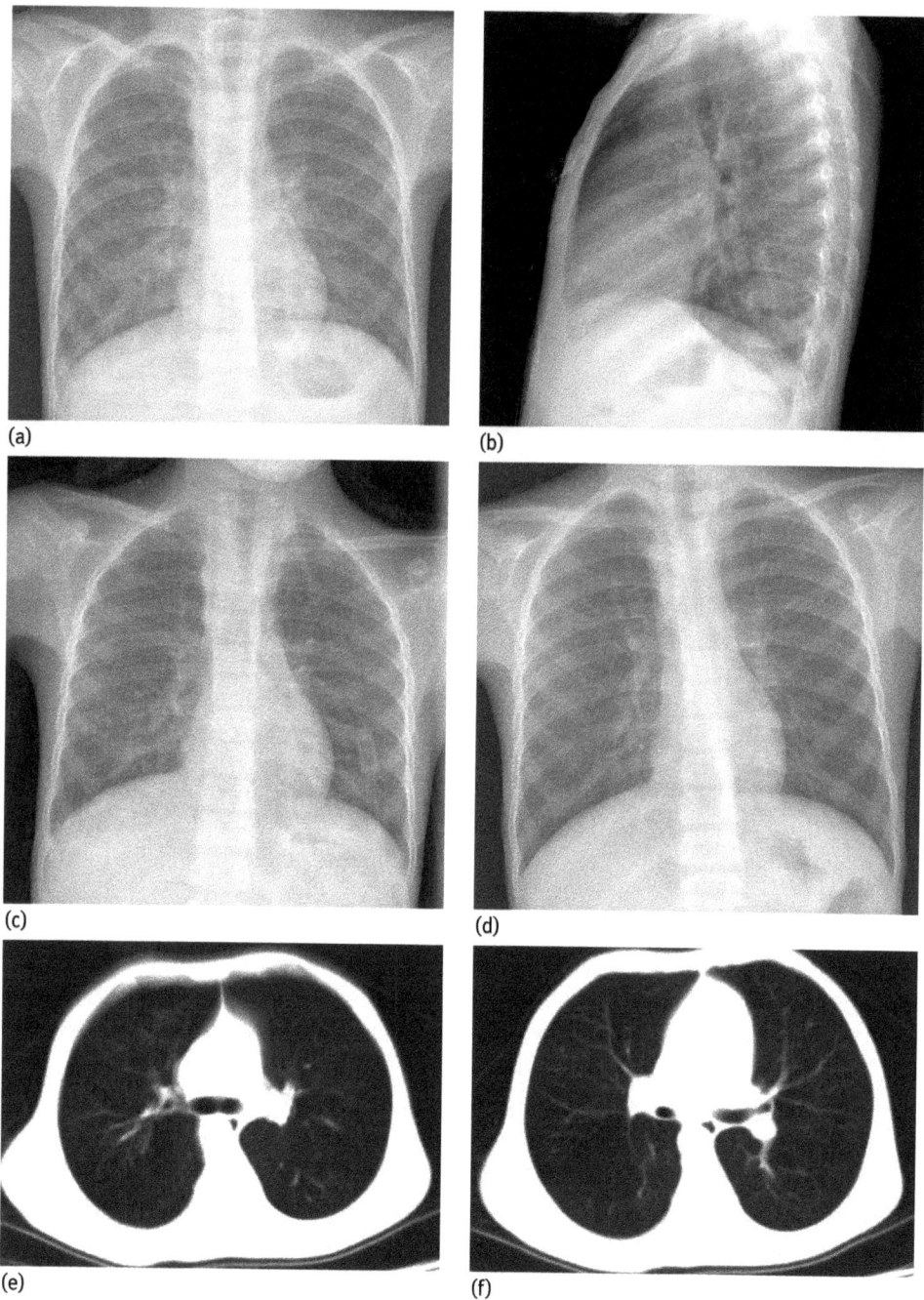

Fig. 15.3 a–i: Pulmonary infection (PCP, bacteria) and sepsis (*Penicillium marneffei*, hemolysis staphylococcus).

(g)

(h)

(i)

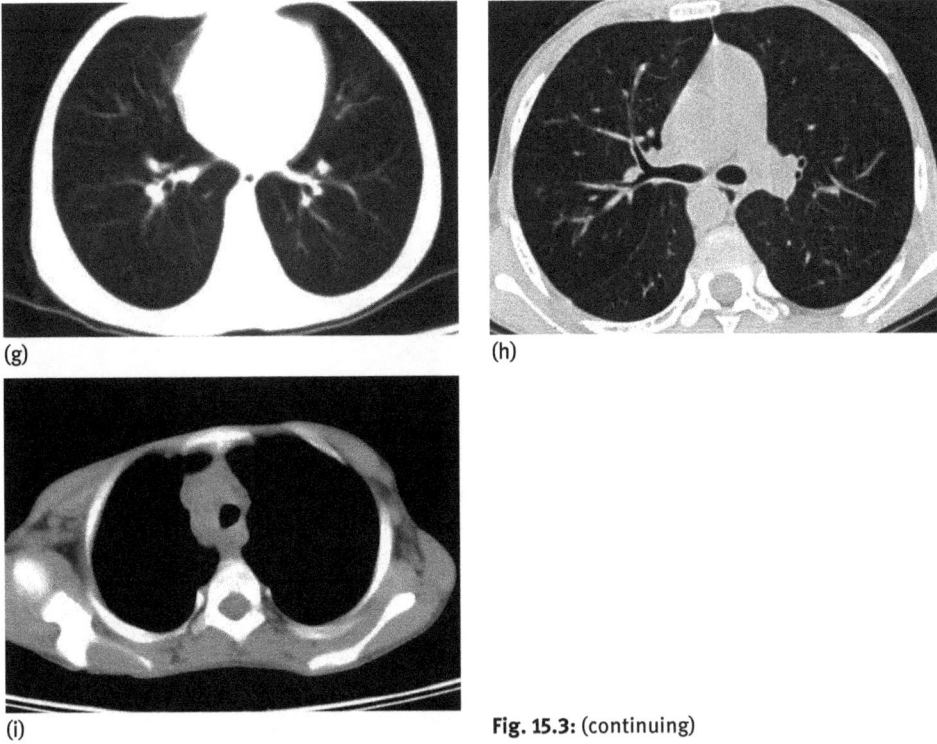

Fig. 15.3: (continuing)

The front and lateral chest radiographs show thickened pulmonary markings, multiple high-density blurring-edged patchy opacities distributed along bronchi in the bilateral lungs and mainly located in lower lobes (a, b) and congenital variations in the right aortic arch and right descending aorta. At reexamination, the front and lateral radiographs (C: 4 days later; D: 10 days later) show gradually absorbed lesions in the bilateral lung and clearer lung fiend than before. The CT scans with lung window at re-check after 6 weeks show mildly blurring-edged markings in the bilateral lungs (e–h) and the CT scans with mediastinal windows show right aortic arch and right descending aorta (i, j).

Case 15.4 (Fig. 15.4 a–d)
A 9-year-old girl presented recurrent tachypnea of unknown origin, worsen after physical activities. She had cough with yellowish mucous, headache, dizziness and vomiting at intervals. The patient was transferred to the Guangzhou Chest Hospital with clinical diagnosis of tuberculosis meningitis. CD4+ cell count was 305/μl, with CD4+/CD8+: 0.1. The cerebrospinal fluid (CSF) examination indicated tuberculosis meningitis. The patient was diagnosed with AIDS (B3) combined with tuberculosis meningitis, tuberculous lymphadenitis in cervical, supraclavicular and mediastinal regions and hematogenous pulmonary tuberculosis.

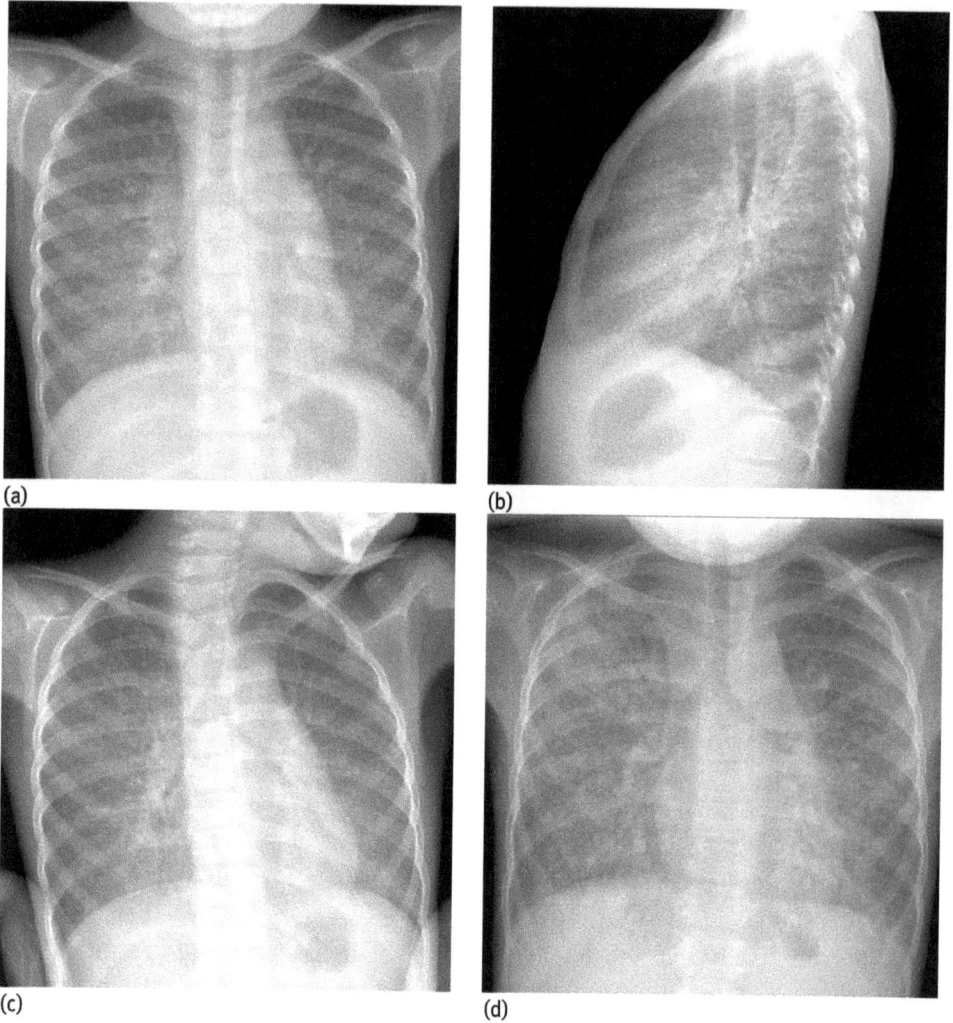

Fig. 15.4 a–d: Hematogenous pulmonary tuberculosis.

The front and lateral chest radiographs show diffuse miliary nodules in the bilateral lungs, broadened mediastinum and obscure pulmonary hilum structures (a, b). The chest radiograph at recheck after 3 weeks shows worsened miliary nodules in the bilateral lung (c). The chest radiograph at recheck after 4 weeks, shows evidently aggravated lesions and extensive patchy opacities in the bilateral lungs (d).

Case 15.5 (Fig. 15.5 a–d)

A 8-year-old boy presented recurrent fever, cough and expectoration for 4 months and tachypnea for 1 month. The weight was 16 kg with clear mind, anemic face, but no rash. Some lymph nodes of soybean size in the patient's cervical and submandibular region were palpated to be soft in nature, smooth and mobile. There was bean-curd-like substance on the tongue surface and congestion in the pharynx. He had a mild shortness in breath and the breath sounds in the left lung were rough and weakened with fine moist rales in the right lower lung. CD4+ cell count was 1/µl, CD4+/CD8+: 0.01. Sputum smear examination was acid-fast bacilli positive, fecal smear fungi positive and scatologic culture *Candida albicans* positive. The patient was diagnosed with AIDS (C3) combined with pulmonary infection, tuberculosis, fungal infection (in oral cavity and intestinal tract).

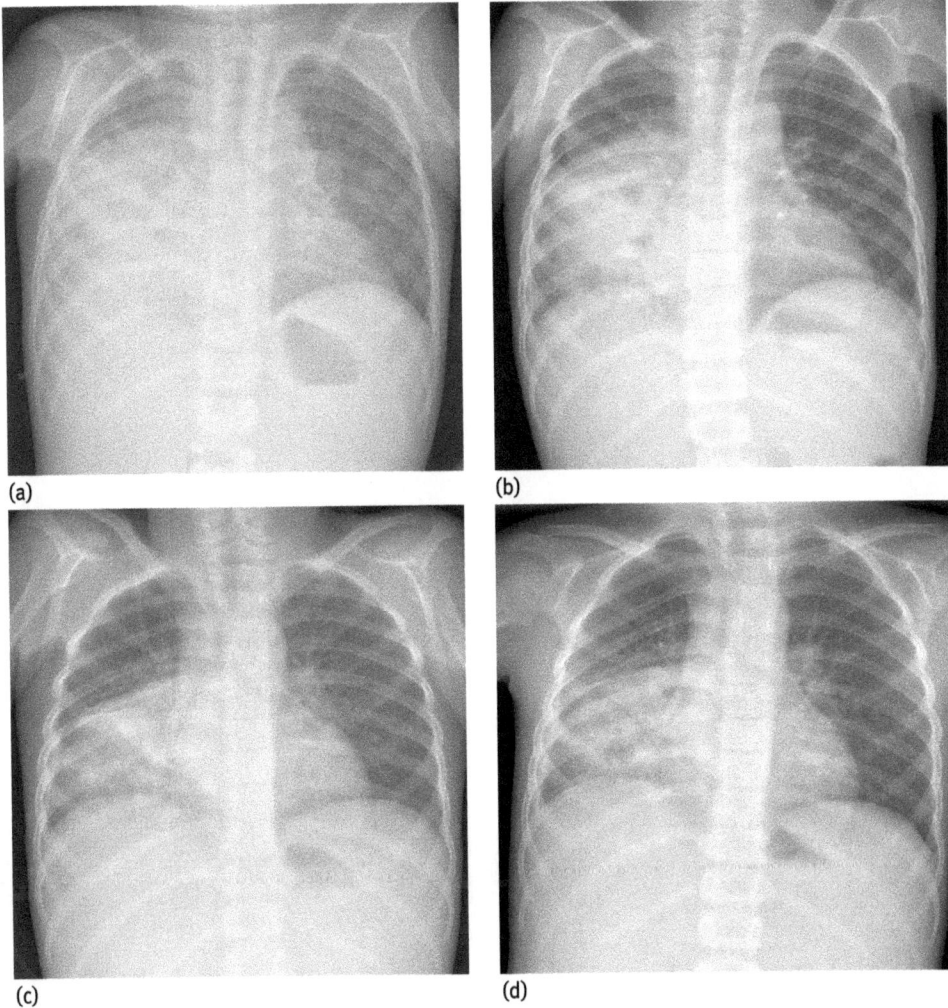

Fig. 15.5 a–d: Pulmonary Infection, Tuberculosis.

Chest radiograph shows a patchy consolidation with a cavity in it, obscure markings and diffuse spotty opacities in the bilateral lungs (a). Chest radiograph at recheck after 1 week shows the shrinking consolidation in the right lung and obviously absorbed diffuse spotty opacities in the bilateral lungs (b). Chest radiographs at rechecks after 1 month and 4 months show gradually absorbed lesions in the right lung (c, d).

Case 15.6 (Fig. 15.6 a–l)

A 5-year-old boy patient was admitted to hospital with recurrent fever, dysphagia and cough for more than 10 months. There was a lot of bean-curd-like substance on the surface of his tongue. CD4+ cell count was 8/μl, CD4+/CD8+: 0.01. Sputum culture was *Klebsiella* bacillus positive. The patient was diagnosed with AIDS (C3) combined with pulmonary infection (*Klebsiella* bacillus), oral fungal infection, esophagus.

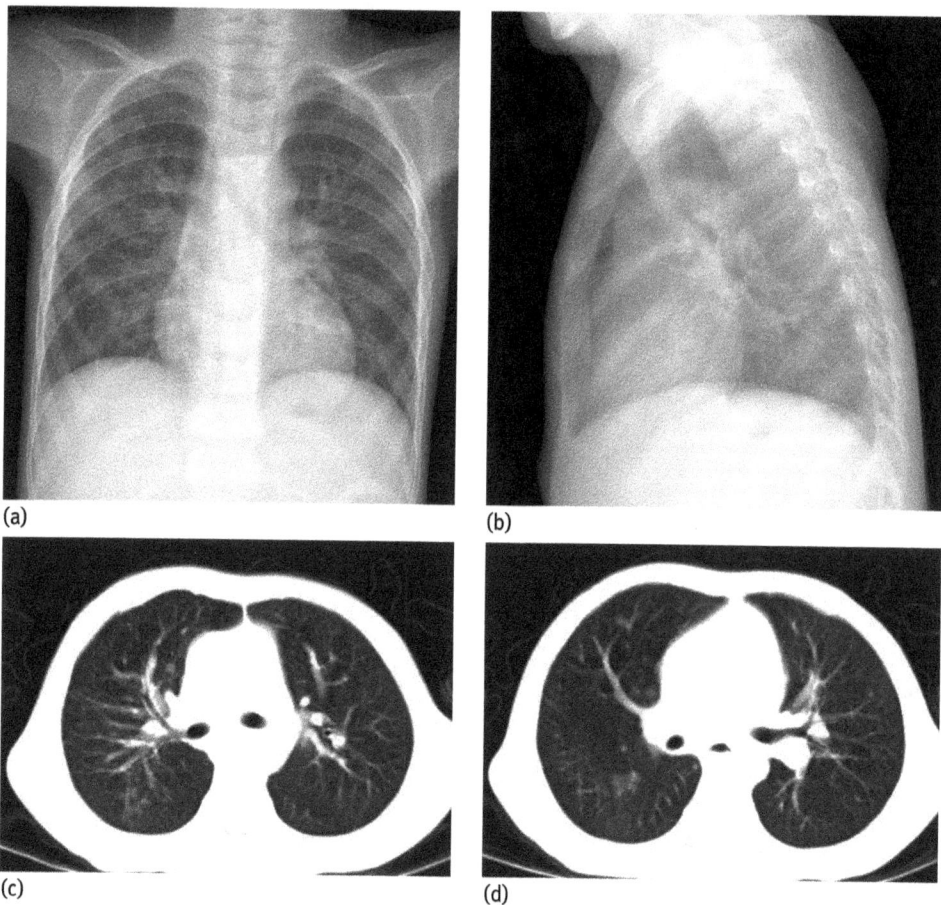

Fig. 15.6 a–l: Pulmonary infection (acid production *Klebsiella* bacillus) and esophageal fungal infection.

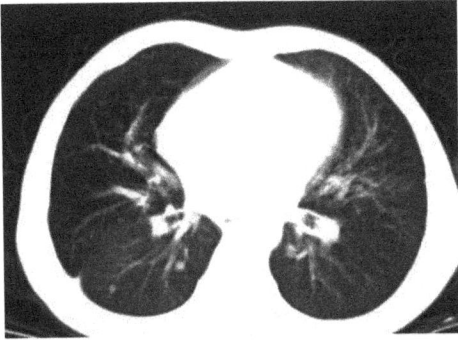

(e)

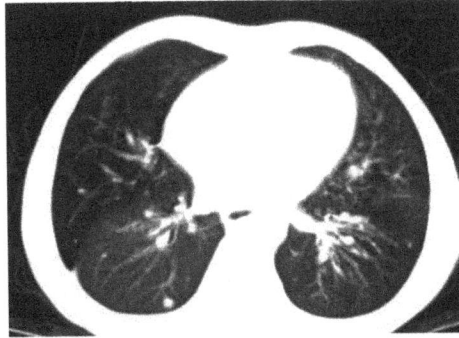

(f)

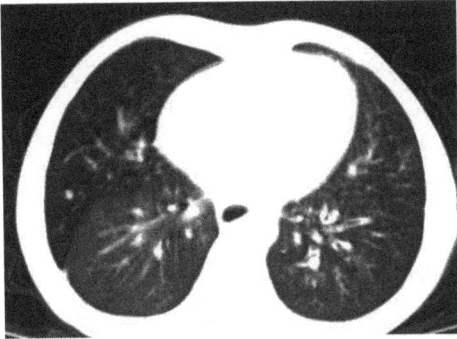

(g)

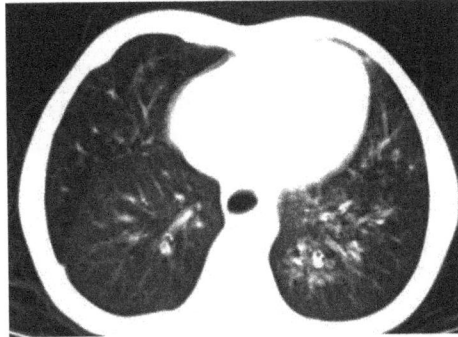

(h)

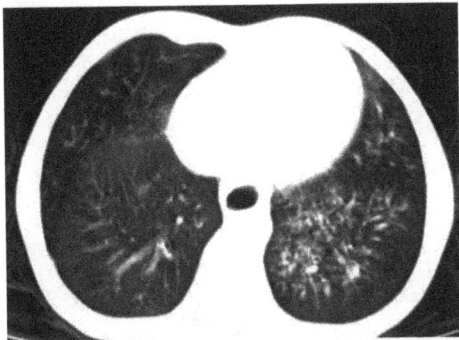

(i)

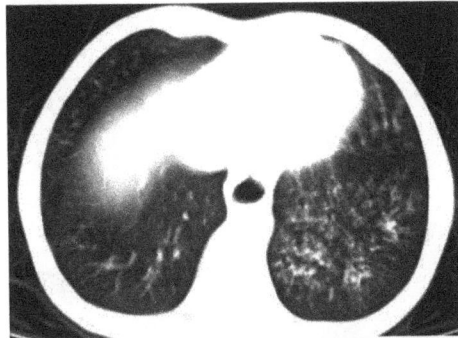

(j)

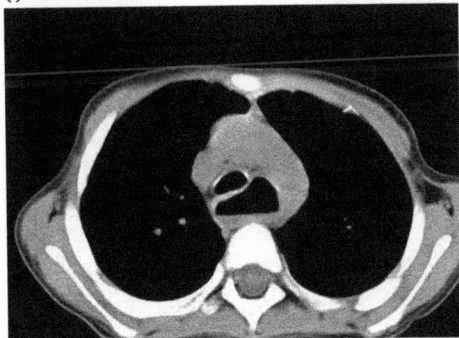

(k)

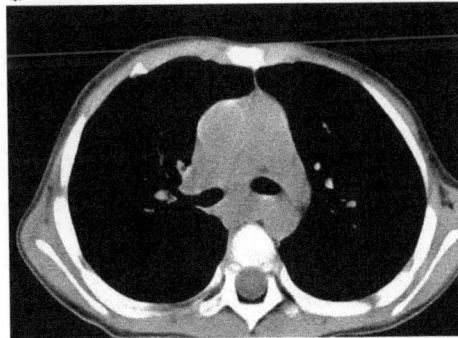

(l)

Fig. 15.6: (continuing)

Chest radiographs show obscure markings in the bilateral lungs, multiple small patchy and nodular opacities with blurring edges in the bilateral lung, and obstructed esophagus at the subcarinal level with obviously dilated esophagus above it, indicating a liquid-air interface (a, b). CT scans with lung window show multiple small patchy and nodular opacities with blurry edges in both lobes, mainly in the left lower lung and obscure tracheal and bloodvessel bundles in the bilateral lung (c–j). CT scans with mediastinal window show obstructed esophagus at the subcarinal level with obviously dilated esophagus above it, indicating a liquid-air interface (k, l).

Case 15.7 (Fig 15.7 a–l)

A 11-year-old girl presented recurrent diarrhea and cough for 6 months, got worsening for 1 day, and fever for 12 hours. In her both armpits and groins several enlarged lymph nodes were palpated to be moderate in nature, smooth on the surface and mobile. The left armpit was partly enlarged and the lymph nodes were tender. The breath sounds in the bilateral lungs were rough, with some dry and moist rales in the left lower lung. CD4+ cell count was 43/μl, CD4+/CD8+: 0.12. The patient was diagnosed with AIDS (C3) combined with pulmonary infection, HIV wasting syndrome and infectious diarrhea.

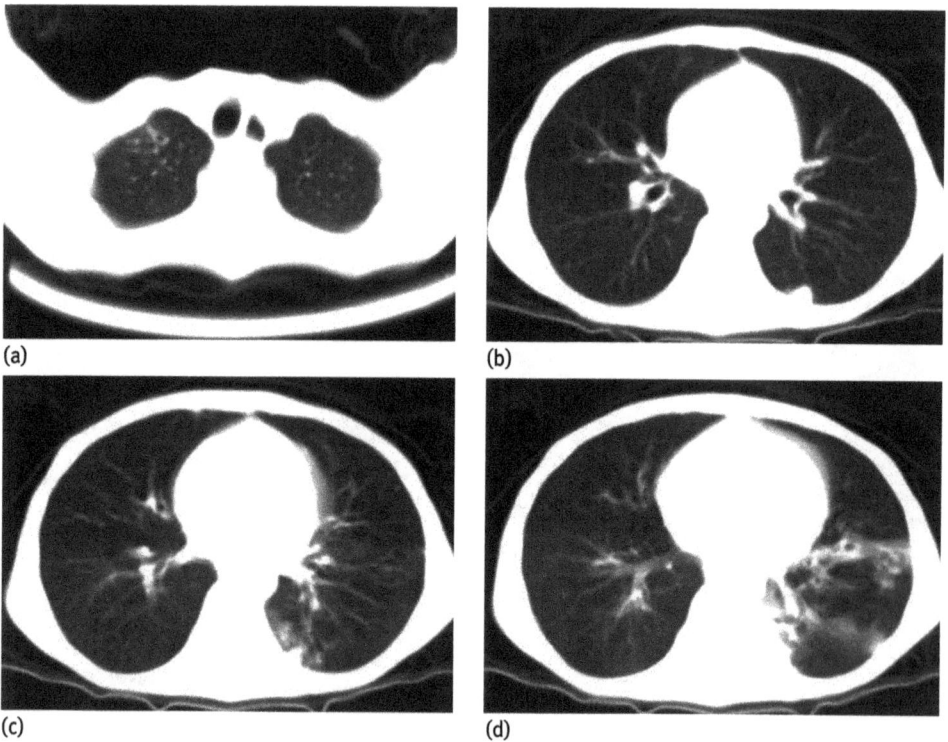

(a)

(b)

(c)

(d)

Fig. 15.7 a–l: Pulmonary infection.

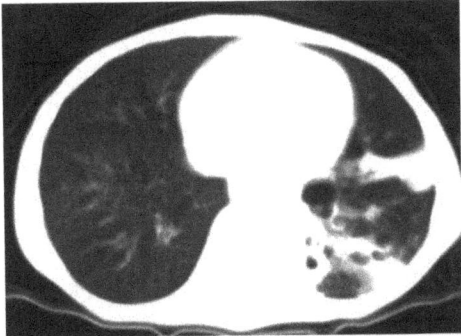
(e)

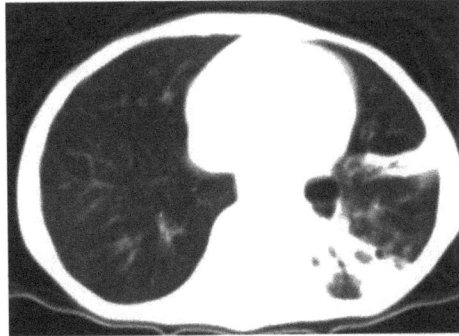
(f)

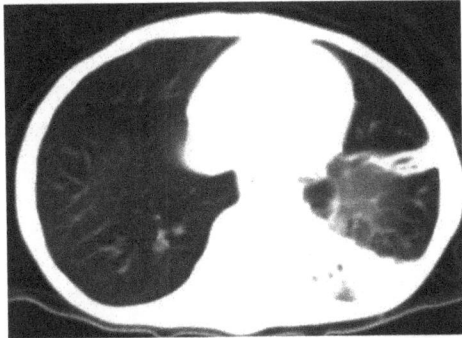
(g)

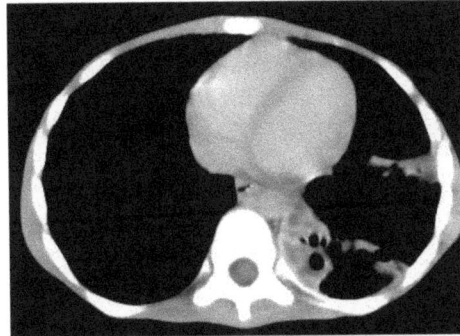
(h)

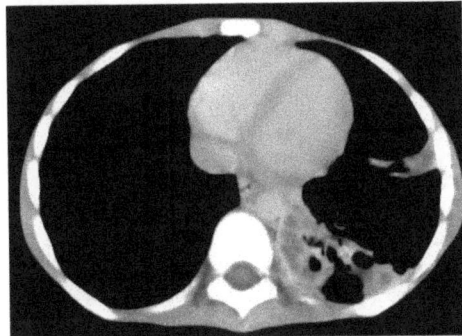
(i)

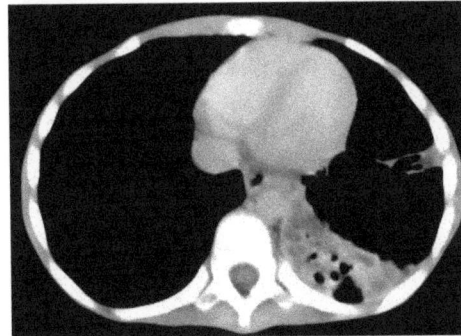
(j)

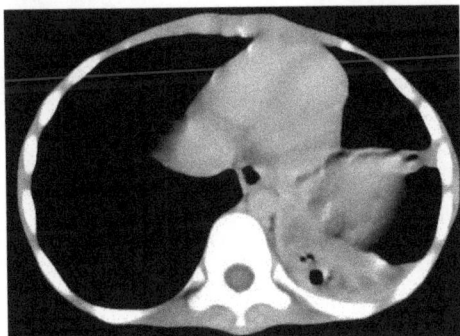
(k)

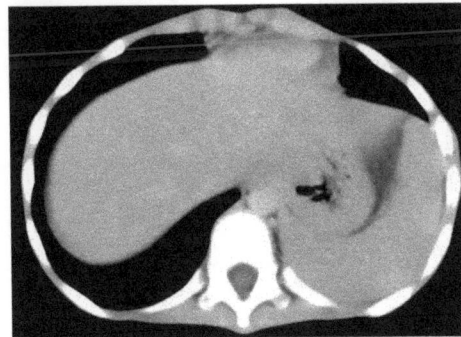
(l)

Fig. 15.7: (continuing)

CT scans with lung window show multiple small patchy consolidations with blurry edges in the right lung apex and the left lower lung (a–g). Enhanced CT scans with mediastinal window show cavities in the lesion, multiple low-density round areas (h–k) and the enlarged spleen (l).

Case 15.8 (Fig. 15.8 a–l)

A 5-year-old boy was admitted to hospital for fever more than 10 days, cough for 5 days and diarrhea for 2 days. His father was HIV infected. He had 5 kg weight loss in resent month. CD4+ cell count was 6/μl, with CD4+/CD8+: 0.03. Sputum culture was *Candida albicans* positive. Blood culture was streptococcus agalactiae positive. The patient was diagnosed with AIDS (C3) combined with severe pneumonia (bacteria, fungi), sepsis, oral fungal infection, infectious diarrhea and HIV wasting syndrome.

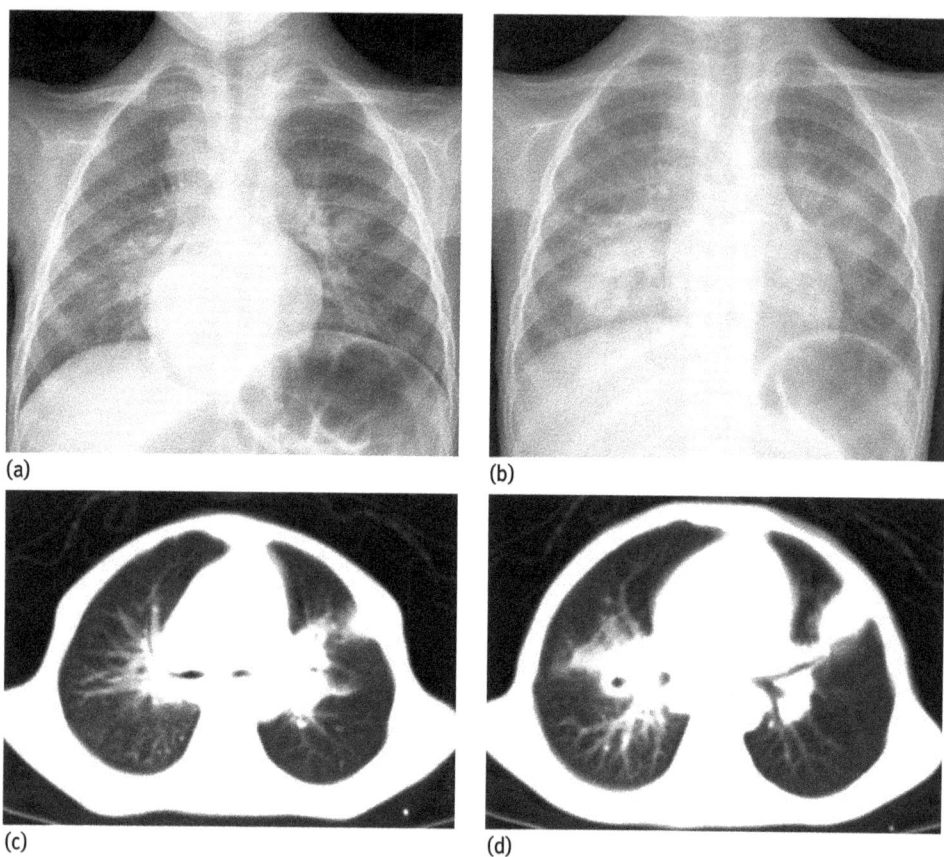

(a)

(b)

(c)

(d)

Fig. 15.8 a–l: Severe pneumonia (bacteria, fungi).

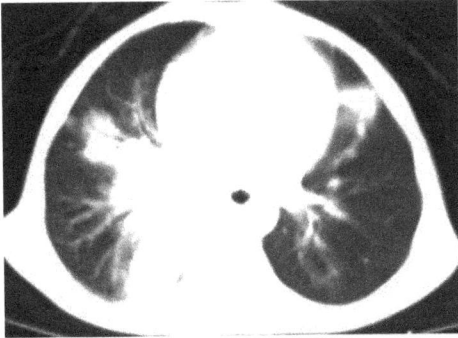
(e)

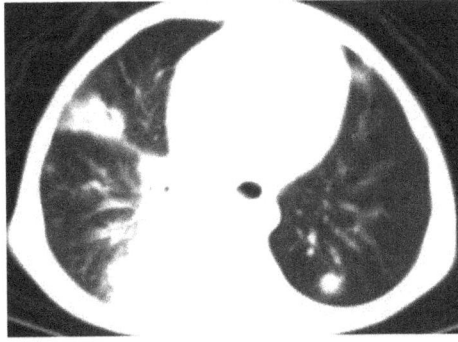
(f)

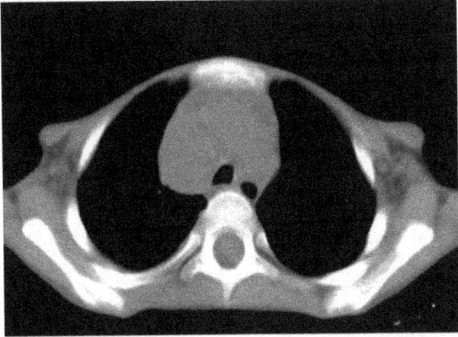
(g)

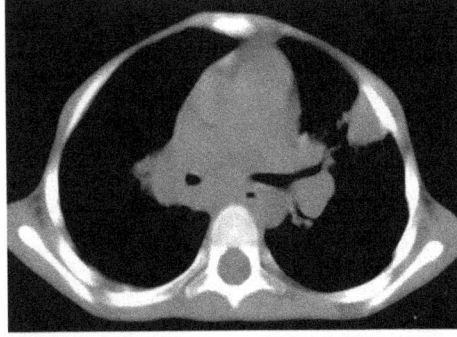
(h)

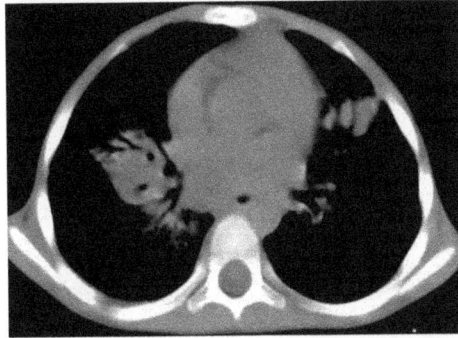
(i)

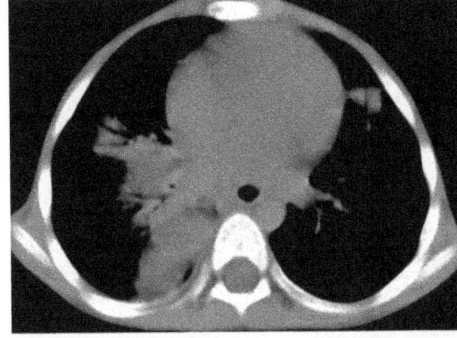
(j)

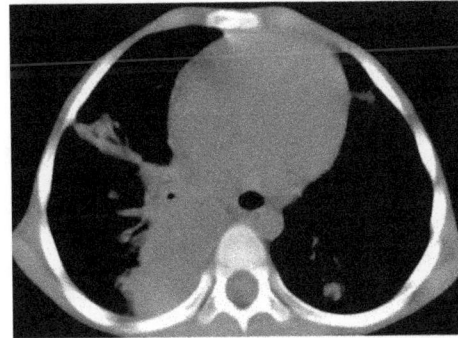
(k)

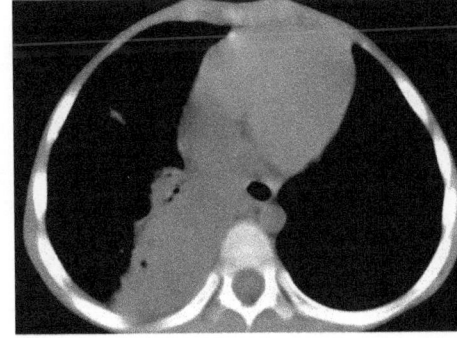
(l)

Fig. 15.8: (continuing)

Chest radiograph showed decreased transparency of the bilateral lungs, multiple patchy opacities with blurry edges in the bilateral lungs, unclear bilateral hilar structures and enlarged lymph nodes in the right upper mediastinum (a). The chest radiograph at the recheck after 5 days showed expanded patchy opacities in the bilateral lung (b). CT scans with lung windows showed multiple patchy and nodular opacities with blurry edges in the bilateral lungs, mainly located in the right lower lung and indicating great flake sign, enlarged bilateral hilums with blurry structures and thickened bronchial blood vessels bundles (c–f). CT scans with mediastinal window showed bronchial air sign in some lesions and evidently enlarged lymph nodes in the mediastinum and right lung hilum (g–l).

Case 15.9 (Fig. 15.9 a–f)

A 5-year-old boy was admitted into hospital for recurrent fever and abdominal distension for 4 months. Multiple lymph nodes in the neck, armpits and some other parts were enlarged by palpation. Abdominal rigidity increased slightly and right lower quadrant had tenderness. CD4+ cell count was 2/μl, CD4+/CD8+: 0.01. Bone marrow culture was *Penicillium marneffei* positive.The patient was diagnosed with AIDS (C3) combined with disseminated penicilliosis marneffei.

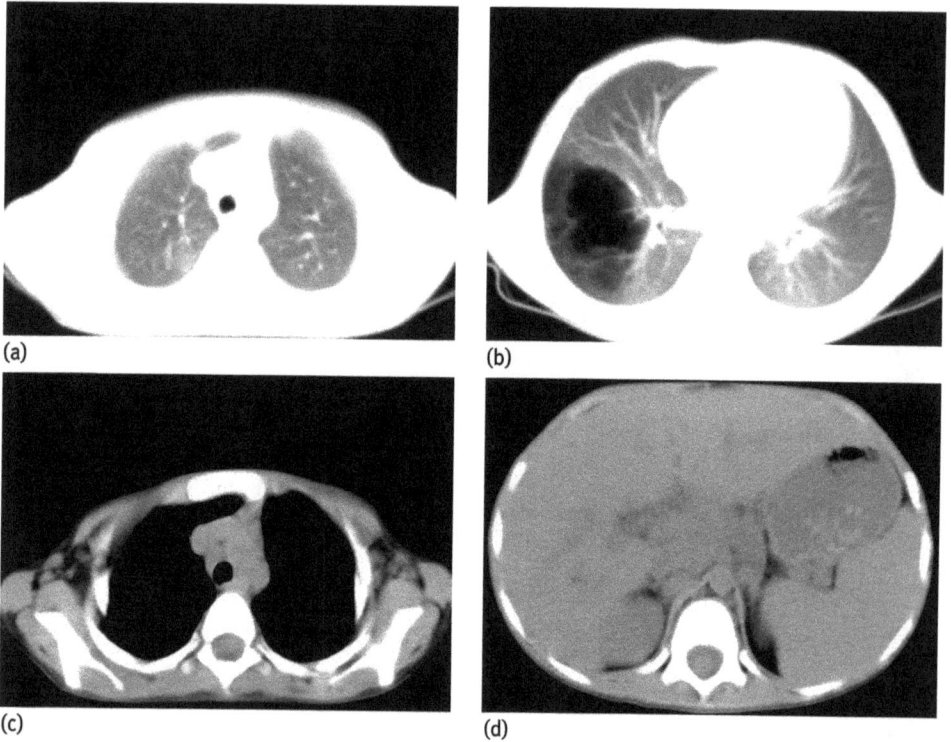

(a)

(b)

(c)

(d)

Fig. 15.9 a–f: Disseminated penicilliosis marneffei.

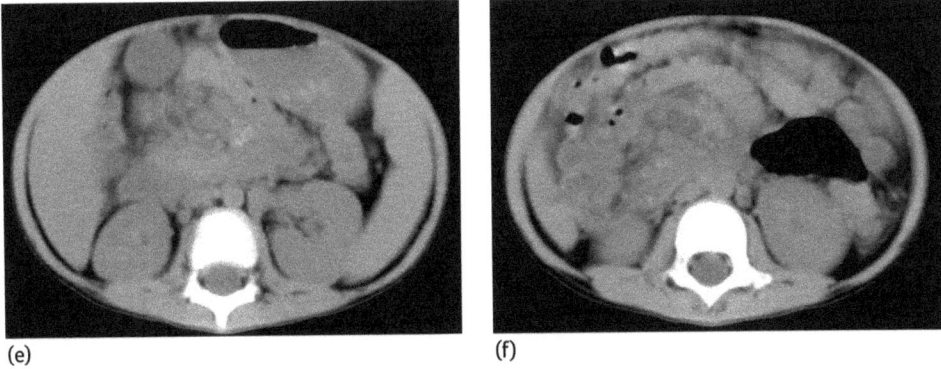

(e)　　　　　　　　　　　(f)

Fig. 15.9: (continuing)

CT scan with lung window showed a small high-density patchy opacity with blurry edge in the apicoposterior segment of right upper lobe (a), a separated giant cystic lesion in the right lower lung (b). CT scan with mediastinal window showed mildly enlarged paratracheal lymph nodes (c). Abdominal CT scans showed hepatospleno-megaly (d) and enlarged lymph nodes with blurry edges in the hepatic hilum and the mesenterium (d–f).

Case 15.10 (Figure 15.10 a-d)

A 3-year-old boy was admitted into hospital for recurrent fever and cough for 1 month, and diarrhea for 1 week. Multiple soybean-sized submaxillary nodes could be palpated. CD4+ cell count was 72/µl, CD4+/CD8+: 0.05. Sputum culture was *Pseudomonas aeruginosa* positive. The patient was diagnosed with AIDS (C3) combined with HIV wasting syndrome, pulmonary infection (*Pseudomonas aeruginosa*) and infectious diarrhea. After one-month treatment, the patient's conditions improved.

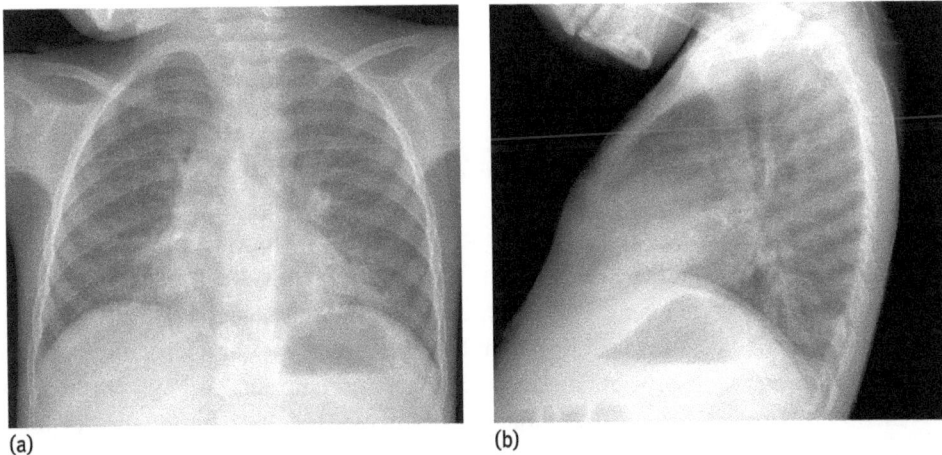

(a)　　　　　　　　　　　(b)

Fig. 15.10 a–d: Pulmonary infection *(Pseudomonas aeruginosa)*.

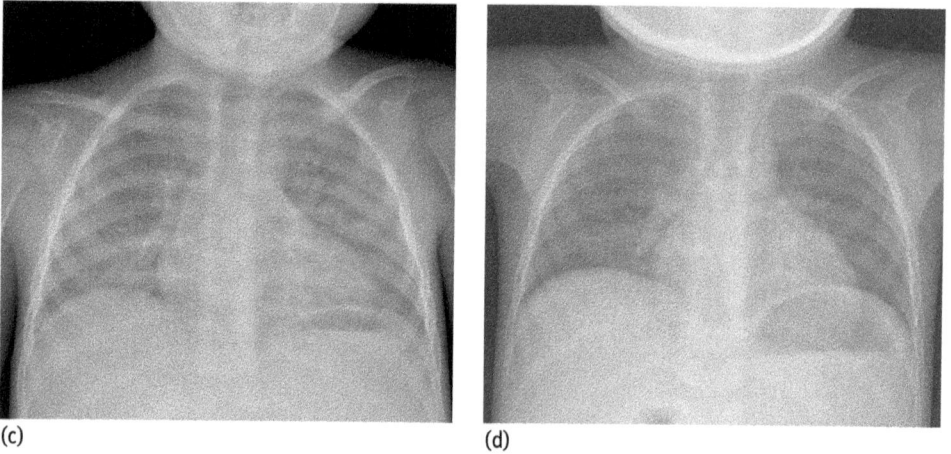

(c)　　　　　　　　　　　　　　　　　(d)

Fig. 15.10: (continuing)

Chest radiographs showed thickened markings in the bilateral lungs and blurry-edged patchy opacities in the lingual segment of left upper lobe and the right middle lobe (a, b). Chest radiographs at the rechecks after 8 weeks and 10 weeks showed gradually absorbed patchy opacities in the bilateral lung, improved interstitial changes and clearer lung fields than before (c, d).

15.3 Imaging features

Pulmonary diseases are one main cause for pediatric AIDS onset and even their deaths. Commonly, the diseases include bacterial pneumonia, pneumocystis pneumonia, tuberculosis, all kinds of fungal pneumonia and lymphoid interstitial pneumonia (LIP). In spite of very few specific findings in imagology, some features in chest radiographs and CT scans may indicate relevant etiological examinations and even diagnostic treatment.

1. Diffuse ground-glass-like shadows are common pulmonary changes in pneumocystis pneumonia.
2. Military diffused nodes are common pulmonary changes in tuberculosis and *Penicillium marneffei*. Importantly, in Southeast Asia and south China, the incidence of *Penicillium marneffei* is higher than in other parts of the world.
3. Lymphoid interstitial pneumonia is a kind of pulmonary disease prevalent in pediatric AIDS patients. Among them, the chest radiographs may display reticular and nodular lesions in pulmonary interstitiums and the chest CT scans display may confirm the small nodules in pulmonary interstitium, bronchiectasis and interstitial fibrosis. From the pathological point of view, these pulmonary lesions are identified to be clustered lymphocytes, plasmacytes infiltration in alveolar interstitial tissue and bronchus and lymphoid follicles with obscure margins in some areas.

Most of the children, normal in immunity, may not contract tuberculosis clinically even though they have bacterial infection. Pathologically, childhood tuberculosis is typical of primary syndrome which is self-healing. But for AIDS children, tuberculosis bacterial infection will fast progress to clinical tuberculosis in a short period of time.

Oral and gastrointestinal fungal infections are often complicated in pediatric AIDS and among those infections the most common is the *Candida albicans* infection. In imaging study, esophagography and CT examination may display esophageal mucosa destruction, different degrees of filling defects, niche and esophageal obstruction. The abdominal CT shows thickening of gastrointestinal tract wall and ulcers in the wall.

The common positive findings of pediatric AIDS by abdominal CT scanning indicate hepatosplenomegaly, enlarged mesenteric and retroperitoneal nodes, peritonitis, ascites and thickening of intestinal wall, which are frequently seen in opportunistic infections. For example, the disseminated penicilliosis marneffei mainly occurs in Southeast Asia and South China.

Editors: Lieguang Zhang, Yi Liang, Xiejie Chen, Weiping Cai

16 CT diagnoses and differential diagnoses of mediastinal hilar lymphadenopathy in AIDS patients

Due to the immunodeficiency caused by HIV infection, the patients are susceptible to opportunistic infections and related neoplasms, which manifest themselves as mediastinal hilar lymphadenopathy on chest CT images.

The lungs as well as hilar lymph nodes are usually involved by opportunistic infections, mostly by mycobacteria and fungal infections, which often turn out to be disseminated infections. On the other hand, lymph nodes are usually affected in lymphoma or Kaposi's sarcoma cases among patients with AIDS. Fishman reported that 55% of the hilar lymphadenopathy seen on CT scans among patients with AIDS (n = 40) was due to infections and 43% due to neoplasms. To our knowledge, hilar lymphadenopathy was mostly affected by opportunistic infections in a review of 178 patients with AIDS based on the pathological and etiological diagnosis study, accounting for 97.8%, among which penicilliosis marneffi and tuberculosis accounted for 67.2% and 24.1%, respectively. Only 2.2% (n = 4) of the cases were carcinomas, including 3 cases of Kaposi's sarcoma and 1 case of lymphoma, which is obviously lower than that reported in the literature.

In Fishman's study, on the other hand, patients with related neoplasms had much higher CD4+ cell count than patients with opportunistic infections. In our series and the previous experience, tuberculosis can be seen in any stage of HIV infection, and the severity of the disease depends on the immunologic status of the host. All the disseminated fungal infections are seen in patients with CD4+ count less than 200 cells/μL, while Kaposi's sarcoma and lymphoma could be seen in patients with CD4+ more than 200 cells/μL.

16.1 The imaging features of mediastinal hilar lymphadenopathy in AIDS patient

16.1.1 Opportunistic infections

Penicilliosis marneffei

Penicillium marneffei prefer the reticuloendothelial system including anaemia, epato splenomegaly and lymphadenopathy. Our previous studies based on the cases from our hospital showed that penicilliosis marneffei in the patients with AIDS manifested itself with mediastinal lymphadenopathy (58.33%), retroperitoneal and mesenteric lymphadenopathy (77.14%) and mesenteric 'Sandwich sign'. Hilar lymphadenopathy is part of systemic lymphadenopathy. In our study based on patients with AIDS who occurred mediastinal hilar lymphadenopathy (n = 178), 65.7% (117/178) of the cases were due to *Penicillium marneffei*. However, the CT images findings were non-specific, characterized by smaller ones with homogeneous density on plain scanning, and mostly mild, occasionally ring or even no enhancement on contrast CT scans. It is hard to distinguish from other opportunistic infections, such as disseminated histoplasmosis, cryptococcosis and tuberculosis. Diagnosis requires culture of the organism from a clinical specimen.

Tuberculosis

It has been reported that tuberculosis lymphadenitis among patients without HIV infection commonly presented with enlarged nodes with hypodense central and peripheral hyperdense enhancing rims, and these findings which are of great value for the differential diagnosis of mediastinal lymphadenopathy. 51% of these patients had active tuberculosis in lungs. Among the 42 cases of tuberculosis lymphadenopathy in our series, 20 cases presented as inhomogeneous density or central low-attenuation, 20 cases as homogeneous, and 2 cases as extremely low-attenuation on plain scans, with enhancing rims seen in 11 cases (11/13) and multilocular appearance in 7 cases. All of these 42 patients had active tuberculosis on both lungs, including diffused miliary small nodules seen in 20 patients. We believe mediastinal and hilar lymphadenopathy with inhomogeneous or central low-attenuation with enhancing rims, especially multilocular appearance may be characteristic appearance of tuberculosis lymphadenitis in patients with AIDS.

Cryptococcosis

Cryptococcosis in patients with ADIS manifests itself in the forms of meningitis, focal pneumonia and systemic infections that involving lymph nodes. In our study, 10 patients had blood culture proven of cryptococcus neoformans, 7 of who showed homogeneous density mediastinal lymph nodes, 3 central low density nodes, and 3 enhancing rims nodes, indicating central necrosis.

Non-tuberculous mycobacteriosis

The clinical features and radiologic performance of non-tuberculous mycobacteria lung disease and mycobacteria tuberculosis infection are similar, mediastinal or hilar lymphadenopathy is commonly seen in patients with AIDS.

16.1.2 Tumors

Kaposis sarcoma

The most common sites of Kaposis sarcoma in patients with AIDS are skin and respiratory tracts. 50% of the patients with HIV-related Kaposis sarcoma from the literature had pleura involvement, and 10–16% of the patients had pulmonary hilar or mediastinal lymph nodes involvement. In our study, 3 patients with AIDS were confirmed to be Kaposis sarcoma by biopsied of the skin, all of who had poorly defined small nodules with a peribronchovascular distribution, and mild enlarged of mediastinal lymphadenopathy. Markedly enhancement of the mediastinal nodes on delay phase of enhanced scans was found in one patient, with high density similar to that of the blood vessels. We believe that the enhancement pattern of the lymph node involved by Kaposis sarcoma is due to the rich of vessels and spindle cells: the more the blood vessels, the higher density is seen in CT scans.

Lymphoma

Different from that in non-AIDS patients, lymphoma in the patients with AIDS seldom involves the mediastinum. In our study, all of the 10 cases of AIDS-associated lymphoma are non-Hodgkin lymphoma, with homogeneous density and uniform enhancement mediastinal lymph nodes seen in only one patient.

16.2 The imaging features and differential diagnosis of mediastinal hilar lymphadenopathy in AIDS patient

16.2.1 Size of lymph nodes

In our study, mediastinal and hilar lymph nodes in patients with tuberculosis measured an average of 1.7 cm on the short axis, larger than nodes in patients with other opportunistic infections. Lymph nodes in lymphoma may grow fast in short time if treatment is unavailable.

16.2.2 Density of lymph nodes and enhancement mode

Xie et al. reported that mediastinal and hilar lymphadenopathy with enhancing rims or multilocular appearance was highly suggestive of tuberculosis lymphadenitis, and our study is coincident with this finding. Homogeneous and mild enhancement nodes are often seen in patients with *Penicillium marneffei* infection, and homogeneous and poorly enhancing nodes due to anergic and necrotizing tissue reaction usually found in patients with Penicilliosis marneffei. Markedly enhancement of the mediastinal nodes was found in one patient with Kaposis sarcoma.

16.2.3 Diffuse miliary lesions

Miliary nodules on both lungs indicate hematogenous infections, which mostly seen in patients with tuberculosis according to literature. In our study, disseminated miliary nodules in bilateral lung were seen in both patients with tuberculosis and penicilliosis marneffei.

16.2.4 Primary complex or similar-primary complex

In our daily clinical practice, pulmonary lesions that accompany affirmative mediastinal and hilar lymphadenopathy are commonly seen in patients with tuberculosis, and occasionally in patients with Penicilliosis marneffei. However, the primary complex sign in the hypoimmunity patients has not been identified to be a true tuberculosis, and what is more, those primary complexes caused by other infections except tuberculosis have not yet been explored comprehensively in the academic sphere, we provisionally define it as 'similar-primary complex'. In our series, the so called "primary complex" are seen in 9 patients with tuberculosis (9/42) and 4 patients with Penicilliosis marneffei (4/117). That means, tuberculosis is primarily considered and Penicilliosis marneffei secondarily once the 'similar-primary complex' is seen on CT scans among patients with AIDS.

16.2.5 Mesenteric lymphadenopathy (Sandwich sign)

Of all the 119 abdominal CT scans in our study, mesareic lymph nodes of "Sandwich sign" were found in 27 patients with Penicilliosis marneffei (27/87), 3 patients with cryptococcosis (3/4), and one patient with tuberculosis only, indicating that differences of locations of lymph nodes between disseminated fungal infections and abdominal tuberculous lymphadenitis. While none of the 10 patients with ADIS-related lymphoma in the same period of this study had mesareic lymph node involved. Therefore, the "Sandwich sign" is highly suggestive of disseminated Penicillionsis marneffei or cryptococcosis, the former predominant in South China.

16.2.6 Pleural effusion and pericardial effusion

Pleural effusion and pericardial effusion are found in patients with all opportunistic infections. Pleural effusion is statistically commonly seen in patients with tuberculosis (45.2%) than in patients with Penicilliosis marneffei. In our study, cultures of pleural effusion were positive in one patient with Penicilliosis marneffei and 2 patients with tuberculosis. And both pleural effusion and pericardial effusion were seen in one patient with Kaposis sarcoma.

In conclusion, opportunistic infections of all sorts and tumors can involve mediastinal lymphadenopathy in patients with AIDS, mycobacterial and fungal infections are the common pathopoiesis. There is a high incidence of Penicilliosis marneffei among

HIV-infected patients in Southern China. CT scans play an importance role in the differential diagnosis of mediastinal lymphadenopathy in AIDS patients.

Case 16.1 (Fig. 16.1 a–h) Disseminated PM.

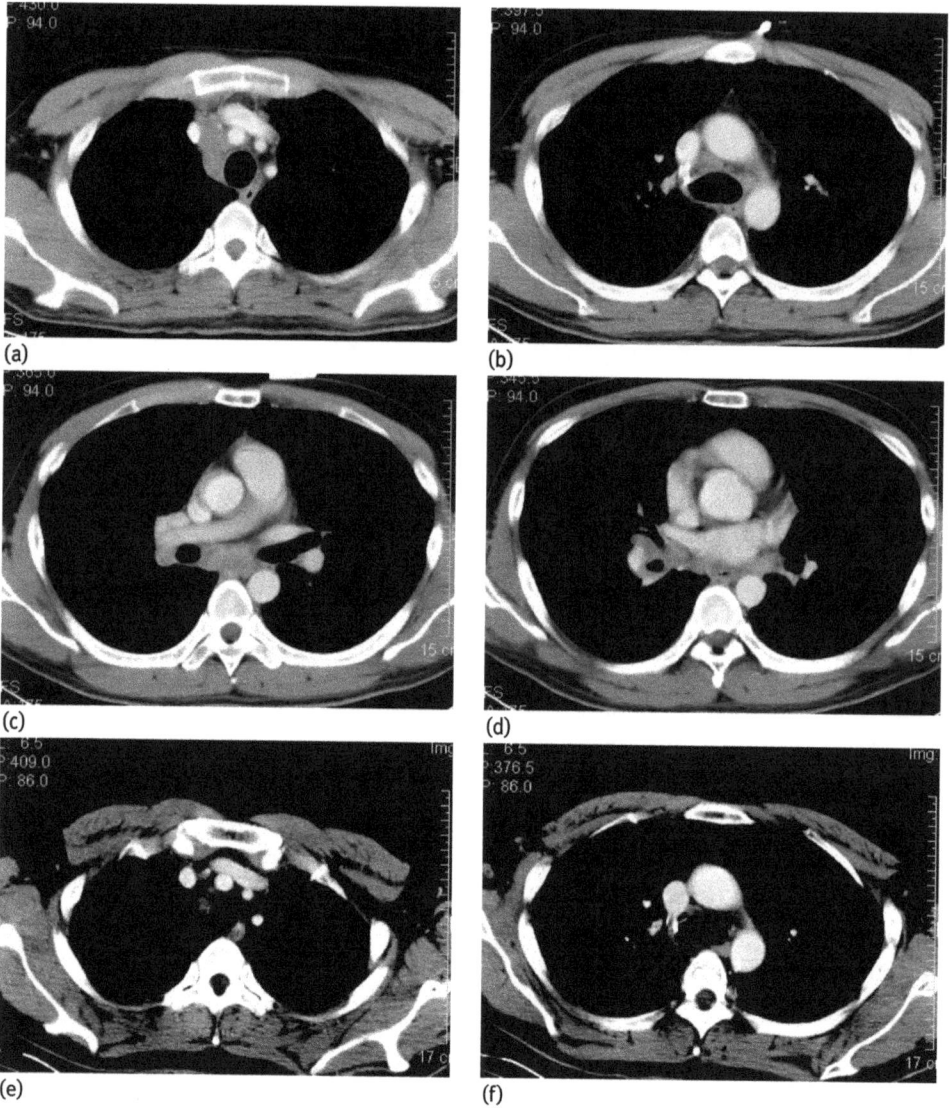

(a)

(b)

(c)

(d)

(e)

(f)

Fig. 16.1 a–h: Disseminated PM.

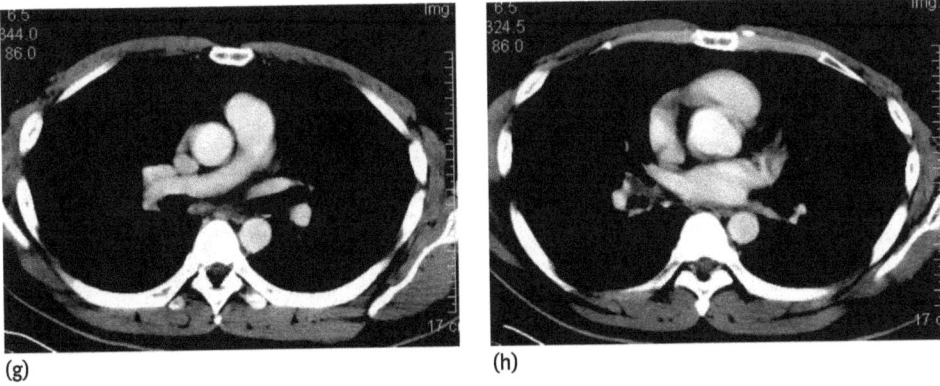

(g) (h)

Fig. 16.1: (continuing)

The enhanced chest CT scans with mediastinal window show the mediastinal and right hilar lymphadenopathy with homogenous enhancement (a–d). The obvious shrinkage of the lymph nodes are seen one month after regular treatment (e–h).

Case 16.2 (Fig. 16.2 a–l) Disseminated PM.

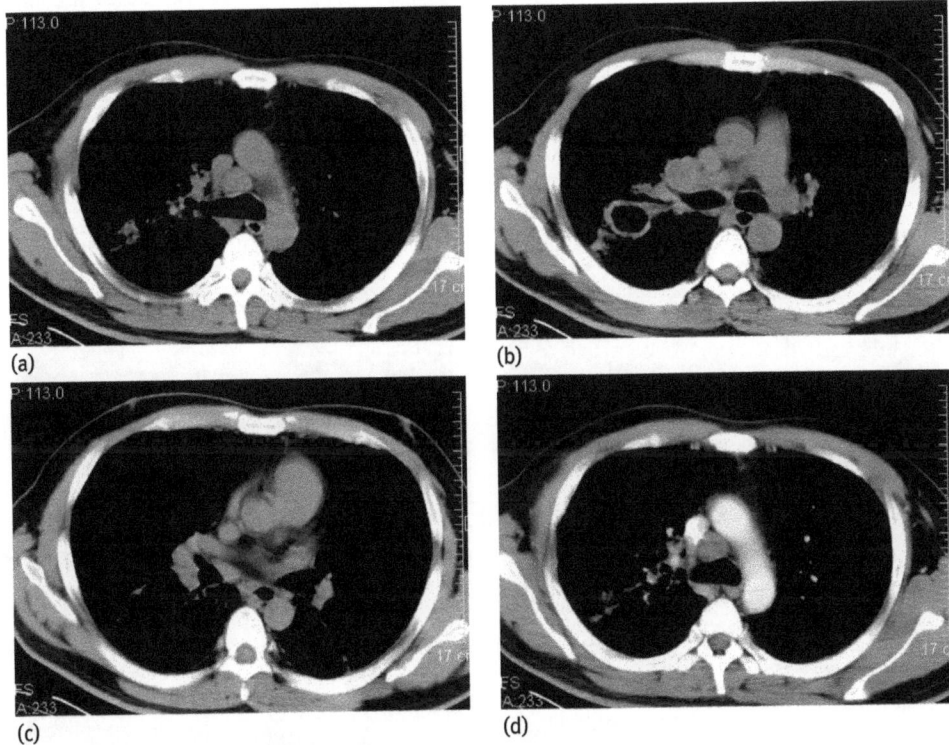

(a) (b)

(c) (d)

Fig. 16.2 a–l: Disseminated PM.

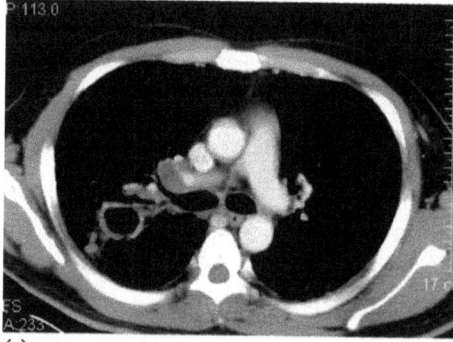

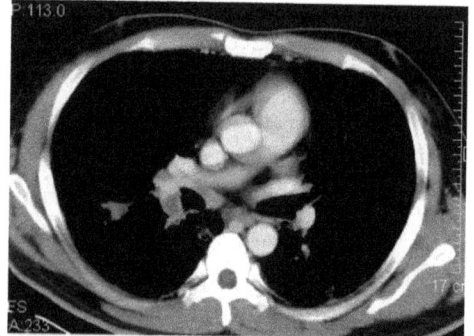

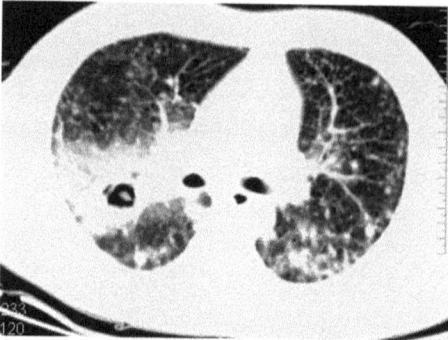

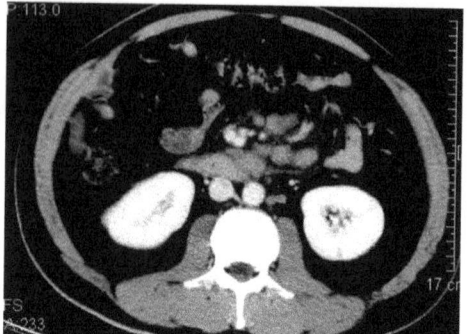

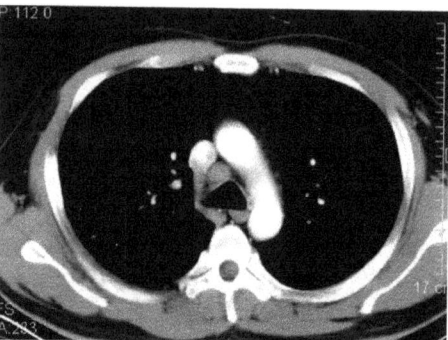

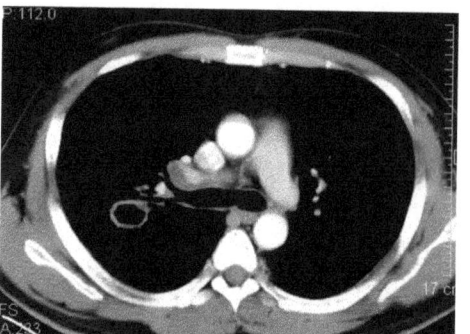

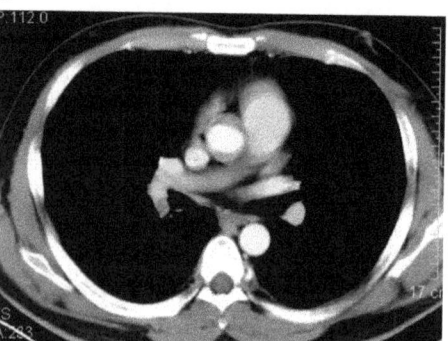

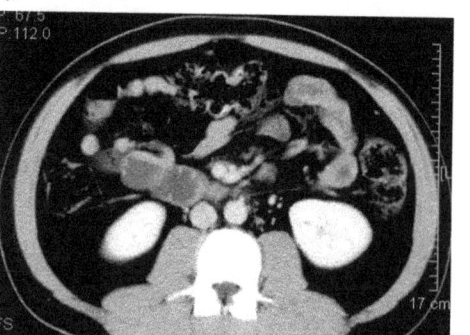

Fig. 16.2: (continuing)

Chest plain CT of mediastinal window (a–c) show mediastinal and right hilar con-glomerate soft-density enlarged lymph nodes. In enhanced CT scan, mediastinal enlarged lymph nodes present with homogeneous enhancement, right hilar lymph nodes present with poorly rim enhanced (d–f), and the 'primary complex' sign is seen (cavitary lesions in the right lung and right hilar lymphadenopathy). The CT scans with lung window (g) shows cavitary lesions on the right upper lung and miliary nodules on both lungs. In the enhanced CT scans (h), mesenteric lymphadenopathy with "Sandwich sign" is seen. The absorption of the cavitary lesion and shrinkage of mediastinal, hilar and mesenteric lymph nodes are seen after 3 weeks of standardized treatment (i–l).

Case 16.3 (Fig. 16.3 a–d) Disseminated PM.

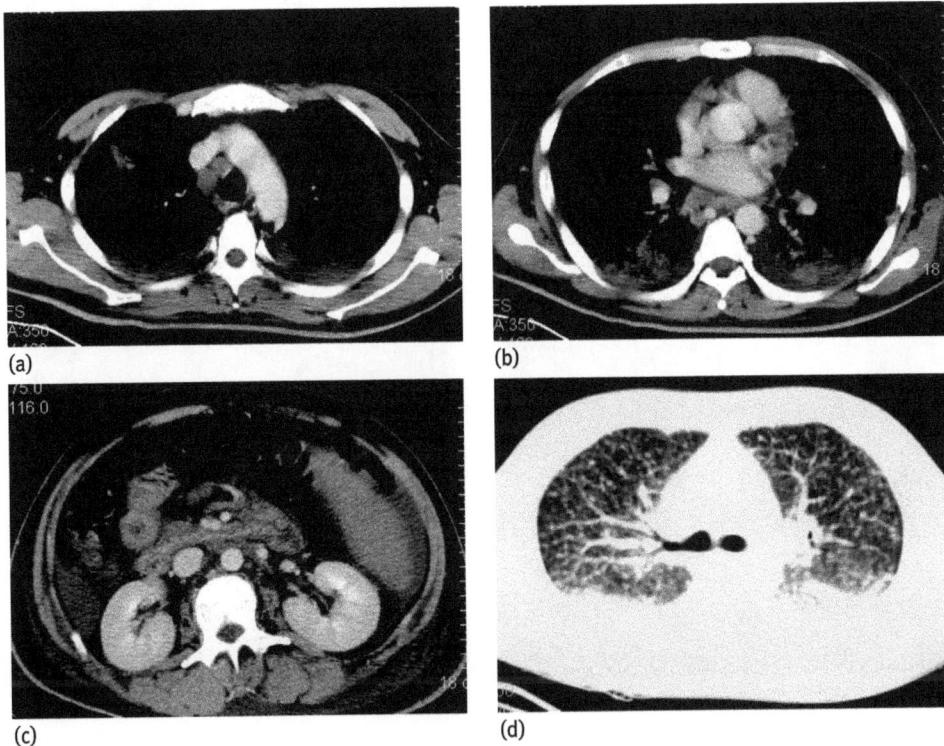

Fig. 16.3 a–d: Disseminated PM.

Enhanced CT scans (mediastinal window) show mild enlarge and homogeneous enhanced nodes on mediastinum and both hilar, bilateral pleural effusion (a–b). Mildly enlarged mesenteric and retroperitoneal lymph nodes and ascites are seen on enhanced CT scans (c). The CT scans with lung window (d) show disseminated miliary nodules in both lungs.

Case 16.4 (Fig. 16.4 a–h) Pulmonary tuberculosis.

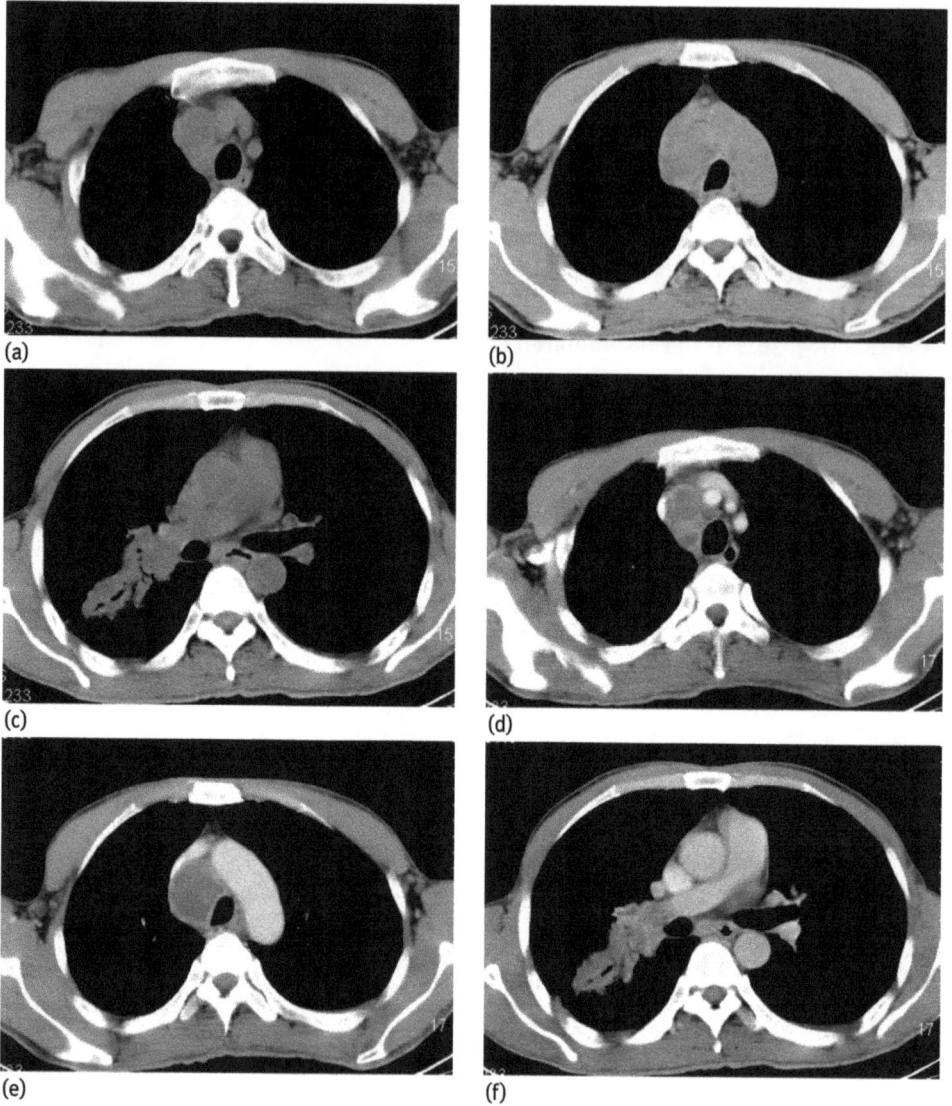

Fig. 16.4 a–h: Pulmonary tuberculosis.

Non-enhanced CT images (a–c) of mediastinal window show conglomerate mixed density nodal masses on mediastinum and right hilar with mixed and central-low density seen; the lesion in the right lung with a density of soft tissue linking to right hilar lymph nodes, presenting 'primary complex' sign. On the enhanced CT scans (d–f), these nodes have multilocular appearance and rim enhanced. The CT scans with lung window (g, h) show patchy lesions on the right upper lung and miliary nodules on both lungs.

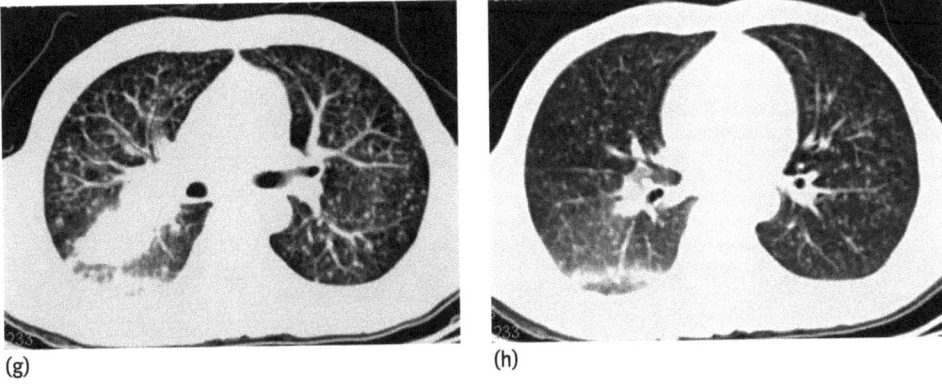

(g) (h)

Fig. 16.4: (continuing)

Case 16.5 (Fig. 16.5 a–f) Pulmonary tuberculosis.

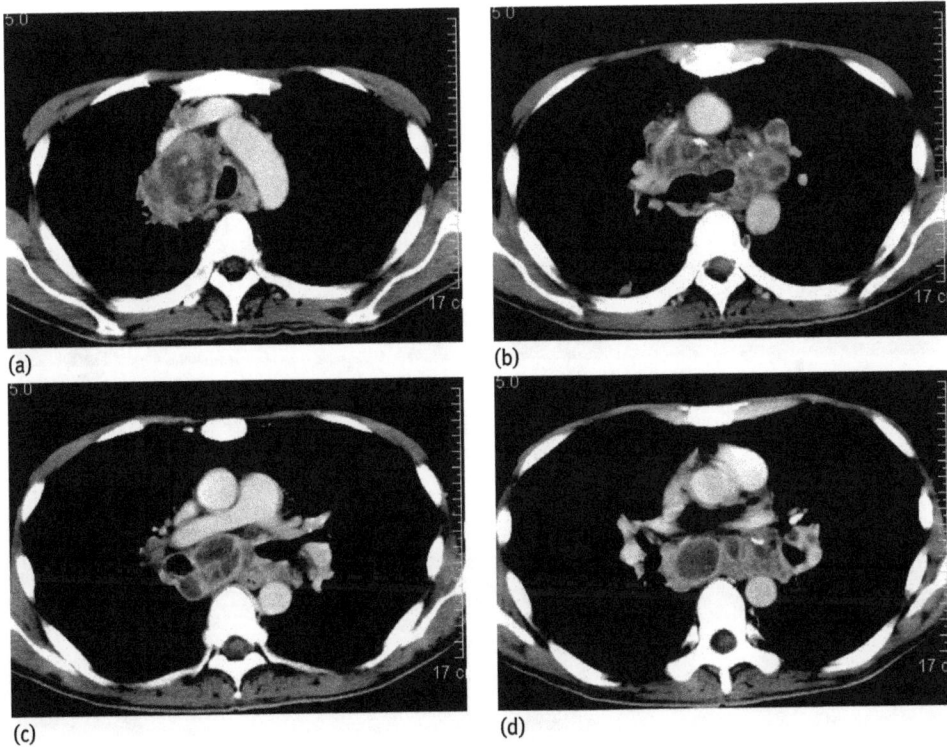

(a) (b)
(c) (d)

Fig. 16.5 a–f: Pulmonary tuberculosis.

The enhanced transverse CT images (a–d) of mediastinal window show conglomerate nodal masses on mediastinum and both hilar, with multilocular appearance and rim enhanced; abdominal CT scans (e–f) show the hepatic hilar region and retroperitoneal lymph nodes of different sizes with rim enhanced, and scattered miliary nodules in the spleen.

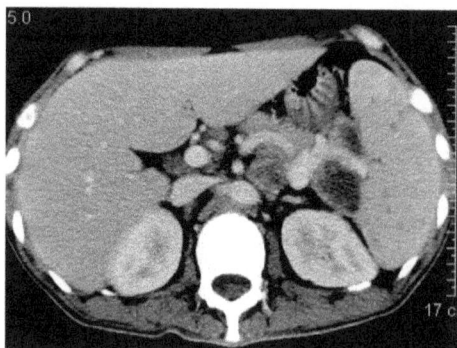

(e)

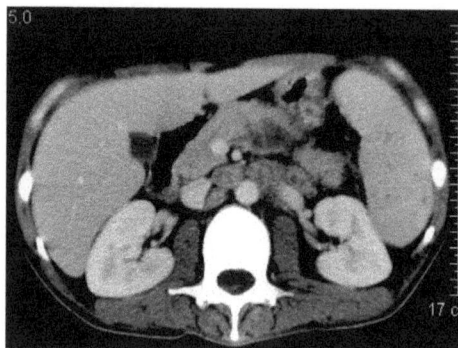

(f)

Fig. 16.5: (continuing)

Case 16.6 (Fig. 16.6 a–f) Pulmonary tuberculosis.

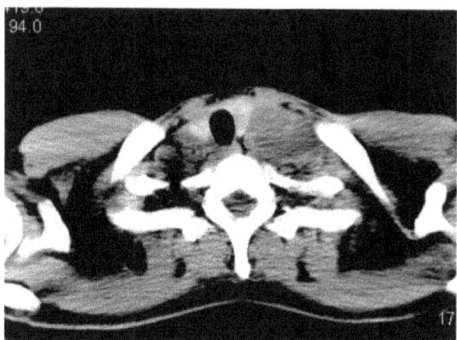

(a)

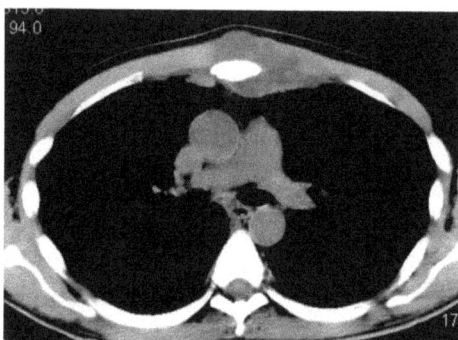

(b)

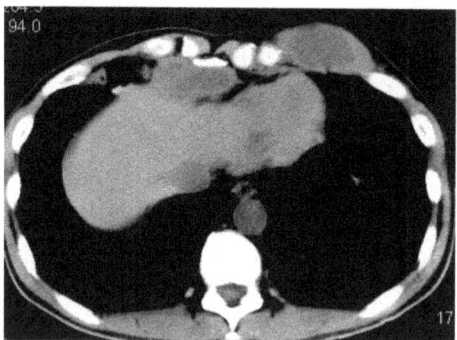

(c)

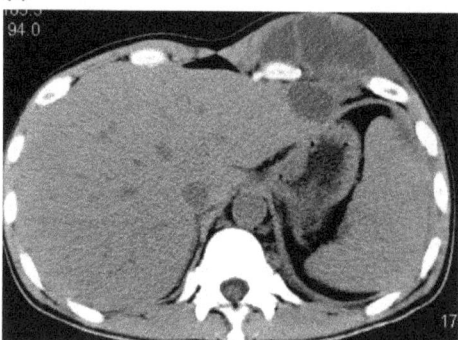

(d)

Fig. 16.6 a–f: Pulmonary tuberculosis.

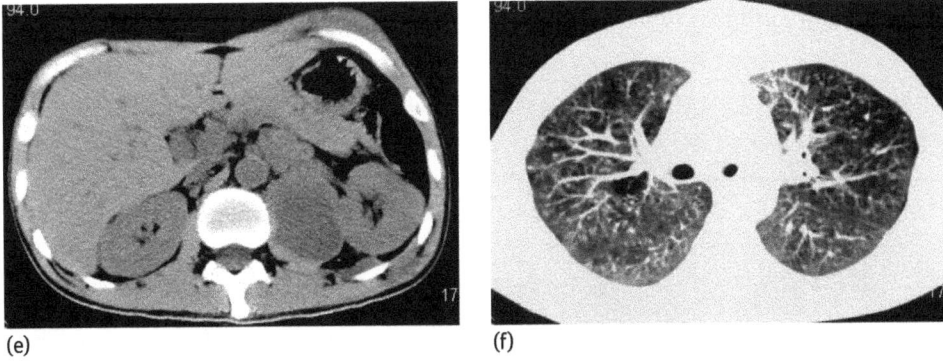

(e)　　　　　　　　　　　　　　　　(f)

Fig. 16.6: (continuing)

Non-enhanced transverse CT images (a–e) of mediastinal window show enlargement of the left upper mediastinal and right cardio-phrenic angle area lymphadenopathy, abscesses in the anterior chest wall and left psoas that all present as central-low density with thin wall, and the hepatic hilar region and retroperitoneal lymph nodes of different sizes. CT image of lung window (f) shows miliary nodules on both lungs.

Case 16.7 (Fig. 6.7 a–d) Non-tuberculous mycobacteriosis pulmonary disease

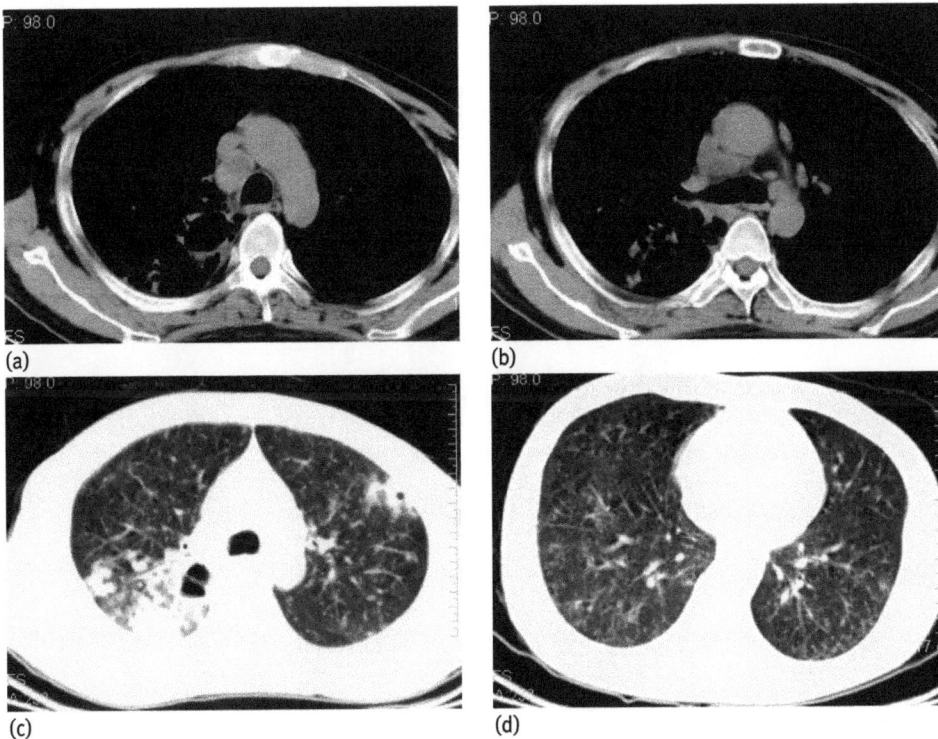

(a)　　　　　　　　　　　　　　　　(b)

(c)　　　　　　　　　　　　　　　　(d)

Fig. 16.7 a–d: Non-tuberculous mycobacteriosis pulmonary disease.

Non-enhanced transverse CT images (a–b) of mediastinal window show mildly enlarged mediastinal lymphadenopathy with central-low density; CT images of lung window (c–d) show cavitary lesions and with scattered miliary nodules with "tree-in-bud" sign on both lungs

Case 16.8 (Fig. 16.8 a–d) Non-tuberculous mycobacteriosis pulmonary disease

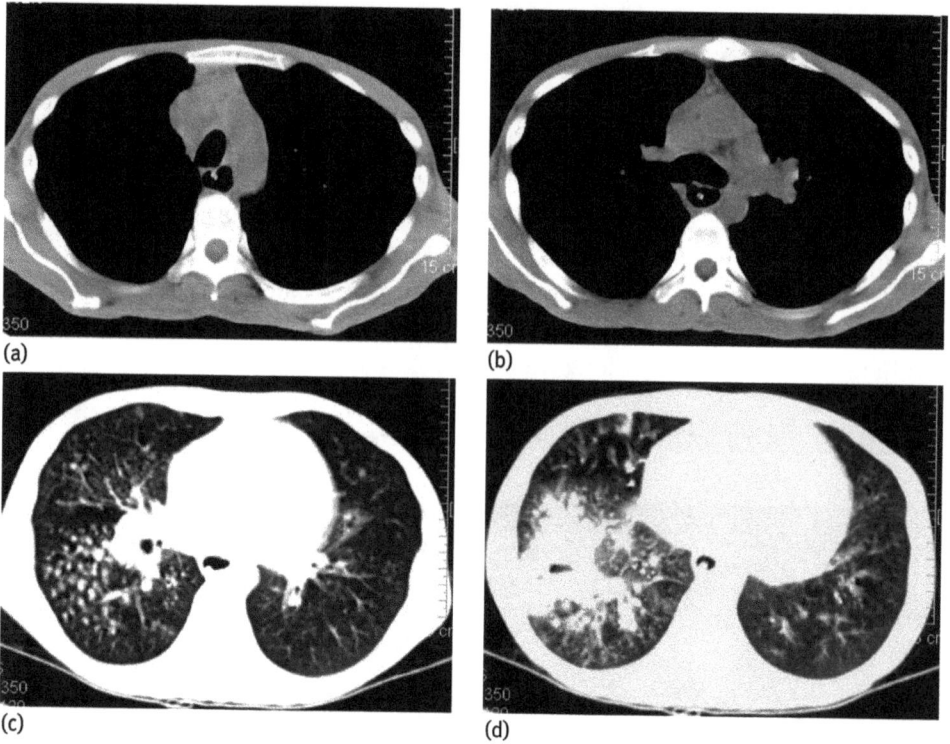

Fig. 16.8 a–d: Non-tuberculous mycobacteriosis pulmonary disease.

Non-enhanced transverse CT images (a–b) of mediastinal window show mildly enlarged mediastinal lymphadenopathy with low density; CT images of lung window (c–d) show a cavitary lesion with nodules of "tree-in-bud" sign seen in the right lower lung and scattered miliary nodules on both lungs.

Case 16.9 (Fig. 16.9 a–d) Cryptococcosis

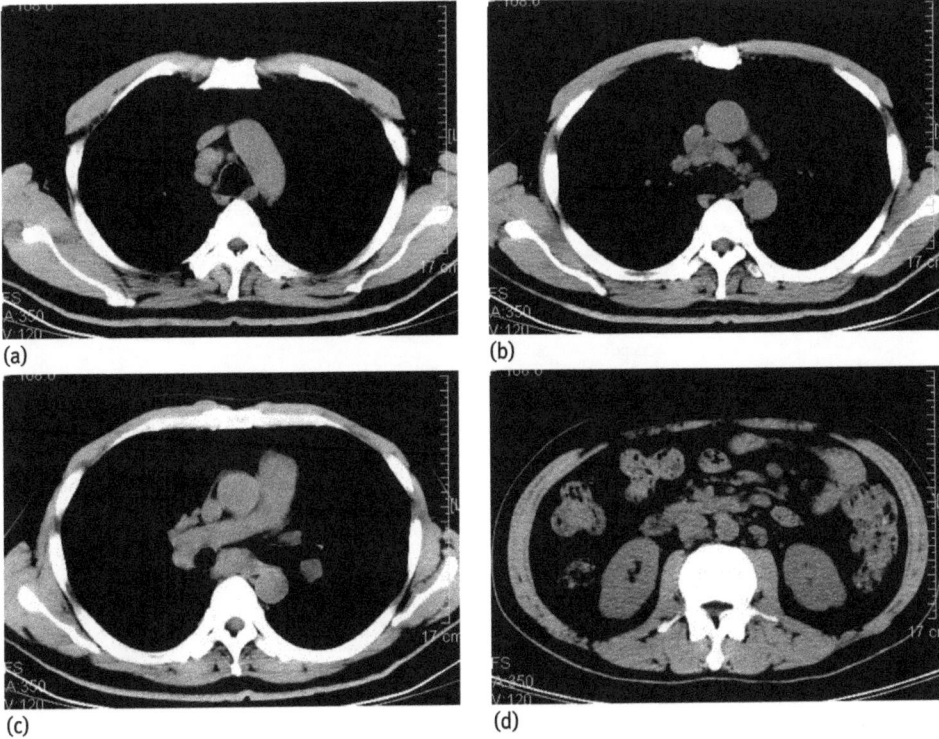

Fig. 16.9 a–d: Cryptococcosis.

Non-enhanced transverse CT images (a–c) of mediastinal window show mildly enlarged mediastinal lymphadenopathy with a density of soft tissue; abdominal CT images (d) shows mild enlarged mesenteric and retroperitoneal lymphadenopathy.

Case 16.10 (Fig. 6.10 a–d) Cryptococcosis

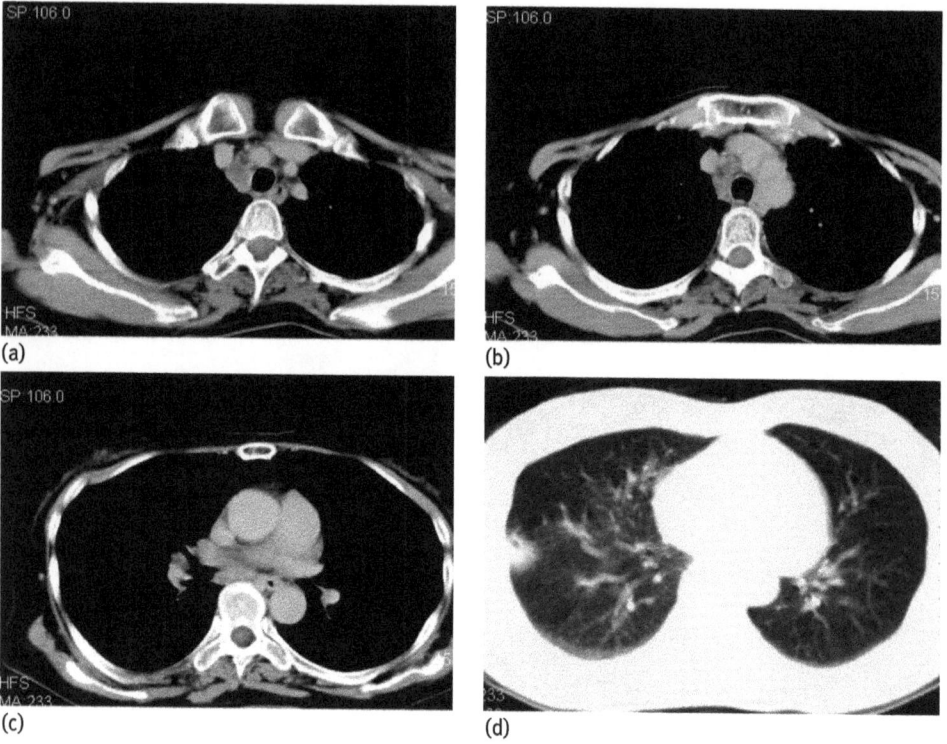

Fig. 16.10 a–d: Cryptococcosis.

Non-enhanced transverse CT images (a–c) of mediastinal window show mildly enlarged mediastinal and right hilar lymphadenopathy with a density of soft tissue; CT image D shows a cavitary nodule in the right upper lung.

Case 16.11 (Fig. 16.11 a–f) Kaposi sarcoma

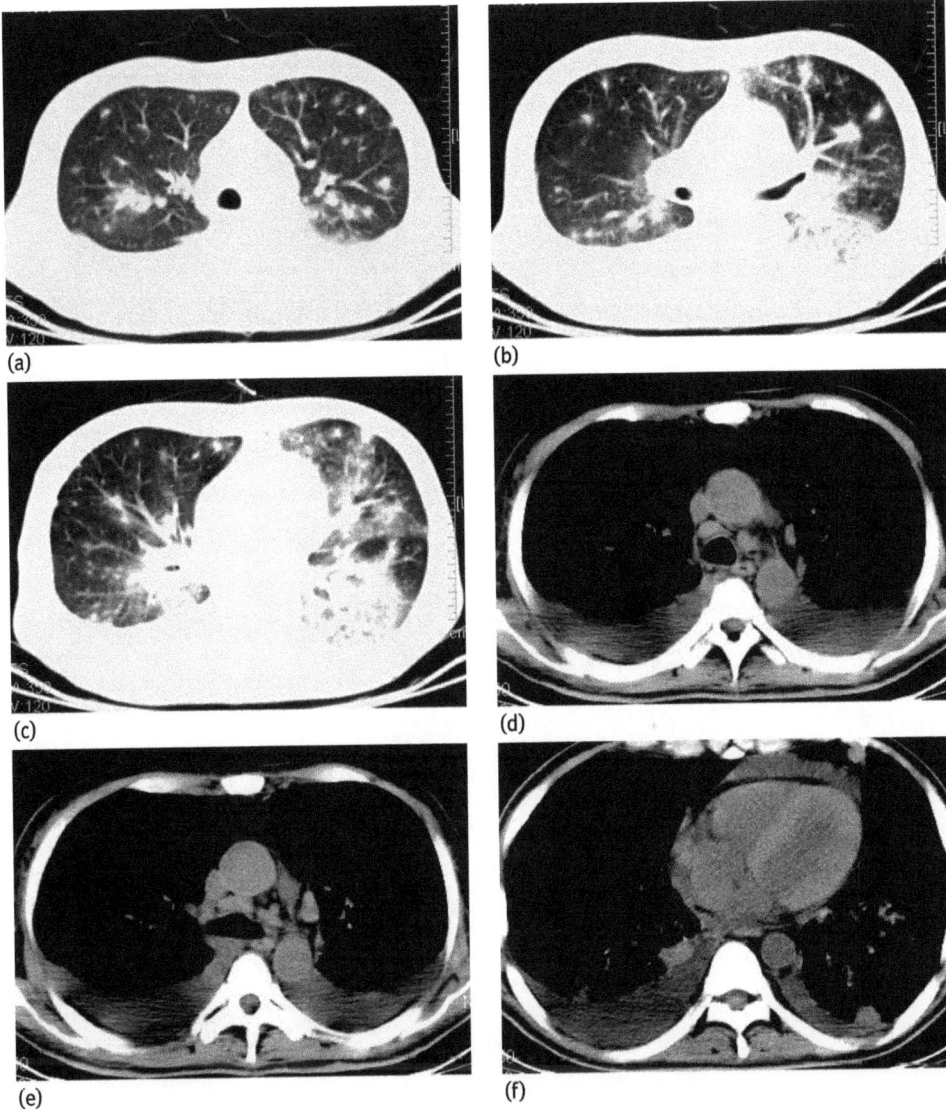

Fig. 16.11 a–f: Kaposi sarcoma.

Non-enhanced transverse CT images (a–c) in a patient with proven show skin KS showed the present of bilateral and symmetric ill-defined nodules in a peribroncho-vascular distribution (flame-shaped lesions). CT images of mediastinal window (d–f) show mildly enlarge of mediastinal lymphadenopathy with a litter higher density, bilateral pleural effusion and pericardial effusion.

Case 16.12 (Fig. 16.12 a–f) Kaposi sarcoma

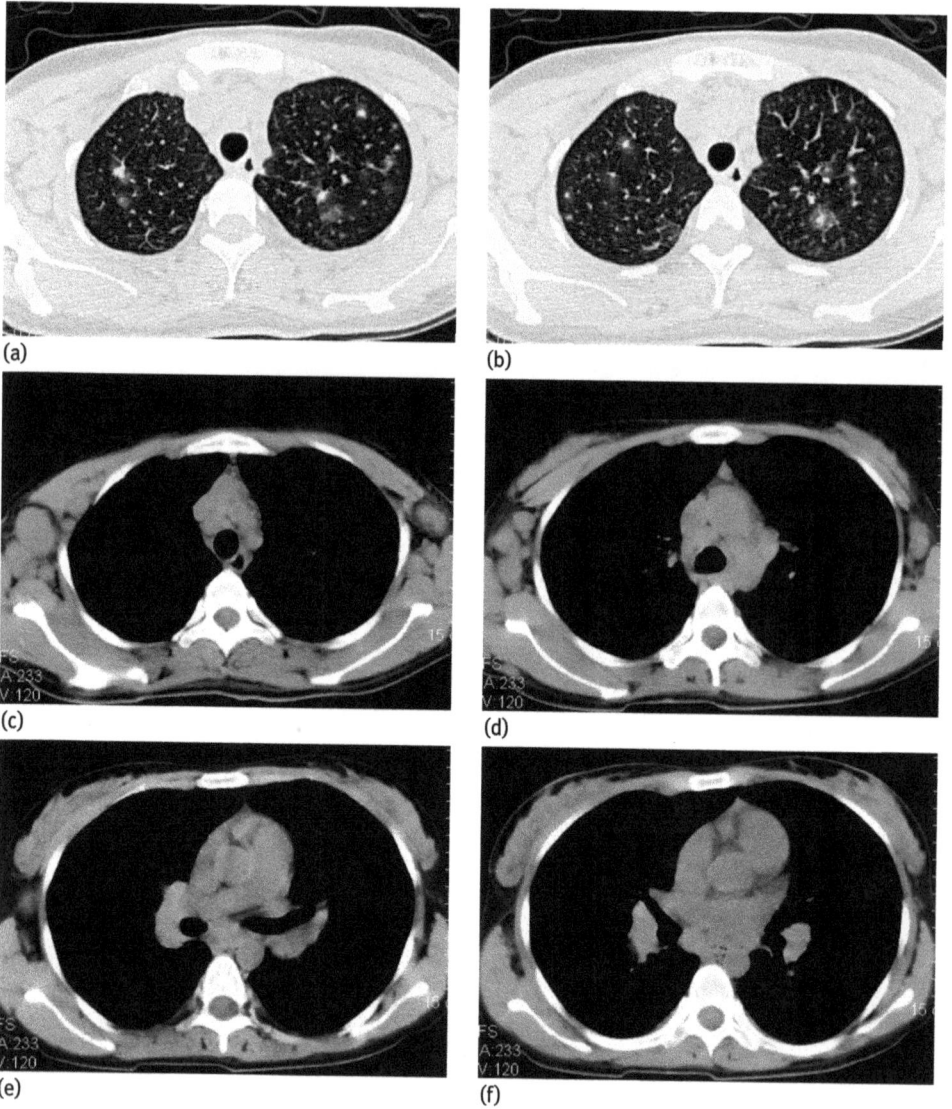

(a) (b) (c) (d) (e) (f)

Fig. 16.12 a–f: Kaposi sarcoma.

Non-enhanced transverse CT images of lung window (a, b) show scattered poorly defined nodules in both lungs; images of the mediastinal window (c–f) show mediastinal and bilateral axillary lymphadenopathy with a density of soft tissue.

Case 16.13 (Fig. 16.13 a–l) Lymphoma

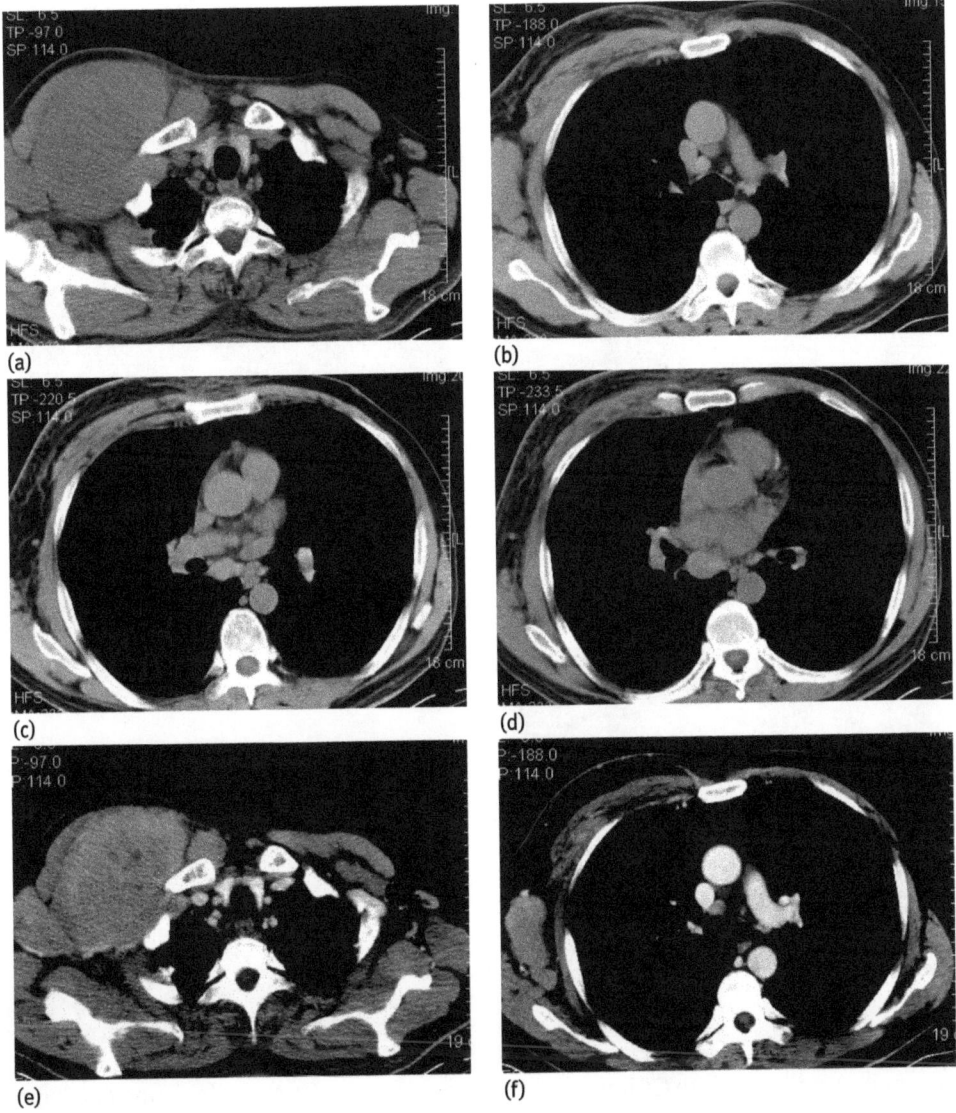

Fig. 16.13 a–l: Non-Hodgkin's lymphoma.

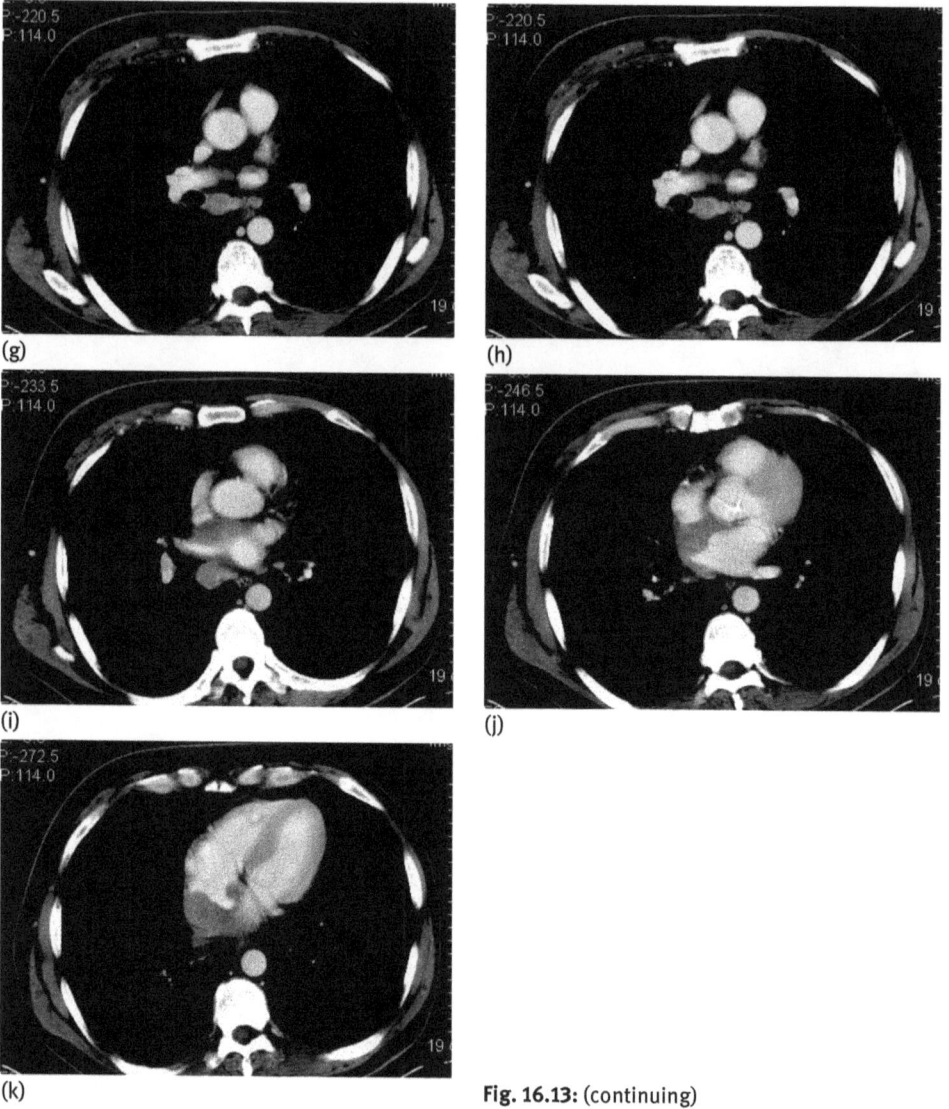

Fig. 16.13: (continuing)

Non-enhanced transverse CT images (a–d) and enhanced CT scans (e–l) show a giant mass with a density of soft tissue in the right anterior chest wall, mediastinal and right axillary lymphadenopathy, and filling defect in the right atrium (a–l).

Editors: Lieguang Zhang, Yi Liang, Deyang Huang

17 CT diagnoses and differential diagnoses of cavitary pulmonary diseases in AIDS patients

Pulmonary opportunistic infection is the most common complication in AIDS, usually manifest with pulmonary cavity. In pathology, cavity results from the introduction of air into the lesions when the liquidized necrotic tissues are expelled via bronchus. In radiology, it presents with airy lacouna with intact wall, generally more than 1mm thick. Most pulmonary complication related with HIV can result in cavity formation. AIDS-associated cavity pulmonary disease (CPD), in most cases, is caused by opportunistic infections by bacteria, Mycobacterium tuberculosis, non-mycobacterium tuberculosis or fungi; relatively, non-infectious cavity pulmonary disease is rare.

We have retrospectively analyzed the imaging data of 85 cases of AIDS-associated CPD treated in our hospital in recent years, concluding the imageological features as followed in Table 17.1.

Table 17.1: The CT sign of 85 cases of AIDS-associated CPD

CT Features		TB	NTM	Pulmonary abscess	Pulmonary mycosis
Cases		28	6	12	39
Superior lobe		27	5	10	19
Focal diameter	≤2 cm	9	3	9	25
	2.4cm	14	1	7	12
	≥4 cm	12	3	7	5
Solitary CPD		15	5	3	33
Thick walled cavity		17	3	9	16
Consolidated cavity		10	3	9	3
Regular cavity		12	3	8	25
Smooth inner wall		17	4	11	28
Coarse outer wall		22	6	8	27
Nodular wall		4	0	0	7
Intra-cavitary liquid-air interface		1	1	4	3
Sublobe		5	0	1	9
Trabs		13	1	1	4
Halo sign		3	1	2	10
Calcification		8	0	0	0

Table 17.1: (continuing)

CT Features	TB	NTM	Pulmonary abscess	Pulmonary mycosis
Satellite foci	21	4	1	5
Bronchiectasis	6	3	0	1
Bronchial drainage	8	0	0	2
Involved pleura	10	1	1	4
Lymphadenectasis	10	1	1	11

The brief points for CT diagnosis and differential diagnosis
1. TB: The CT manifestations of TB are characterized by location at the superior lobe, satellite foci, funicular shadows around the focus, calcified foci on the cavitary wall or around it, shadows of bronchial drainage and affected pleura, which are statistically significantly different from those of non-TB.
2. NTM: The CT signs of bronchiectasis from NTM are significantly different from non-NTM. The difference of satellite foci in NTM, pulmonary abscess and pulmonary fungal disease is statistically significant.
3. Pulmonary abscess: Pulmonary abscess is significantly different from non-pulmonary abscess in terms of three CT signs, including multiple cavities, diameter >4 cm and liquid-air interface in the cavities.
4. Pulmonary fungal disease Solitary cavity is specific for pulmonary mycosis but not for non-pulmonary mycosis.

17.1 AIDS-associated TB

As kind of special inflammation caused by *Mycobacterium tuberculosis*, TB is one of most common opportunistic infections in AIDS patients. Cavities are more tend to happen in patients with AIDS than those patients are non-immunosuppression, in early stage of HIV infection, when the cell immunity are at a high level, it's common that cavity occurs in TB.

The major imaging features of AIDS-associated TB cavity are concluded as followed: most cavities have typical predilection location, like apex of lung, posterior segment of superior lobe and dorsal segment, usually occurs in nodules or consolidation, presenting with irregular thin-walled or thick-walled, liquid-air interfaces is relatively less common. The cavity may be solitary or multiple, multiple cavities located in upper lobe are common, manifest with insect-bite or sclerotized multilocular shape. Besides, calcification foci can be seen in the wall or around, satellite foci around it and funicular shadows; shadow of branchial drainage beside hilum of lung; involved pleura, mediastinal and/or hilar lymph enlarged. HRCT can show small cavity, small calcification and draining branchial. The cavity sign showed in CT scan have less difference in AIDS patients with TB and non-immunosuppression patients with TB.

Case 17.1 (Fig. 17.1 a–c)

Images from a 46-year-old male with AIDS C3 and pulmonary TB infection, clinical history and symptom: recurrent pharyngalgia, cough and fever for 1 month, accompanied with weight loss. Physical examinations at admission: body temperature was 37.8 °C, no superficial lymph nodes enlarged. The CD4+ cell counted 79/µl. Sputum smear: antiacid bacillus tuberculosis, Sputum culture and identification was *Mycobacterium tuberculosis*.

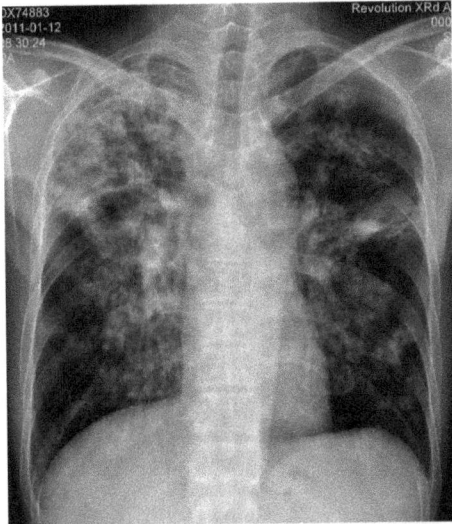

(a)

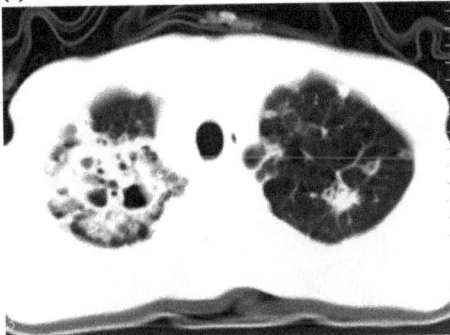

(b)

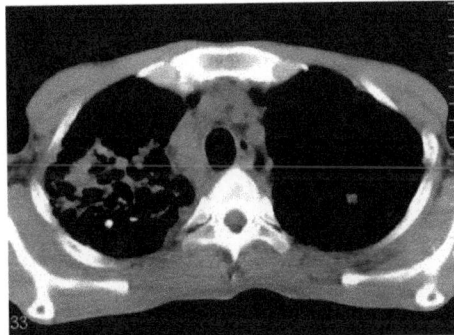

(c)

Fig. 17.1 a–c: Pulmonary *Mycobacterium tuberculosis*.

The plain film showed wide distributed edge-blurred patchy, disseminated lesions in the right upper lung with small multiple irregular patchy opacities with lower density (a). CT scan (lung window) showed large consolidation on the apex of right lung, with multiple small insect-bite cavities in it and adjacent pleural thickening; small patchy shadow on the apex of left lung (b). Mediastinal window showed small calcified lesions in the apex of right lung and right paratracheal lymph nodes enlarged (c).

Case 17.2 (Fig. 17.2 a–c)
Images from a 37-year-old male with AIDS C3 and pulmonary TB infection, clinical history and symptom: cough, expectoration of sputum mixed with blood streaks for 5 months, and afternoon fever for 4 days. Physical examinations: admission body temperature was 38.8 °C, no superficial lymph nodes enlarged. The CD4+ cell count

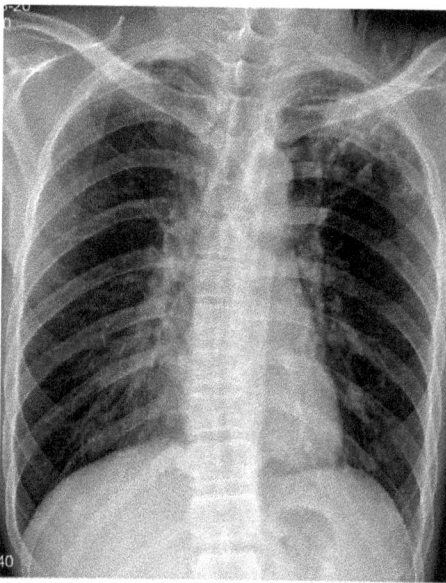

(a)

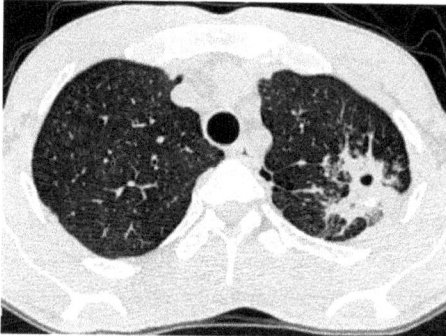

(b)

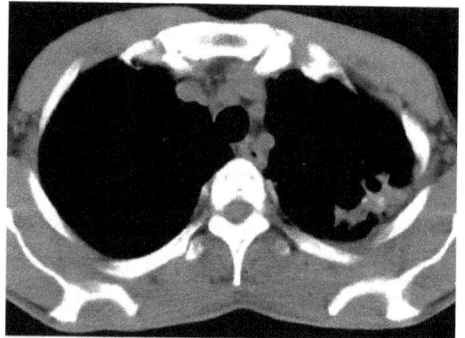

(c)

Fig. 17.2 a–c: Pulmonary *Mycobacterium tuberculosis*.

was 49/µl. Sputum smear: antiacid bacillus tuberculosis, Sputum culture and identification was *Mycobacterium tuberculosis*.

The chest film showed multiple edge-blurring patchy with uneven density (a). HRCT showed the small thick-walled cavity on the apex of left lung, which was uneven in thickness and with smooth inner wall surrounded by funicular shadows and satellite foci (b). CT scan (mediastinal window) showed multiple calcified lesions in the wall of the cavity (c).

Case 17.3 (Fig. 17.3 a–e)

Images from a 32-year-old male with AIDS C3 and pulmonary TB infection. Clinical history and symptom: productive cough for 5 months, sputum mixed with blood streaks and afternoon fever for 4 days. Physical examinations: the highest body temperature reached 37.9 °C. Multiple enlarged lymph nodes were palpated in the bilateral necks and supraclavicular fossa. CD4+ cell counted 239/µl. Sputum smear: antiacid bacillus tuberculosis ; sputum culture and identification was *Mycobacterium tuberculosis*.

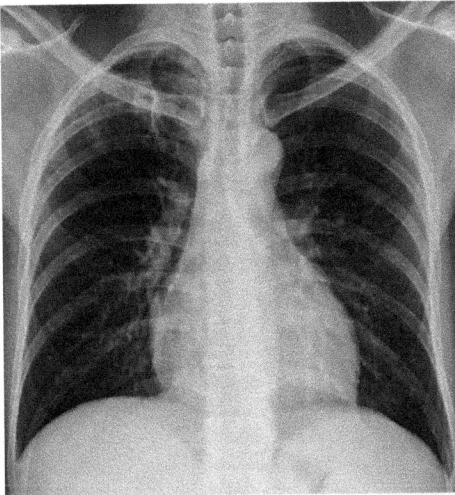

(a)

Fig. 17.3 a–e: Pulmonary *Mycobacterium tuberculosis*.

Chest film showed irregular cavity in right upper lung, with blurring edge, uneven wall, funicular shadows at its margin, and multiple satellite foci around it (a). CT scan (lung window) showed irregular edge-blurring thick-walled cavities, funicular shadows around it, a sign of satellite and adjacent pleural adhesions (b). HRCT showed the smooth inner wall of the cavity (c). CT scan (mediastinal window) showed small calcification in the lesion, mild mediastinal lymph nodes enlarged (d–e).

(b)

(c)

(d)

(e)

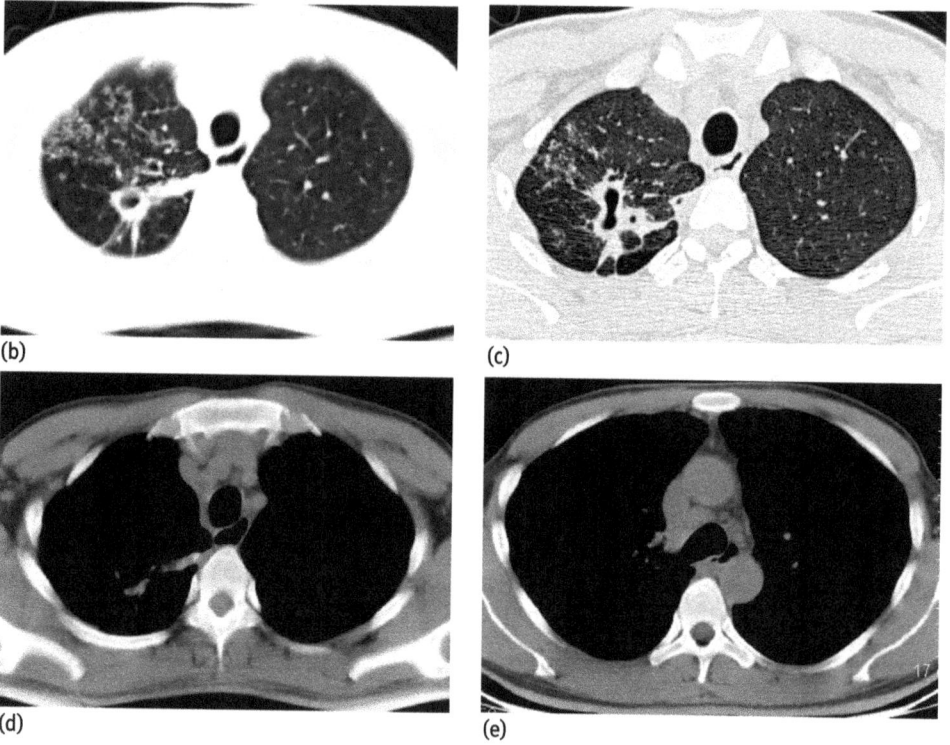

Fig. 17.3: (continuing)

Case 17.4 (Fig. 17.4 a–g)

Images from a 38-year-old male with AIDS C3 and pulmonary TB infection. Clinical history and symptom: recurrent productive coughs for over 2 months, accompanied with blood streaks sputum. Physical examinations: the admission body temperature was 36.8 °C. Multiple enlarged lymph nodes of the left neck and armpit can be palpated. The CD4+ cell count was 188/μl. BALF culture and identification: *Mycobacterium tuberculosis.*

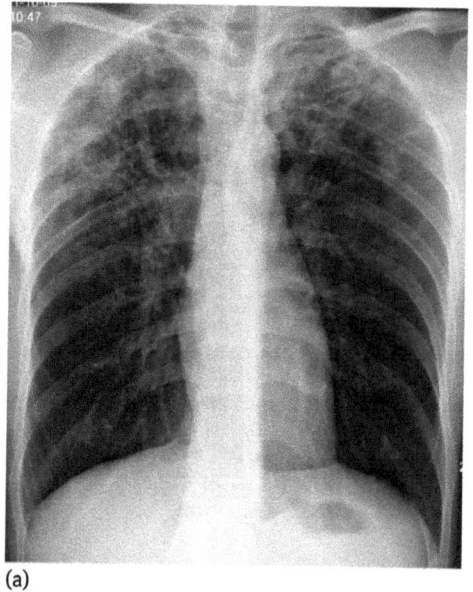

(a)

Fig. 17.4 a–g: Pulmonary *Mycobacterium tuberculosis.*

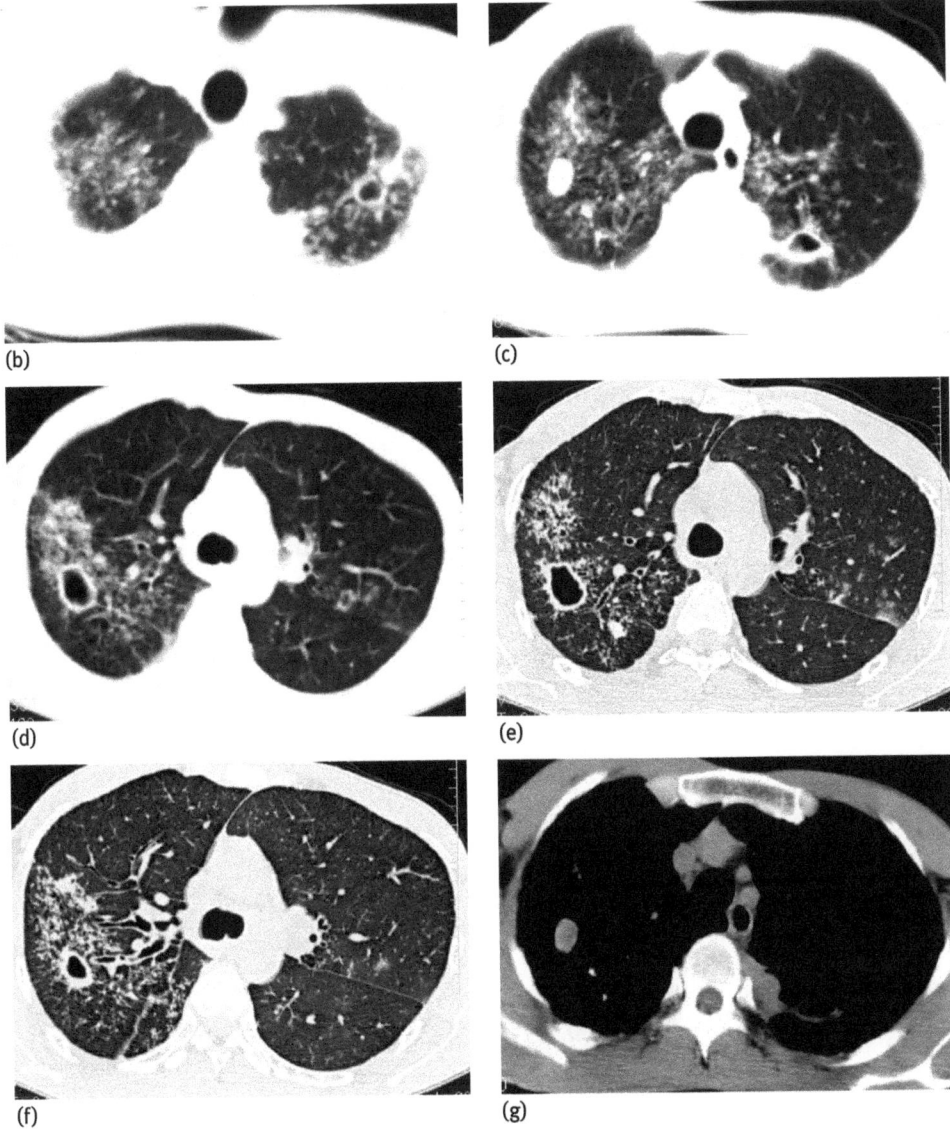

(b)

(c)

(d)

(e)

(f)

(g)

Fig. 17.4: (continuing)

The chest film showed the widespread edge-blurred nodular, patchy and funicular high density shadows of varied size, with multiple thin-walled cavities of different sizes in it (a). CT scan (lung window) showed multiple thin-walled cavities, with regular formation, blurring edge, smooth inner wall, satellite foci, and adjacent pleural thickening and adhesions (b–d). HRCT showed Isolated bronchiectasis in the superior lobe of right lung (e, f). CT scan (mediastinal window) showed the small calcification in the lesion of right upper lobe, and liquid-air interfaces in posterior segment of superior lobe of left lung (g).

17.2 AIDS-associated NTM diseases

Non-tuberculous mycobacteria (NTM) is referred to as mycobacteria excluding *Mycobacterium tuberculosis* complex (MTC) and mycobacterium leprae (ML). AIDS-associated NTM pulmonary disease is caused by *Mycobacterium avium* complex (MAC), with a higher incidence of cavities.

The major image features of AIDS-associated NTM pulmonary disease are concluded as followed: a higher rate of solitary or multiple cavitary lesions located at upper lobe; location of cavities in lung consolidation or in the nodules with regular or irregular shapes; diffusive foci of bronch; bronchiectasis which increases in incidence during focal absorption. Its final diagnosis depend on bronchofibroscopic lavage (BALF) culture or lung biopsy culture of NTM.

Case 17.5 (Fig. 17.5 a–e)

Images from a 38-year-old male with AIDS C3 and NTM pulmonary disease. Clinical history and symptom: an abscess at the left elbow for half a year, herpes at the left abdomen for 2 month, fever for 1 month. Physical examinations: the admission body temperature was 38.6 °C and no superficial lymph nodes was palpated enlarged. The CD4+ cell count was 3/μl. BALF culture and identification: NTM.

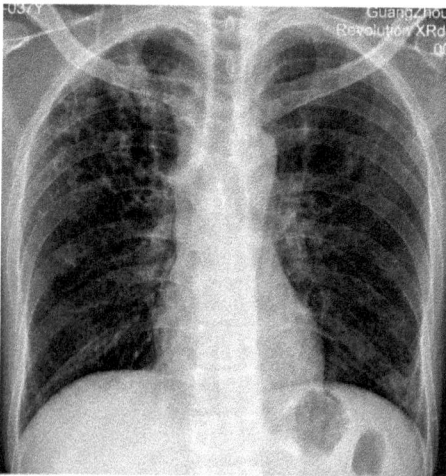

(a)

Fig. 17.5 a–e: NTM pulmonary disease.

The chest radiograph showed the multiple blurring-edge opacities in bilateral upper lobes, with multiple varied size cysts in right upper lesion (a). CT scans (lung window) showed multiple thin-walled cavities of different sizes in the superior lobe of both lungs with blurring edges and smooth inner wall, a satellite lesion around them, sig-

(b) (c)

(d) (e)

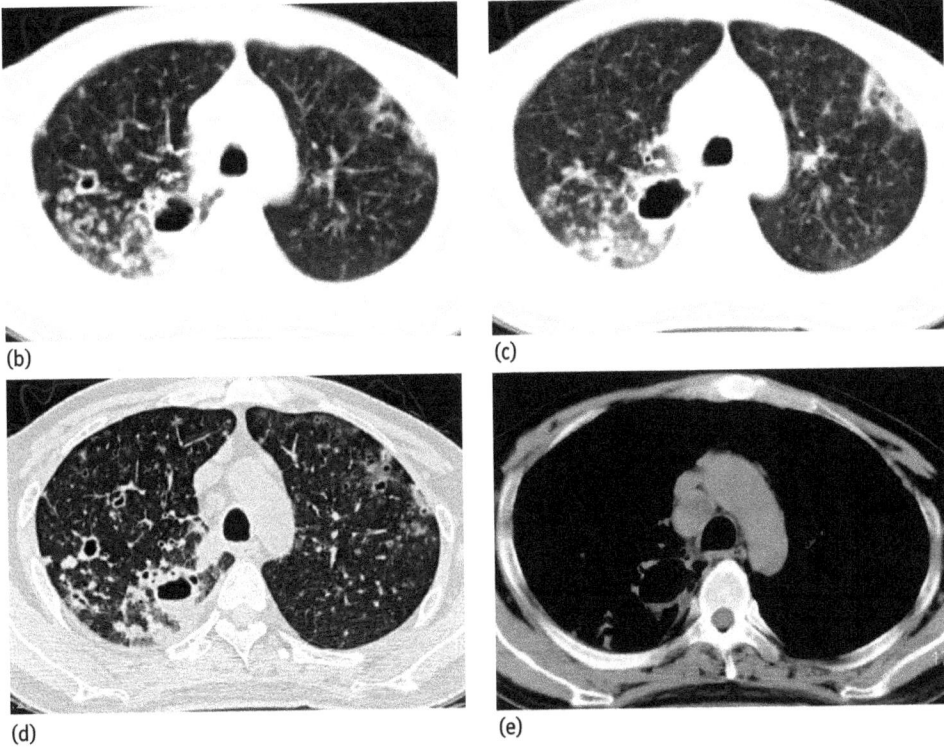

Fig. 17.5: (continuing)

nificantly in right lung (b–d). CT scan (mediastinal window) showed the liquid-air interface in the superior lobe of right lung and paratracheal lymphadenectasis on the right size (e).

Case 17.6 (Fig. 17.6 a–g)

Images from a 25-year-old male with AIDS C3 and NTM pulmonary disease. Clinical history and symptom: recurrent fever for one month, productive cough, short breath for two weeks, Physical examinations: the admission body temperature was 39.5 °C. No obvious chilliness and shivers, no rash. No superficial lymph nodes was palpated enlarged. The CD4+ cell count was 16/µl. BALF culture and identification: NTM.

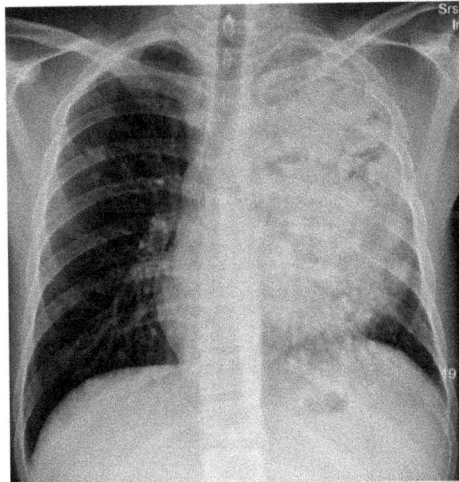

(a)

Fig. 17.6 a–g: NTM pulmonary disease.

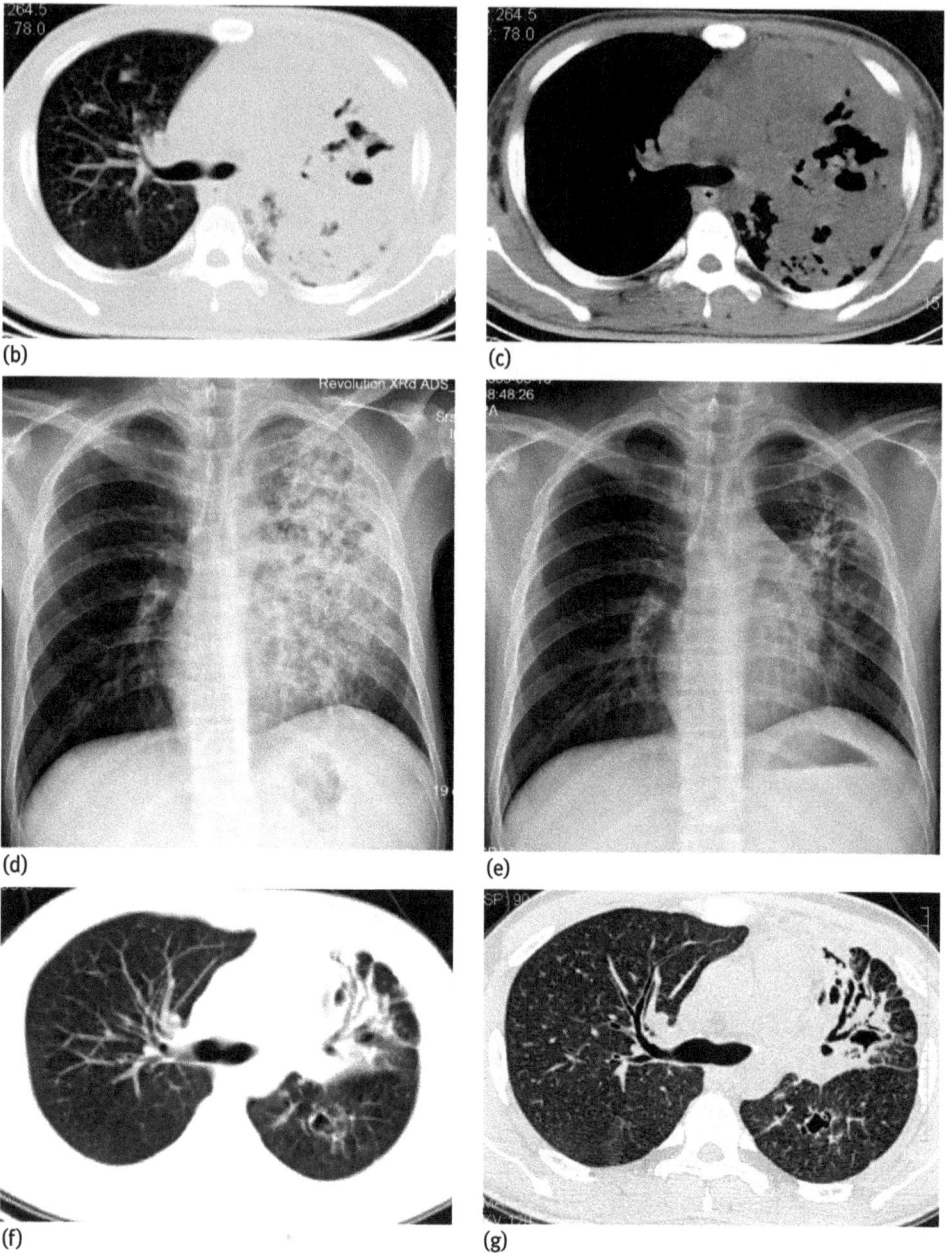

Fig. 17.6: (continuing)

The chest radiograph showed large consolidation in the left lung, with air-filled bronchi and cavitation in it, multiple edge-blurring nodules in the right lung (a). CT scan demonstrated the same manifestations. The CT scan with mediastinal window show massive consolidation in the left lung with air pronchogram in it. The CT scan 2 weeks after treatment shows obvious absorption with multiple cavities in it (d). The chest radiograph at recheck 7 weeks after that shows further absorption of the lesions in the left lung, the funicular lesions of the residuals and the shrinkage of left lung (e). The CT scans with lung window at recheck 8 weeks after treatment show obvious absorption of the lesion in the lungs, evident bronchiectasis as well as the fibrosis, and the elimination of nodular lesions in the right lung (f–g).

17.3 AIDS-associated pulmonary abscess

Some bacterial pneumonia are always complicated with cavities, which proceed into pulmonary abscess. *Staphylococcus aureus* and bacillus pyocyaneus are most common pathogen that cause lung abscess. Nocardia asteroids and rhodococcus are relatively less common, but with high incidence of cavity.

The major imaging features of lung abscess in AIDS patient can be concluded as follow: the multiple lung abscess are usually caused by *Staphylococcus aureus* septicemia, presenting with multiple irregularly diffused distributed cavities, which may show different size and thick-walled, liquid-air interfaces can be seen in cavity sometimes; besides, multiple patchy infiltrates and blurry nodular are always accompanied by. The solitary lung abscess is usually caused by pneumococci, gram negative bacilli (e. g., *Klebsiella pneumoniae*) and rhodococcus, which cavity rate is higher than the immunocompetent normal people. CT can show large cavity in the lung consolidation, with smooth inner wall, liquid-air interface in the cavity. AIDS-associated pulmonary abscess in radiology include: for multiple pulmonary abscess, *Staphylococcus aureus* being the major pathogens, disseminated multiple foci, thick-walled cavities of different sizes with possible liquid-air interfaces in them and patchy blurry nodular foci in the lung.

Case 17.7 (Fig. 17.7 a–d)

Images from a 32-year-old male with AIDS C3 and staphylococci aureus pneumonia. Clinical history and symptom: irregular fever with no inducing factors for 1 month, the highest body temperature was 40 °C, accompanied by chilliness and shivers, severe cough in daytime, productive sticky yellow mucus mixed with a little blood streaks occasionally, the symptom of night sweat was obvious.No superficial enlarged lymph nodes were palpated. The CD4+ cell count was 508/μl. BALF and blood culture and identification: *Staphylococcus aureus*.

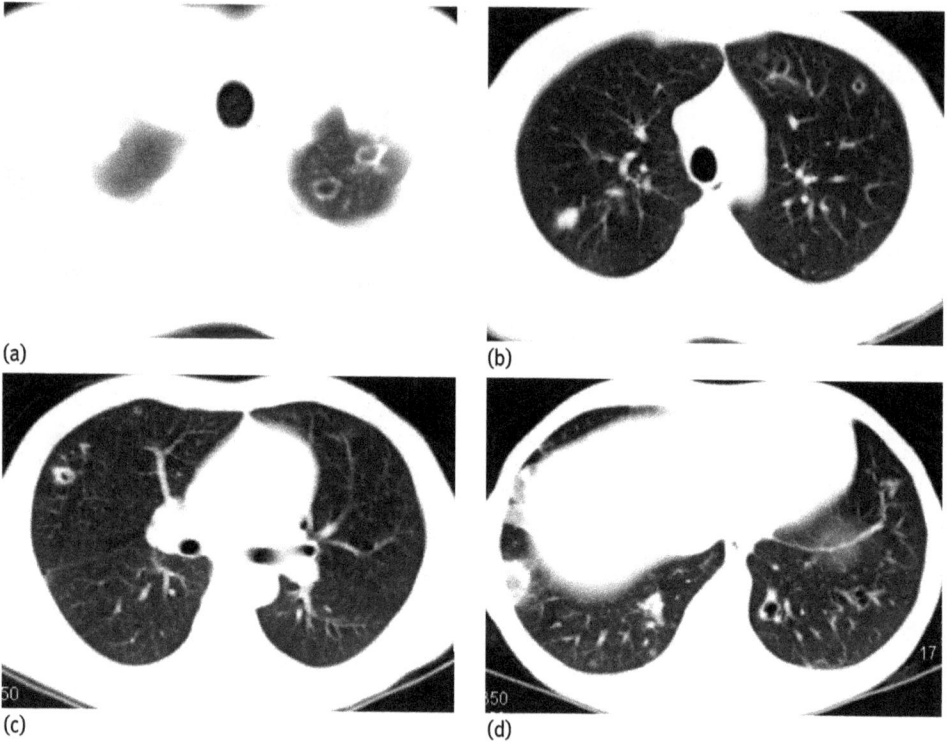

Fig. 17.7 a–d: *Staphylococci aureus* pneumonia.

CT scans showed multiple different size nodules in bilateral lungs, with blur edge, cavities can be seen formed in most lesions, which wall were uneven and inner wall was smooth (fig. a–d).

Case 17.8 (Fig. 17.8 a–d)

Images from a 32-year-old male with AIDS C3 and staphylococci aureus pneumonia. Clinical history and symptom: fever for half a month, the highest body temperature was 40.1 °C, accompanied by chilliness and shivers. Physical examinations: enlarged lymph nodes were palpated in the right mandibule. The CD4+ cell count was 47/μl. BALF culture, blood and bone marrow culture: *Staphylococcus aureus*.

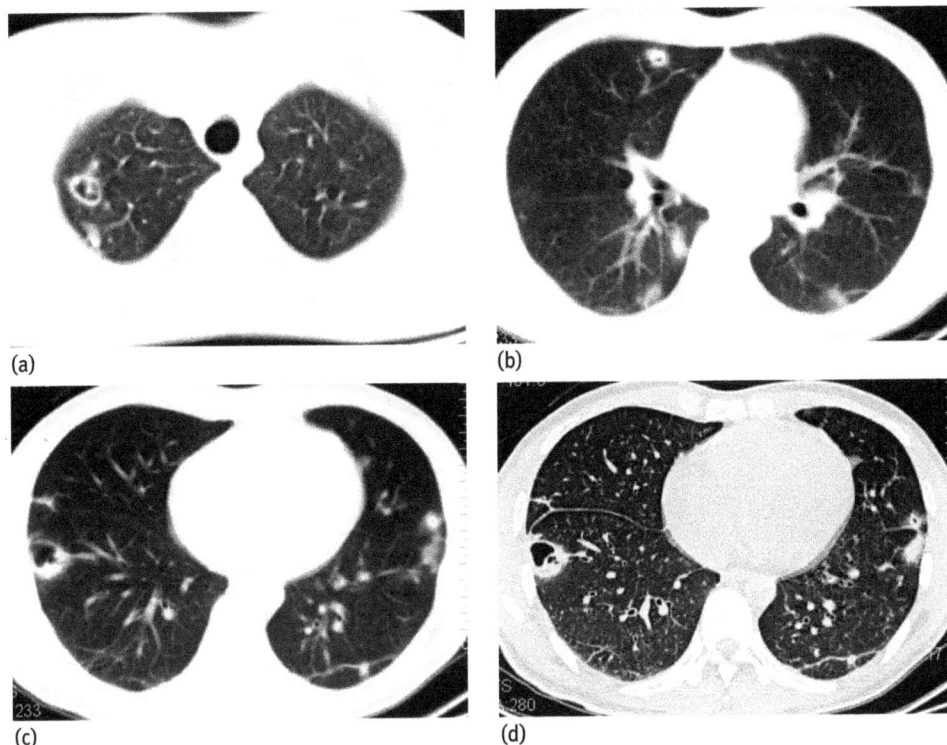

(a)

(b)

(c)

(d)

Fig. 17.8 a–d: *Staphylococci aureus* pneumonia.

CT scans showed multiple various size nodules in bilateral lungs, with blur edge, cavities formed in the most lesions, cavity wall were uneven, most inner wall were smooth, small septation can be seen in some cavity (a–d).

Case 17.9 (Fig. 7.9 a–e)

Images from a 41-year-old male with AIDS C3 and *Rhodococcus equi* pneumonia. Clinical history and symptom: recurrent coughs, hemoptysis and occasional fever for 3 months, the admission body temperature was 38.3 °C. Physical examinations: dry and moist rales in the bottom of left lung were heard by auscultation. No superficial enlarged lymph nodes were palpated. The CD4+ cell count was 77/μl. BALF and blood culture and identification: rhodococcus.

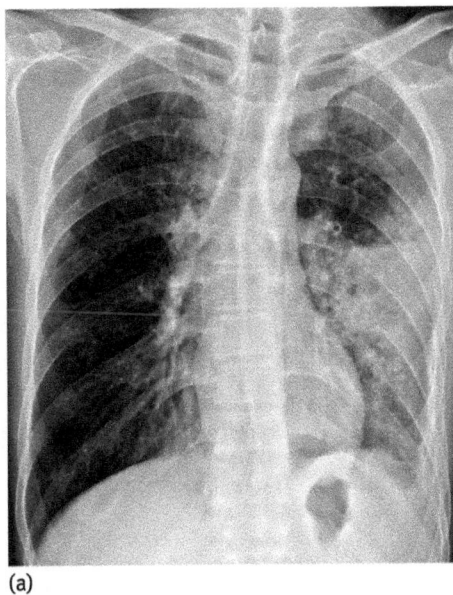

(a)

Fig. 17.9 a–e: *Rhodococcus equi* pneumonia in the inferior lobe of left lung.

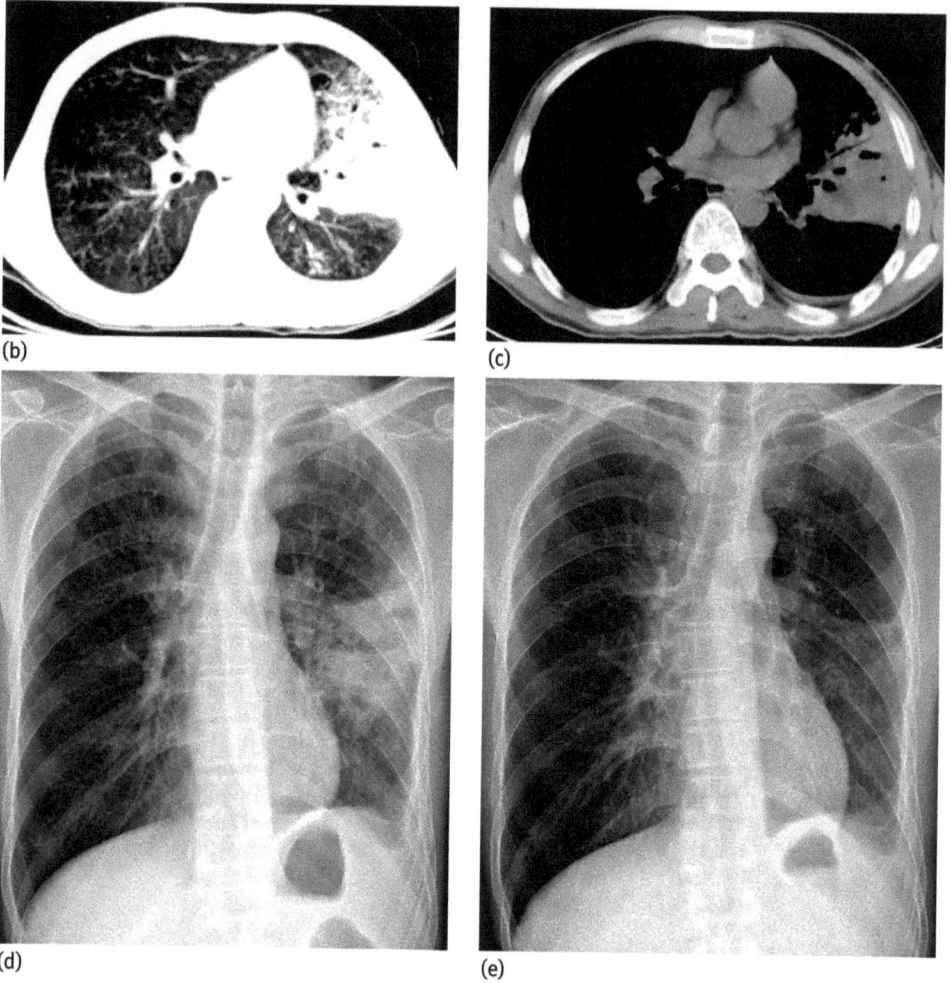

Fig. 17.9: (continuing)

The chest radiograph showed a massive patchy shadow of high density, with blurring edges and spotty opacities in it and thickened pleura on the left (a). The CT scans showed massive consolidation in the lingular superior segment of left lung, with spotty opacities of lower density and small cavities in which there are liquid-air interfaces, a little hydrothorax on the left side, and the spotty opacity of high density in the interior lobe of left lung (b–c). The chest radiographs at recheck 13 days after treatment showed obvious shrinkage of the lesions in the left lung, with sharp edge, and the extended low-density area in the lesion (d). The radiograph of 5 months later that showed the further shrinkage of the lesions as well as the local funicular shadow of higher density (e).

17.3.1 AIDS-associated pulmonary mycosis

Pulmonary fungal infections usually occur secondary to chronic consumptions (e. g. pulmonary TB, diabetes, tumor and hemopathy) and those people of suppressed immune function due to long-term uses of antibiotics, hormones and immunosuppressives. AIDS patients are reported to be susceptible to fungal infections when the CD4+ T lymph cell counting is lower, blastomyces albicans and cryptococcus are most common pathogen, aspergillus is in the second place. The incidence of cavities caused by invasive aspergillus infections is higher up to 36 % to 42 %, with superior lung lobe predilection. The fungal infections are epidemic in South China where *Penicillium marneffei* is one of the most common conditioned fungal pathogen.

The main image features of AIDS-associated pulmonary mycosis are included as follow:

CT manifestations of pulmonary mycosis cavities are complex and various, it can be solitary or multiple, it can arise up and be formed in consolidation, nodule or mass, surrounded by halo sign, with different size, uneven walled, inner wall is usually smooth while outer wall is rough . All the fungi are nonspecific in radiology. Anyhow, we consider that pulmonary mycosis is primarily suggestive when CT scan detects solitary regular cavity in the nodule with smooth inner wall.

Pneumocystis jiroveci belongs to fungal, Pneumocystis carinii pneummonia is kind of common opportunistic infection in AIDS patients. Its treatment is different from other fungal infection, and has some characteristic in radiology, presented with ground-glass opacity in bilateral lungs, or patchy opacities frequently at bilateral upper lobes,or solitary or multiple nodular shadow, thin-walled aerocyst and pneumothorax, cavity is less seen in the lesion. The final diagnosis depends on the finding of PCP cyst/trophozoite from cultures of sputum or BALF or on biopsy of pulmonary tissues.

Case 17.10 (Fig. 17.10 a–b)

Disseminated cryptococcus neoformans disease in a 52-year-old female with AIDS C3. Clinical history and symptom: recurrent pharyngodynia, fever and cough for a month, the highest body temperature was 39 °C, body check: no superficial enlarged lymph nodes were palpated. The CD4+ cell count was 13/μl.Culture of blood, bone marrow and CSF detected cryptococcus neoformans.

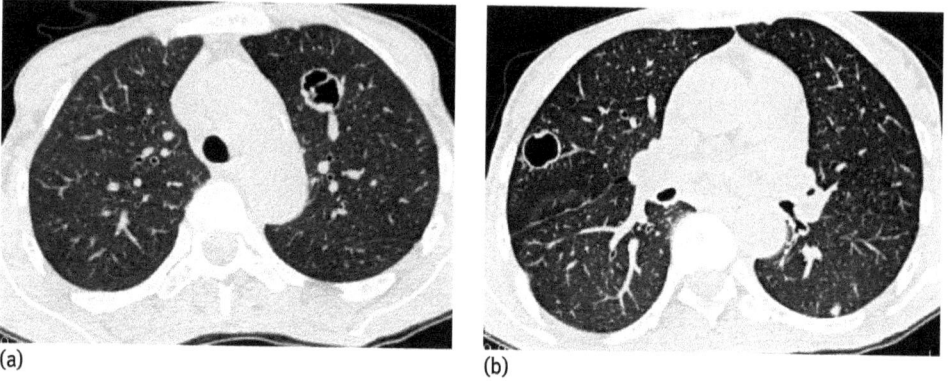

(a)　　　　　　　　　　　　　　　　　(b)

Fig. 17.10 a–b: Pulmonary cryptococcosis.

The CT scans showed thin-walled cavity with smooth edge, mural nodule in the inner wall located in the inferior lobe of bilateral lungs, hole interval can be seen in left lung cavity, sharp-edge small nodule in subpleura of inferior lobe of left lung (a, b obtained from HRCT).

Case 17.11 (Fig. 17.11 a–c)

Pulmonary aspergillosis in a 41-year-male with AIDS C3.Clinical history and symptom: recurrent cough for 1 month, fever with headache for over 10 days and weight loss of 10 kg recently. The body temperature fluctuated between 38 °C–39 °C. Physical examinations: enlarged lymph nodes were palpated in the right neck. The CD4+ cell count was 46/µl. Culture of BALF: aspergillus.

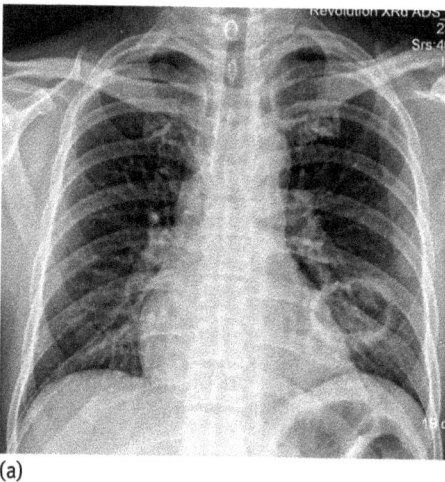

(a)

Fig. 17.11 a–c: Pulmonary aspergillosis.

(b)

(c)

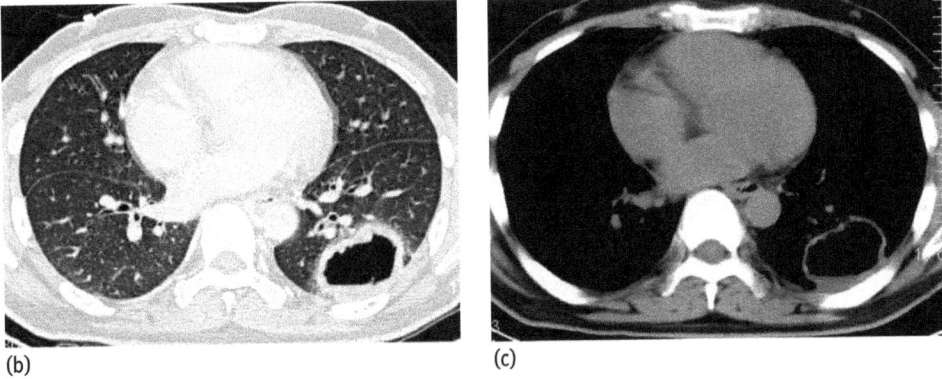

Fig. 17.11 (continuing)

The chest radiographs showed the thick-walled cavity with blurring edge (a). CT scans showed thick-walled cavity with halo sign, with uneven inner wall and liquid-air interface in the cavity (b, c).

Case 17.12 (Fig. 17.12 a–e)

Disseminated penicilliosis marneffei in a 45-year-old male with AIDS C3. Clinical history and symptom: cough and fever for 2 months, expectoration of white sputum and weight loss of 10 kg. The highest body temperature was 40 °C. Physical examinations: skin rashes on the face and trunk, tenacious and painless, presented with notch sign. The CD4+ cell count was 56/μl. Culture of sputum, blood and bone marrow: *Penicillium marneffei.*

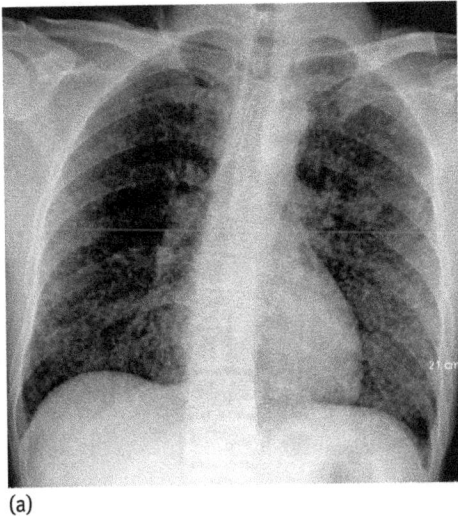

(a)

Fig. 17.12 a–e: Penicilliosis marneffi disease.

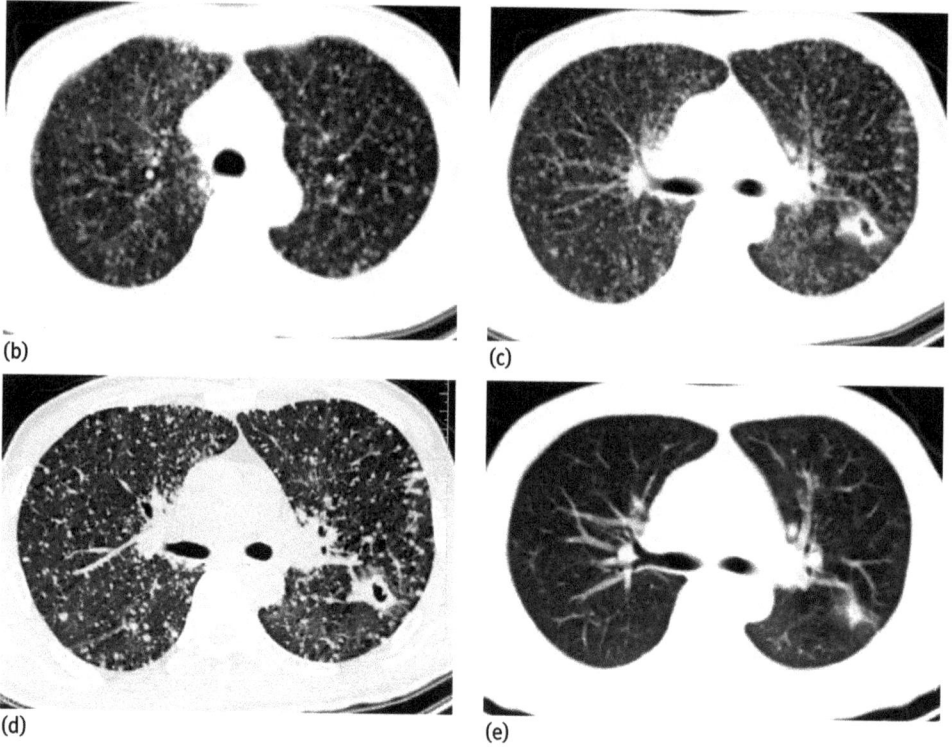

(b)

(c)

(d)

(e)

Fig. 17.12 (continuing)

Chest radiograph showed disseminated miliary nudoles of different sizes in both lungs (a). CT scans showed the thick-walled cavity with regular shape, the wall was uneven, with small mural nodule in the inner wall, the outer wall was rough disseminated miliary lesions in the bilateral lungs (b–d, d obtained from HRCT). CT scans rechecked after 5 weeks treatment showed the miliary lesion of both lungs were completely absorbed, the opacity in the inferior lobe of left lung shrinking and the cavity closed (e).

Case 17.13 (Fig. a–b)

Pulmonary mycosis in a27-year-old male with AIDS C3. Clinical history and symptom: recurrent fever, cough for over 3 months, mainly happen at dusk, and weight loss of 10 kg during the recent 3 months. The body temperature was between 38 °C–39.3 °C. Physical examinations: maculopapules on the forehead, back and neck, with a sized of 2×2 mm and a scab in the center, and multiple small cervical lymph nodes were palpated. The CD4+ cell count was 20/μl. BALF culture and lung tissues pathology: Mucors and *Penicillium marneffei*.

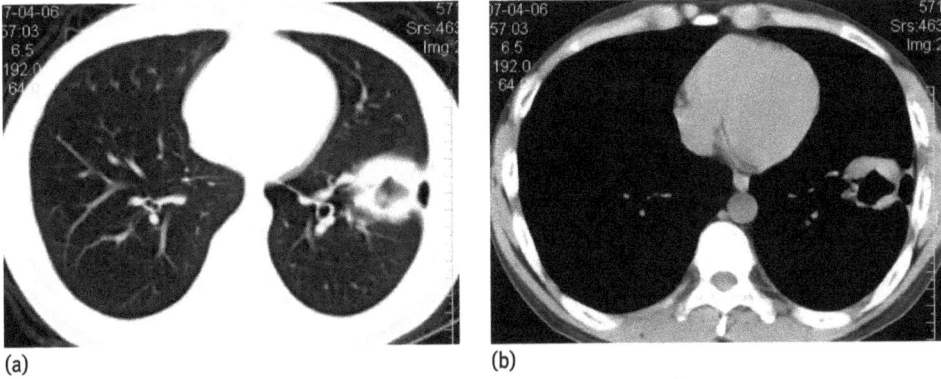

Fig. 17.13 a–b: Pulmonary mycosis (mucors and *Penicillium marneffei* mixed infection).

The CT scans showed thick-walled cavity with smooth inner wall in the inferior lobe of left lung, and adjacent pleural adhesions (a–b).

Case 17.14 (Fig. 17.14 a–e)

PCP in a 33-year-old male with AIDS C3. Clinical history and symptom: recurrent fever, cough and expectoration for over 1 month. The highest body temperature was 39.3 °C. Physical examinations: no systemic superficial lymphadenectasis. The CD4+ cell count was 15/μl. Lung tissues pathology by bronchoscopy: Pneumocystis carinii pneummonia.

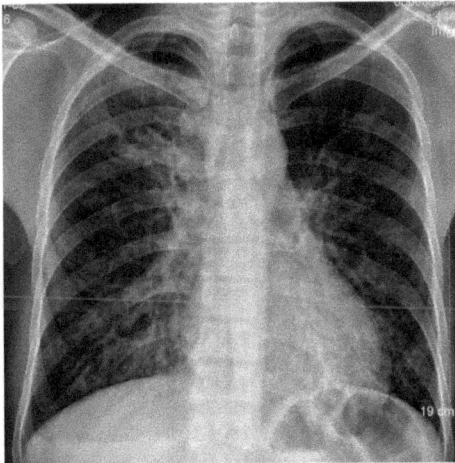

Fig. 17.14 a–e: Pneumocystis carinii pneumonitis.

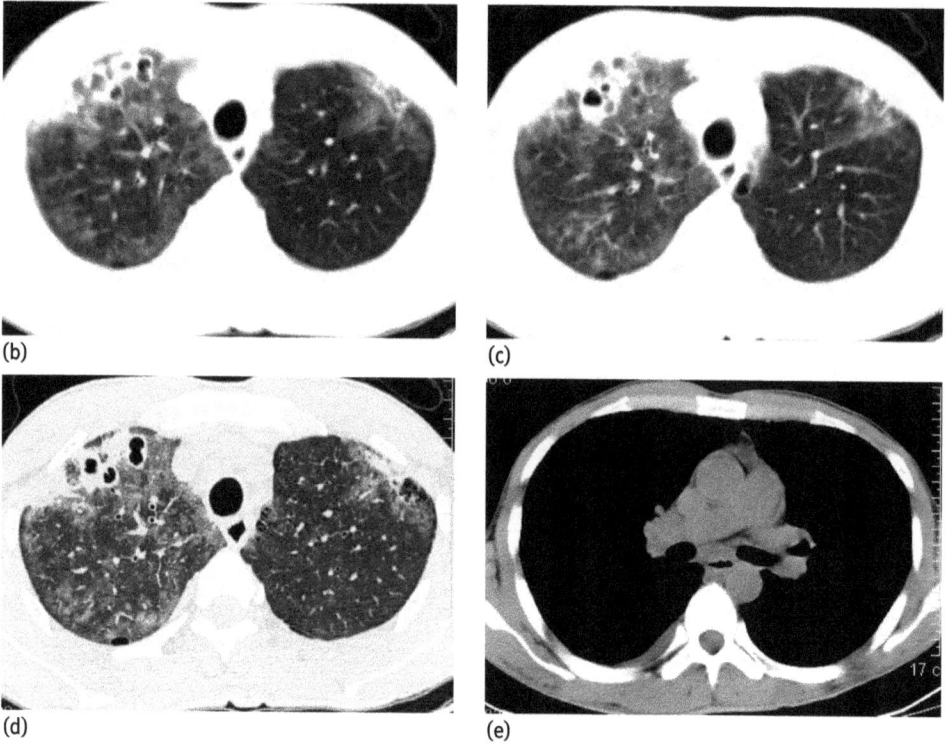

(b)

(c)

(d)

(e)

Fig. 17.14 (continuing)

The chest plain film showed the widespread ground-glass shadow, scattering patchy opacities and multiple capsular low-density areas in the lesions of the right superior lung. The CT scans (lung window) showed widespread ground-glass shadow, scattering patchy opacities, multiple cavities in the upper lobe of right lung, the cavity walls were uneven, with smooth inner wall.Thin-walled aerocysts (b–c) can be seen subpleural. Mediastinal window showed a little pleural effusion on the right side (e).

Editors: Songfeng Jiang, Yan Ding, Zhoukun Ling, Tianli Hu

18 The CT diagnosis and differential diagnosis of disseminated miliary nodules in AIDS patients

18.1 Introduction

Miliary nodules, as a kind of pulmonary opportunistic infect sign, is one pathological manifestation in AIDS patients. Disseminated pulmonary miliary nodules (DPMN), including the nodular lesions less than 10 mm in diameter and the tiny miliary ones less than 3 mm in diameter in the lung, result from different pathogeneses, and are distributed in random in the lung or around the lobule generally, or following both distribution regularities in some cases: the random distribution indicates hematogenous dissemination, the distribution around the lobule indicates bronchial dissemination, and both distribution regularities in combination indicates the combination of those two kinds of dissemination. According to recent literature, the disseminated miliary nodules in the non-AIDS patients are mostly due to pulmonary metastasis, TB, sarcoidosis and pneumoconiosis, and those in the AIDS patients are attributed to hematogenous acute miliary pulmonary tuberculosis (AMPT) and hematogenous fungal infections. In a retrospective study on the HRCT manifestations of 112 DPMN patients affirmatively diagnosed by bacterial culture and histopathological examination, we found that DPMN were mostly caused by *Mycobacterium tuberculosis* and penicillium marneffi.

TB, as another kind of pulmonary opportunistic infection, may occur in AIDS patients at any stage of HIV infection. AIDS-associated AMPT, however, often occur when CD4+ cell counting is lower than 200/uL and even manifest itself with disseminated pulmonary miliary nodules in most cases. In our study, 57 cases of mycobacterial infections combined with disseminated miliary nodules, most miliary nodules were randomly distributed, part of them around the center of lobules. and part of them are distributed in mixed (both) regularities Among them, 38 cases infected mediasetinal and hilar lymphadenectasis, and 31 cases infected hydrothorax. In our previous study in 2014, we found that AIDS-associated mycobacterium intracellulare (MAC) also caused disseminated miliary nodules in the bilateral lungs which were randomly distributed in most cases.

AIDS-associated disseminated miliary fungal nodules, as a kind of invasive fungal infections tend to be predominant in a certain regions. For example, penicilliposis marneffei (PM) as a special opportunistic infection is confined in Southeast Asia and South China. Our investigations based on the data from our hospital discovered the fact that PM is a common conditional pathomycete. In the study, 34 cases out of the entire 45 ones contracting fungal infections and presenting the lesions of disseminated miliary nodules in the bilateral lungs resulted from PM, 9 cases from aspergillus and 2 from mucor. Similarly, the majority of disseminated miliary nodules by fungal infection were randomly distributed in the lung, some of them around the lobule and some were distributed in mixed (both) regularities. They were evidently absorbed after 3–4 weeks of anti-fungi therapy, which is quite different from miliary tubercles.

In radiological diagnosis, the sign of 'bud-in-tree' presents centrilobular nodules and a linear shadow connecting them by the thin-layer CT scanning, which highly indicates inflammatory diseases in the small airways. Meanwhile, the sign is frequently observed as well in the patients with bronchial disseminated TB, bacterial infections, immunologic derangement or neoplastic diseases. In our study, 10 cases with disseminated miliary nodules in the bilateral lungs from bacterial infections presented a distribution around lobules and same with those cases of the disseminated miliary nodules in the bilateral lungs due to the infections of *Mycobacterium tuberculosis* and fungi like PM, which suggests that the bronchus may perform as an accessible route to disseminated miliary nodules from *Mycobacterium tuberculosis* and fungal infections.

The differential diagnosis of disseminated miliary nodules
Our study showed that, it is difficult to perform a confirmative diagnosis of disseminated miliary nodules differentially only based on the detection of their size and forms, but it may help to the diagnosis if their signs are considered.

Specifically, disseminated miliary nodules together with hydrothorax and mesenteric lymphadenectasis by CT scanning are closely related to AIDS-associated pulmonary *Mycobacterium tuberculosis* and penicilliosis marneffei, respectively.

For the examination of disseminated miliary nodules, HRCT is most valuable, (because) it is able to elaborate the morphological characteristics, scope, distribution and dissemination of the lesions as well as basic diseases in the patients, especially for those patients who cannot stand bronchoscopic alveolar wash examination. The combined examination with CT, HRCT and MIP may lead to the accurate diagnosis of the lesions.

Case 18.1 (Fig. 18.1 a–e) Disseminated PM

The patient, a 51-year-old male, was admitted to the hospital because of dyspnea for 3 months, cough and fever for 2 months, and then he was confirmatively diagnosed with PM infections by bone marrow culturing. The CD4+ cell count was 58/μl. Consequently, he was diagnosed with AIDS (C3) and PM infections.

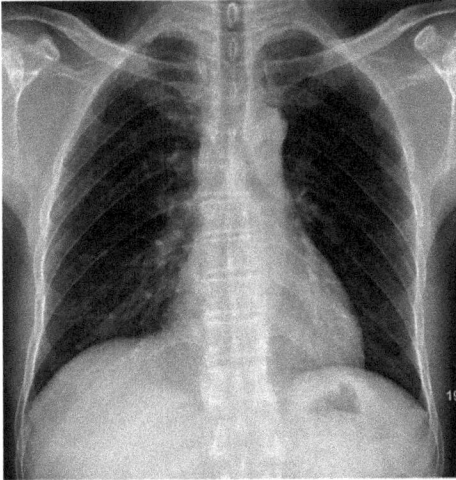

(a)

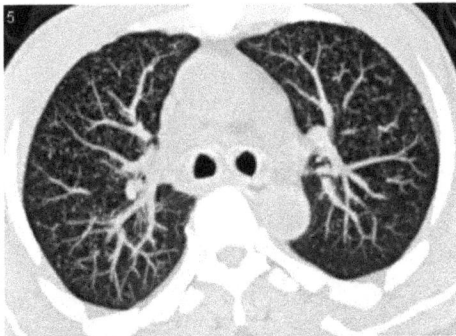

(b)

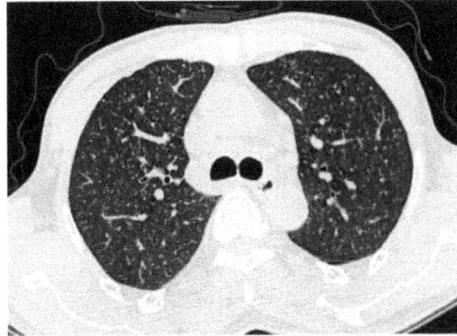

(c)

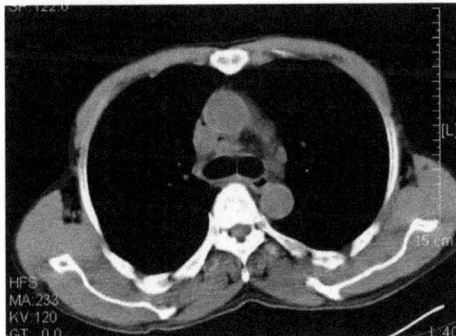

(d)

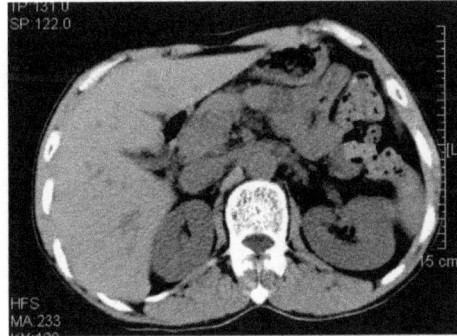

(e)

Fig. 18.1 a–e: Disseminated PM.

The chest X-ray shows disseminated miliary lesions in bilateral lungs (a). MIP and HRCT scans show random miliary lesions in the bilateral lungs (b, c). Mediastinal lymphadenectasis (d). Multiple retroperitoneal lymphadenectasis (e).

Case 18.2 (Fig. 18.2 a–e) Disseminated PM

The patient, a 38-year-old male, was admitted to the hospital because of fever, cough and expectoration for 1 month, and then he was diagnosed with PM infections by spinal marrow culturing. The CD4+ cell count was 36/µl. Consequently, he was diagnosed with AIDS (C3) and PM infections.

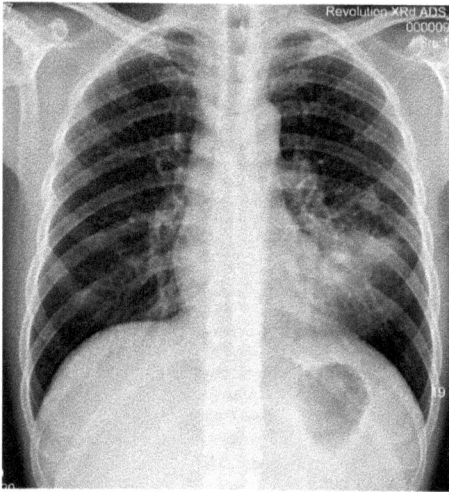

(a)

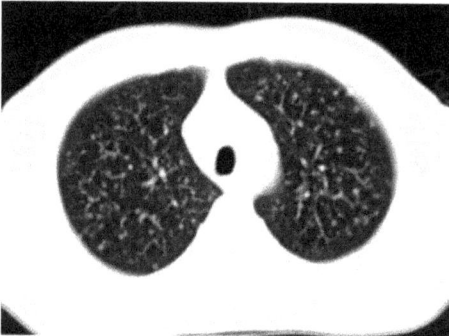

(b)

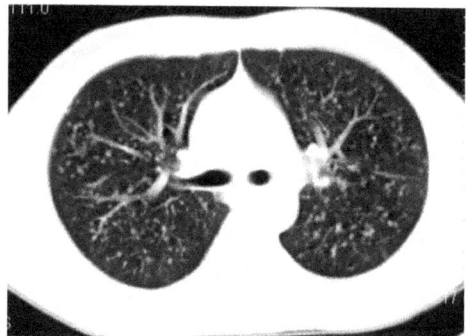

(c)

Fig. 18.2 a–e: Disseminated PM.

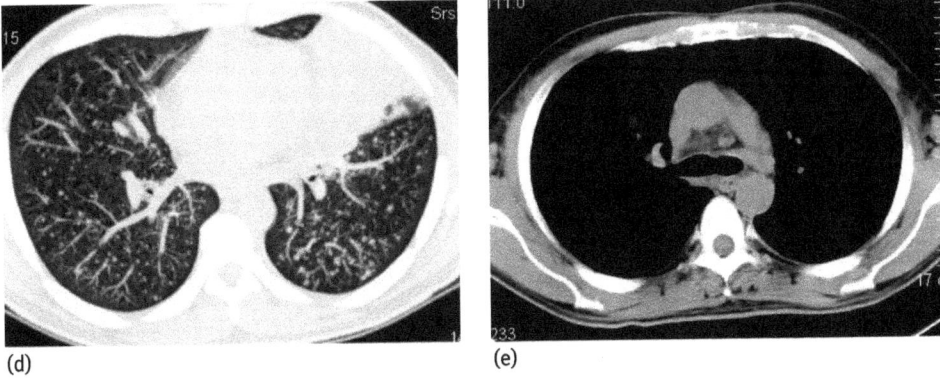

(d)　　　　　　　　　　　　　　　　(e)

Fig. 18.2: (continuing)

The chest X-ray shows disseminated miliary lesions in bilateral lungs combined with patchy shadows in the left lower lung field (a). Chest CT, HRCT and MIP scans show disseminated and random miliary lesions combined with inferior lingular consolidation of the left upper lobe (b–d). Mediastinal lymphadenectasis (e).

Case 18.3 (Fig. 18.3 a–e) Disseminated PM

The patient, a 45-year-old male, was admitted to the hospital because of fever, cough and skin rashes for 2 months, and then he was diagnosed with PM infections by spinal marrow and blood culturing. The CD4+ cell count was 56/μl. Consequently, he was diagnosed with AIDS (C3) and PM infections.

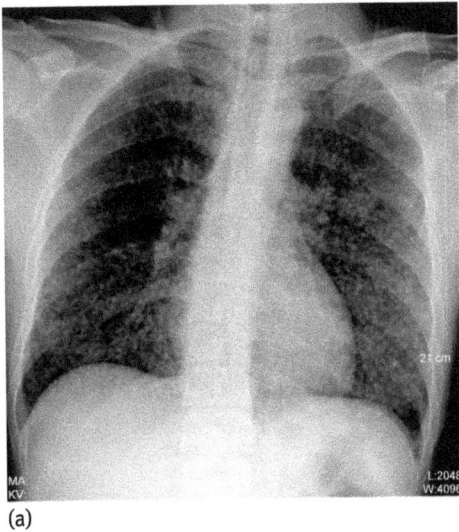

(a)

Fig. 18.3 a–e: Disseminated PM.

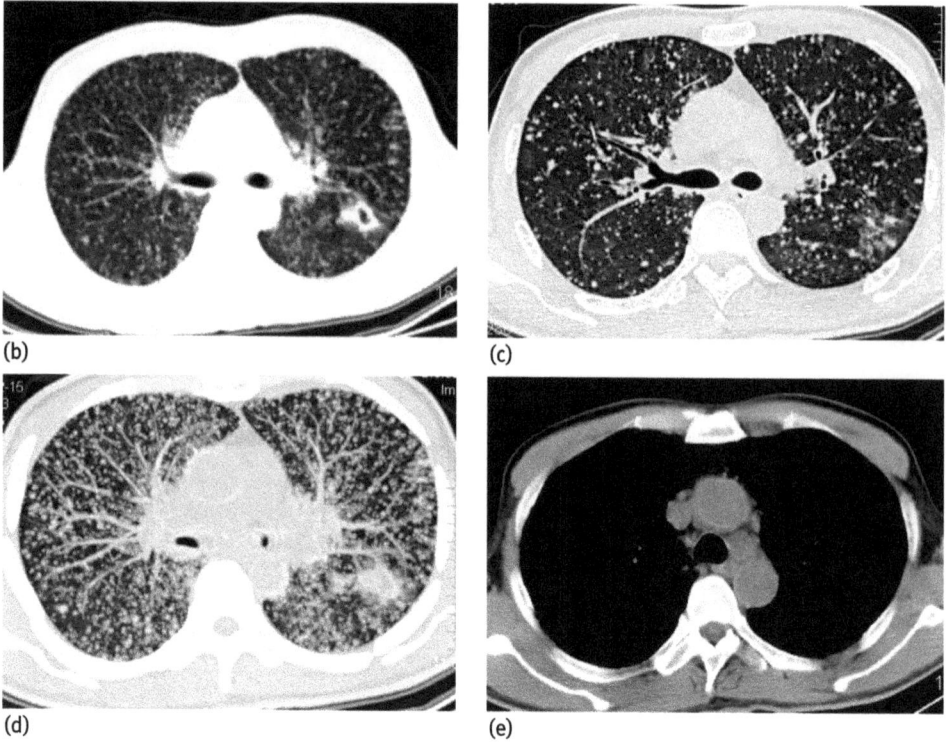

Fig. 18.3: (continuing)

Chest X-ray shows disseminated miliary lesions in bilateral lungs combined with patchy shadows in left upper lobe (a). Chest CT, HRCT and MIP scans show disseminated and random miliary lesions combined with patchy exudative lesions and cavitation in the posterior segment of the left upper lobe (b–d). Mediastinal lymphadenectasis (e).

Case 18.4 (Fig. 18.4 a–e) Disseminated PM

The patient, a 33-year-old male, was admitted to the hospital because of fatigue, cough and fever for over 1 month, and then he was diagnosed with PM infection by bronchoalveolar lavage fluid culturing. The CD4+ cell count was 5/μl. Consequently, he was diagnosed with AIDS (C3) and PM infections.

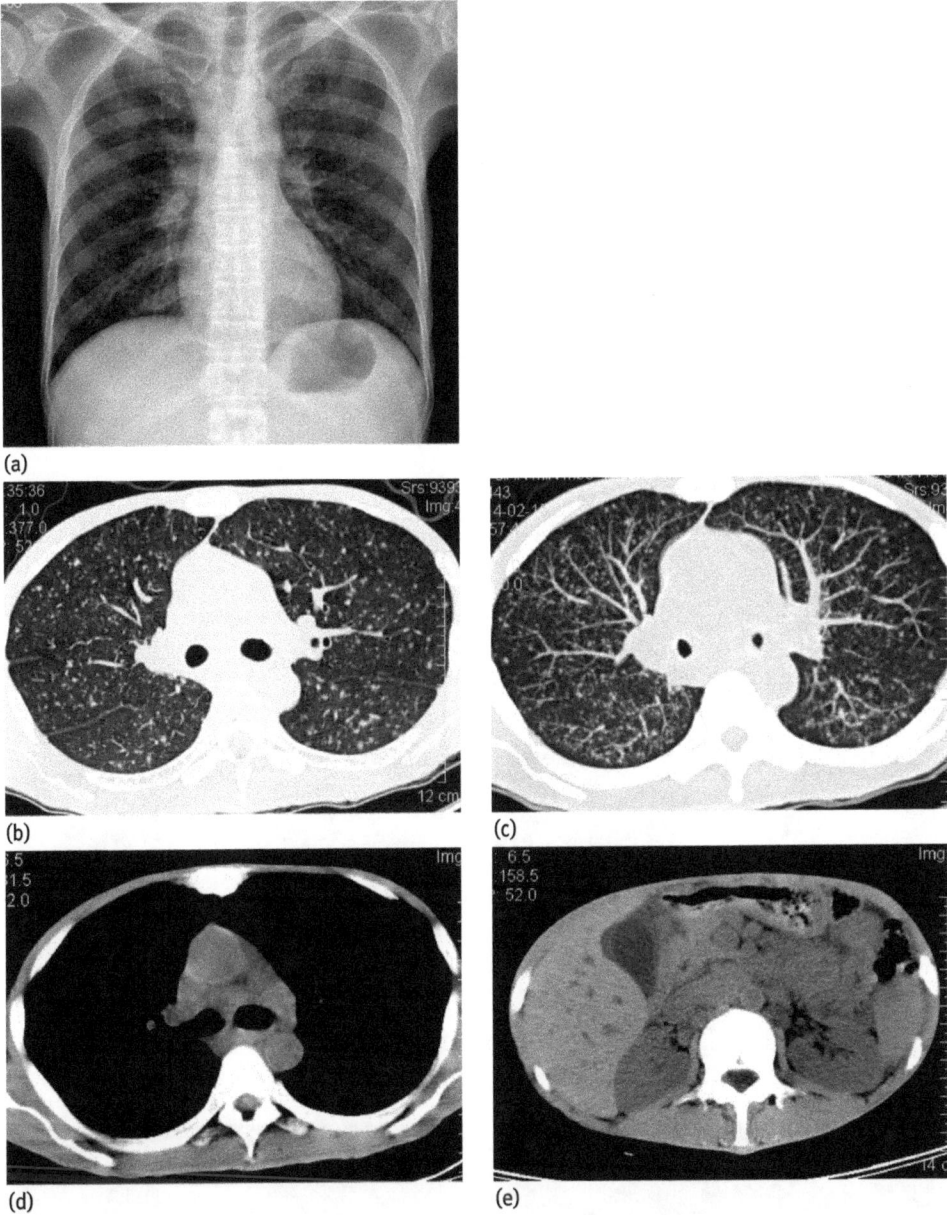

Fig. 18.4 a–e: Disseminated PM.

The chest X-ray shows disseminated miliary lesions in bilateral lungs (a). The chest HRCT and MIP scans show disseminated and random miliary lesions in bilateral lungs (b, c). Multiple mediastinal and retroperitoneal lymphadenectasis (d, e).

Case 18.5 (Fig. 18.5 a–e) Pulmonary tuberculosis

The patient, a 44-year-old male, was admitted to the hospital because of fever for 10 days, and he was then diagnosed with *Mycobacterium tuberculosis* infection by bronchoalveolar lavage fluid culturing. The CD4+ cell count was 71/μl. Consequently, he was diagnosed with AIDS (C3) and pulmonary tuberculosis.

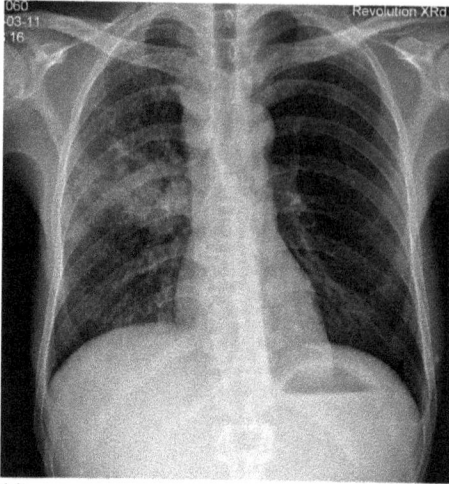

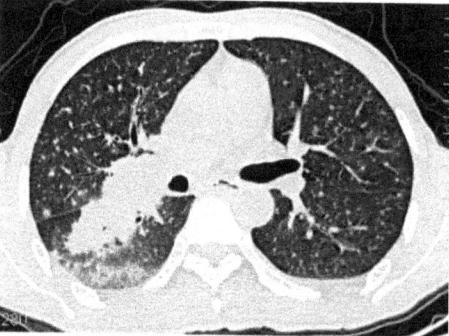

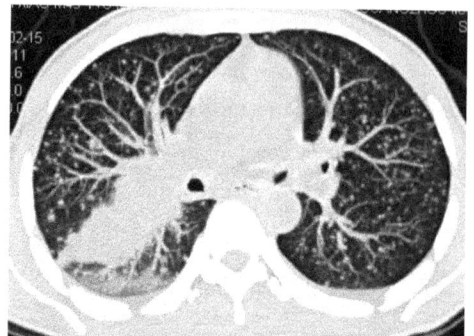

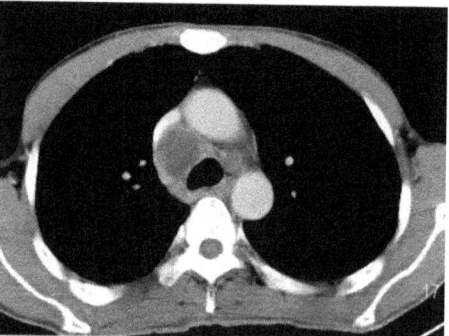

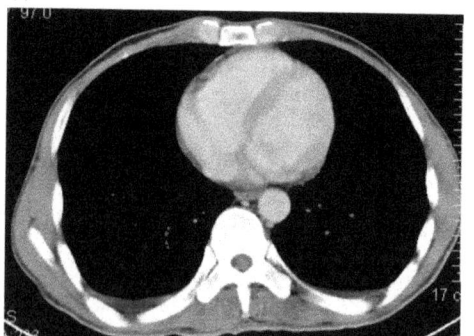

(a)

(b)

(c)

(d)

(e)

Fig. 18.5 a–e: Pulmonary tuberculosis.

The chest X-ray shows disseminated miliary lesions in the bilateral lungs combined with patchy shadows in the right lung (a). The HRCT and MIP scans show disseminated and random miliary lesions in the bilateral lungs and exudative lesions in the dorsal segment of the right lower lobe (b, c). The CT scans with mediastinal window show mediastinal lymphadenectasis with lower density in the center, considered as changes after central necrosis of lymph nodes (d). A small quantity of hydrothorax in the bilateral thoraxes (e).

Case 18.6 (Fig. 18.6 a–e) Tuberculosis

The patient, a 32-year-old male, was admitted to the hospital because of progressive enlargement of bilateral neck tumors for half a year along with fever for 2 months, and he was then diagnosed with *Mycobacterium tuberculosis* infection by secretion culturing. The CD4+ cell count was 36/μl. Consequently, he was diagnosed with AIDS (C3) and pulmonary tuberculosis.

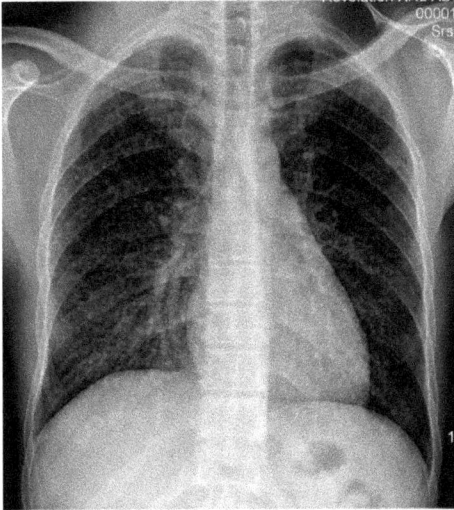

(a)

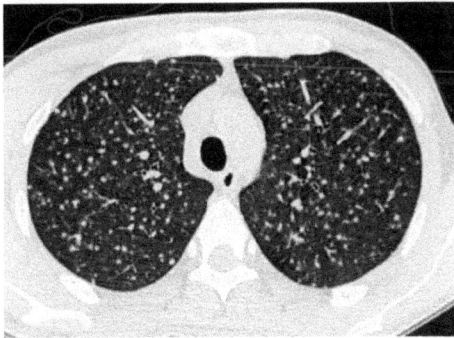

(b)

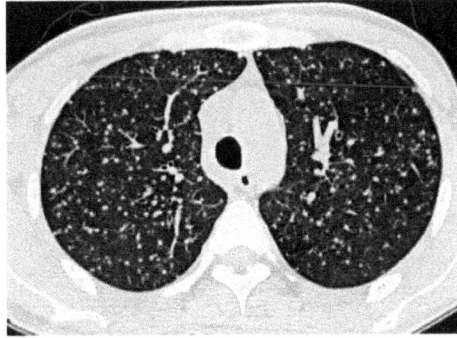

(c)

Fig. 18.6 a–e: Tuberculosis.

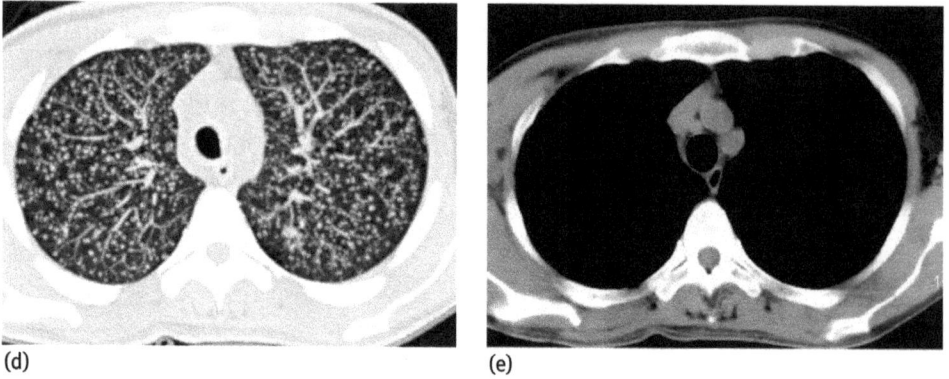

(d) (e)

Fig. 18.6: (continuing)

The chest X-ray shows disseminated miliary lesions in the bilateral lungs (a). The HRCT and MIP scans show disseminated and random miliary lesions in the bilateral lungs (b–d). The CT scans with mediastinal window show right axillary lymphadenectasis (e).

Case 18.7 (Fig. 18.7 a–e) Tuberculosis
The patient, a 26-year-old male, was admitted to the hospital because of recurrent diarrhea, and fever for over 1 month, and he was then diagnosed with *Mycobacterium tuberculosis* infections by sputum smear culturing. The CD4+ cell count was 18/μl. Consequently, he was diagnosed with AIDS (C3) and pulmonary tuberculosis.

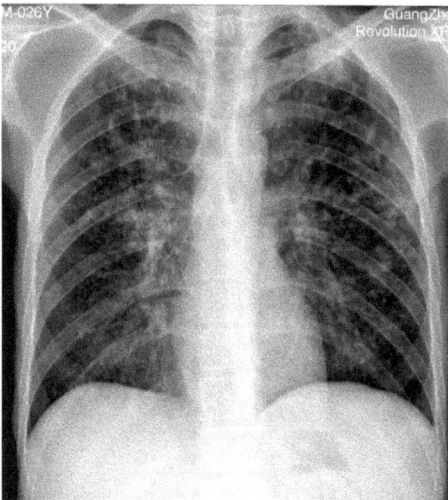

(a)

Fig. 18.7 a–e: Tuberculosis.

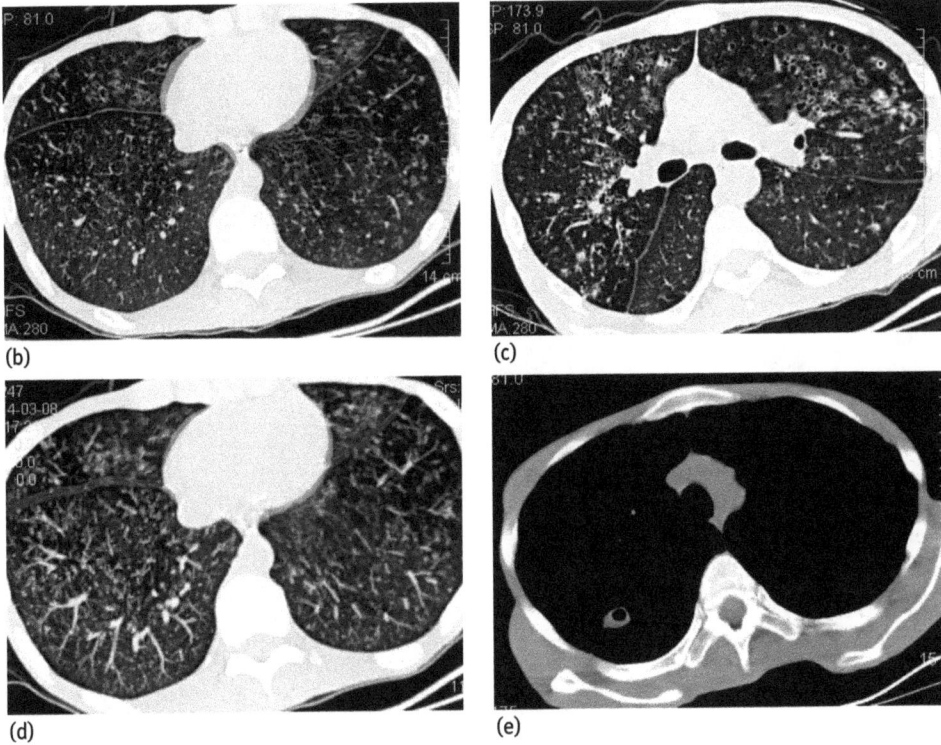

(b)

(c)

(d)

(e)

Fig. 18.7: (continuing)

The chest X-ray shows miliary lesions in the bilateral lungs combined with minor patchy shadows (a). The HRCT and MIP scans show disseminated and random miliary lesions in the bilateral lungs combined with superior lobar bronchiectasis in the bilateral lungs (b–d). The CT scans with mediastinal window show cavitation in the superior lobe of right lung (e).

Case 18.8 (Fig. 18.8 a–e) Tuberculosis
The patient, a 30-year-old male, was admitted to the hospital because of left supraclavieular mass for over one month and fever for 24 days, and he was then diagnosed with *Mycobacterium tuberculosis* infection by sputum smear culturing. The CD4+ cell count was 14/μl. Consequently, he was diagnosed with AIDS (C3) and pulmonary tuberculosis.

The chest X-ray shows disseminated miliary lesions in the bilateral lungs (a). The HRCT and MIP scans (b–d) show disseminated and random miliary lesions in the bilateral lungs combined with patchy shadows and bronchiectasis in the superior lobe of the left lung. The CT scans with mediastinal window show multiple lymphadenectasis and the enhanced scanning shows circular enhancement of the mediastinal lymphadenectasis with lower liquid density in the center, considered as changes after central necrosis (e).

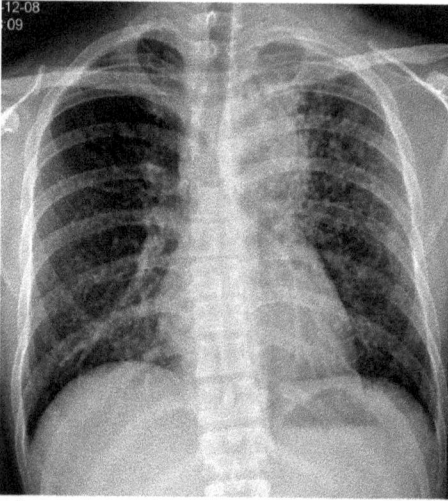

(a)

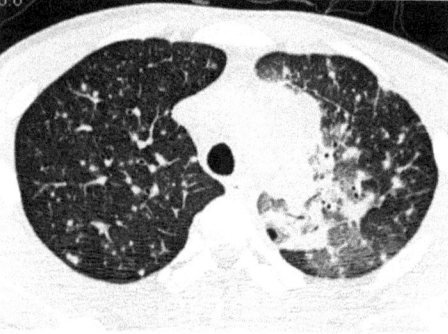

(b)

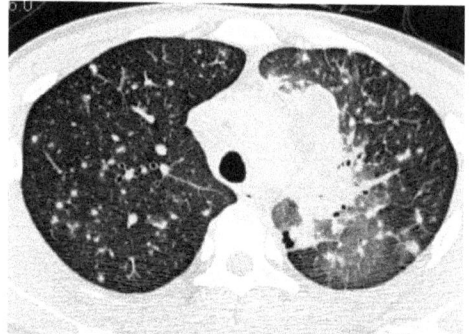

(c)

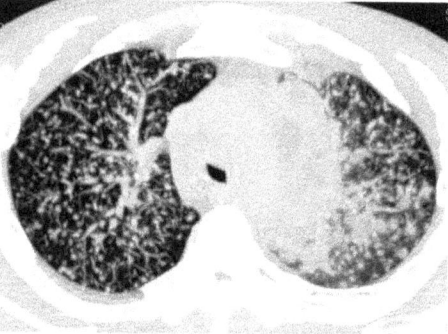

(d)

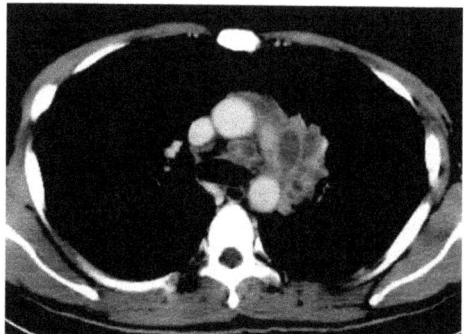

(e)

Fig. 18.8 a–e: Tuberculosis.

Case 18.9 (Fig. 18.9 a–e) Streptococcus pneumonia

The patient, a 38-year-old female, was admitted to the hospital because of fever and a right cervical mass for 3 months, and he was then diagnosed with AIDS (C3)-associated infections by viridans streptococcus confirmed by bronchoalveolar lavage fluid culturing. The CD4+ cell count was 17/μl. Consequently, she was diagnosed with AIDS (C3) and viridans streptococcus pneumonia.

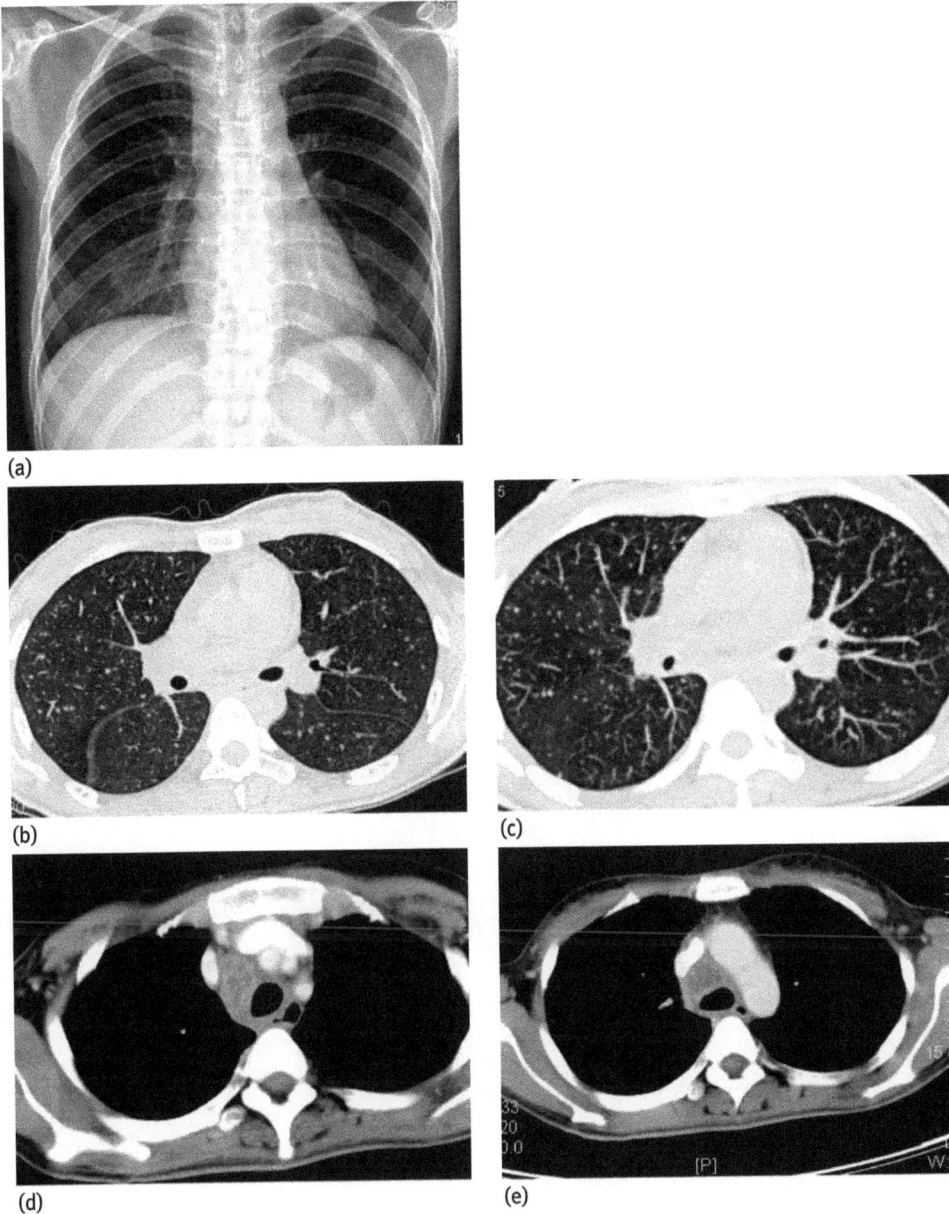

Fig. 18.9 a–e: Viridans streptococcus pneumonia.

The chest X-ray shows miliary lesions in the bilateral lungs (a). The HRCT and MIP scans (b, c) show miliary lesions in the bilateral lungs. The CT scans with mediastinal window (d, e) show multiple lymphadenectasis, the enhanced scanning show rim enhancement of the mediastinal lymphadenectasis with lower density in the center.

Case 18.10 (Fig. 18.10 a–e) *Klebsiella pneumoniae* pneumonia

The patient, a 34-year-old female, was admitted to the hospital because of recurrent fever and cough for 1 month, and he was then diagnosed with infections by *Klebsiella pneumoniae* by way of sputum culturing. The CD4+ cell count was 36/µl. Consequently, she was diagnosed with AIDS (C3) and *Klebsiella pneumoniae* pneumonia.

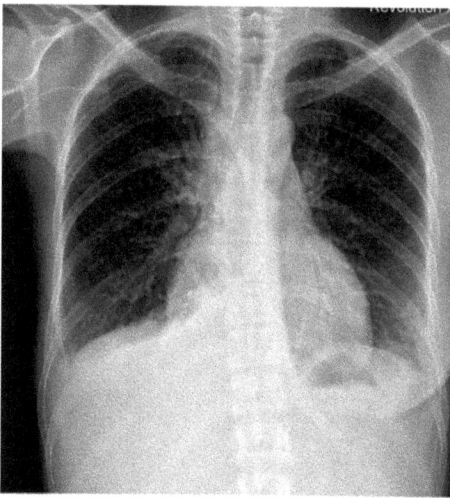

(a)

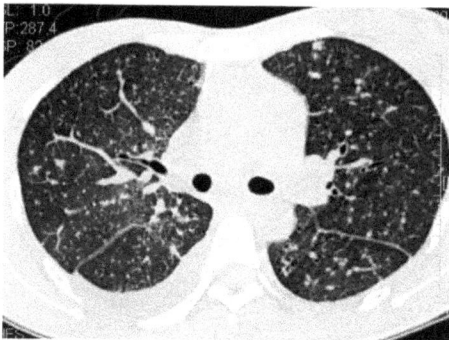

(b)

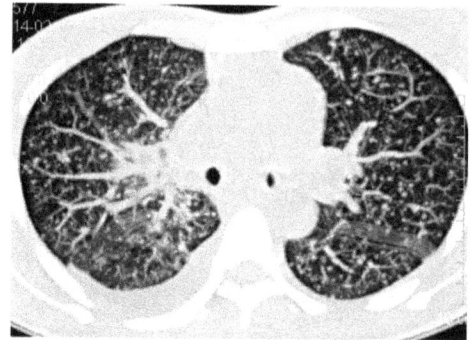

(c)

Fig. 18.10 a–e: *Klebsiella pneumoniae* pneumonia.

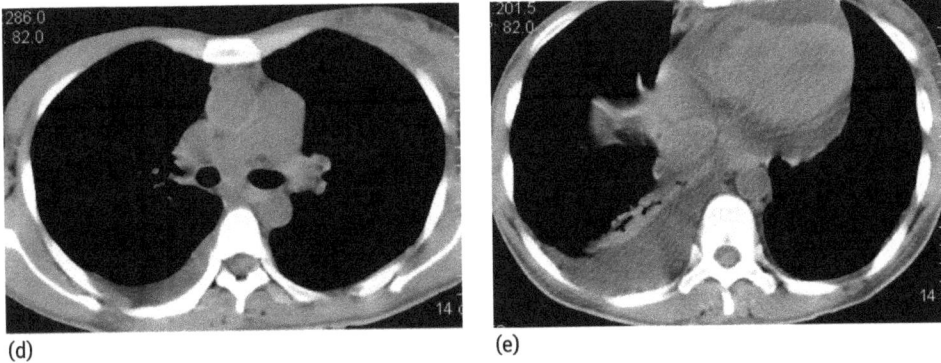

(d)　　　　　　　　(e)

Fig. 18.10: (continuing)

The chest X-ray shows disseminated miliary lesions in the bilateral lungs (a). The HRCT and MIP scans (b, c) show miliary lesions in the bilateral lungs. The CT scans with mediastinal window (d, e) show mediastinal lymphadenectasis with lower density in the center, accompanied with a small quantity of hydrothorax and hydropericardium in the right thorax.

Case 18.11 (Fig. 18.11 A-E) *Klebsiella pneumoniae* Pneumonia

The patient, a 36-year-old female, was admitted to the hospital because of recurrent fever, abdominal pain for 1 month, and anhelation for 2 weeks, and he was then diagnosed with *Klebsiella pneumoniae* infections by bronchoalveolar lavage fluid culturing. The CD4+ cell count was 21/μl. Consequently, she was diagnosed with AIDS (C3) and *Klebsiella pneumoniae* pneumonia.

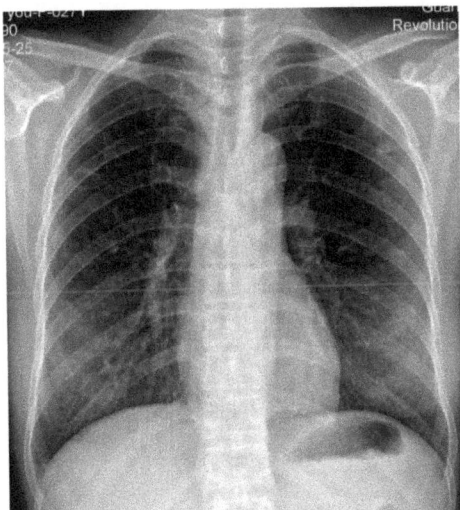

(a)

Fig. 18.11 a–e: *Klebsiella pneumoniae* pneumonia.

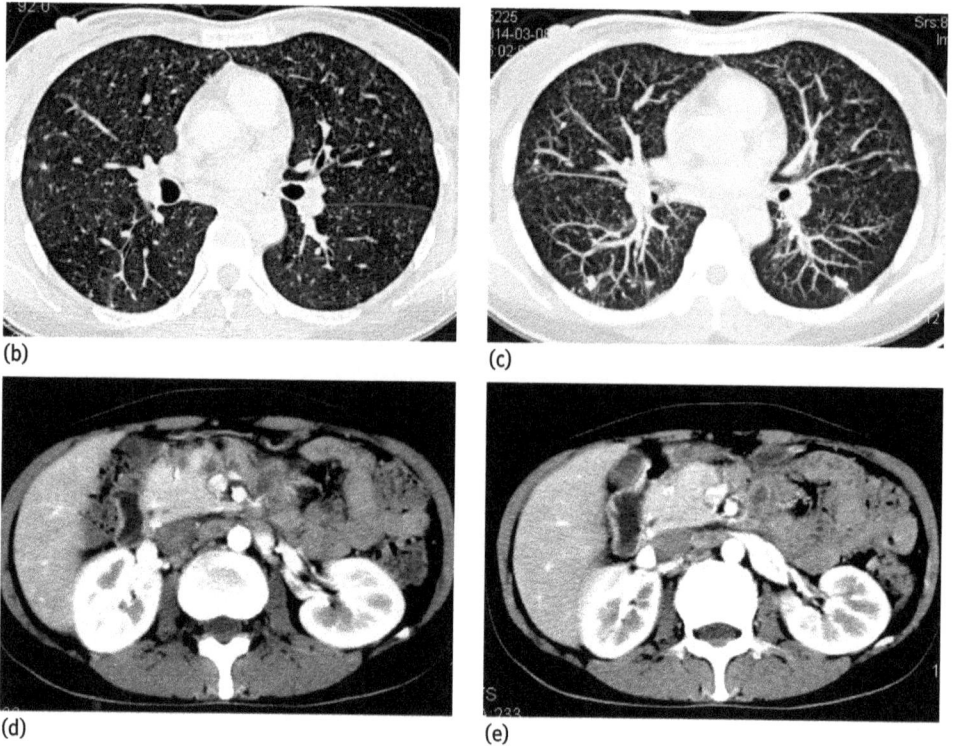

(b)

(c)

(d)

(e)

Fig. 18.11: (continuing)

The chest X-ray shows disseminated miliary lesions in the bilateral lungs (a). The HRCT and MIP scans (b, c) show miliary lesions in the bilateral lungs with partial fusion. The CT scans with mediastinal window (d, e) show multiple retroperitoneal and mesenteric lymphadenectasis, the enhanced scanning show circular enhancement of the retroperitoneal lymphadenectasis with lower density in the center.

Case 18.12 (Fig. 18.12 a–e) Pulmonary Mucormycosis

The patient, a 26-year-old male, was admitted to the hospital because of fever, cough, and anhelation for over 1 month, and diarrhea for over 10 days, and then he was diagnosed with mucor infections by bronchoalveolar lavage fluid culturing. The CD4+ cell count was 11/μl. Consequently, he was diagnosed with AIDS (C3) and pulmonary mucormycosis.

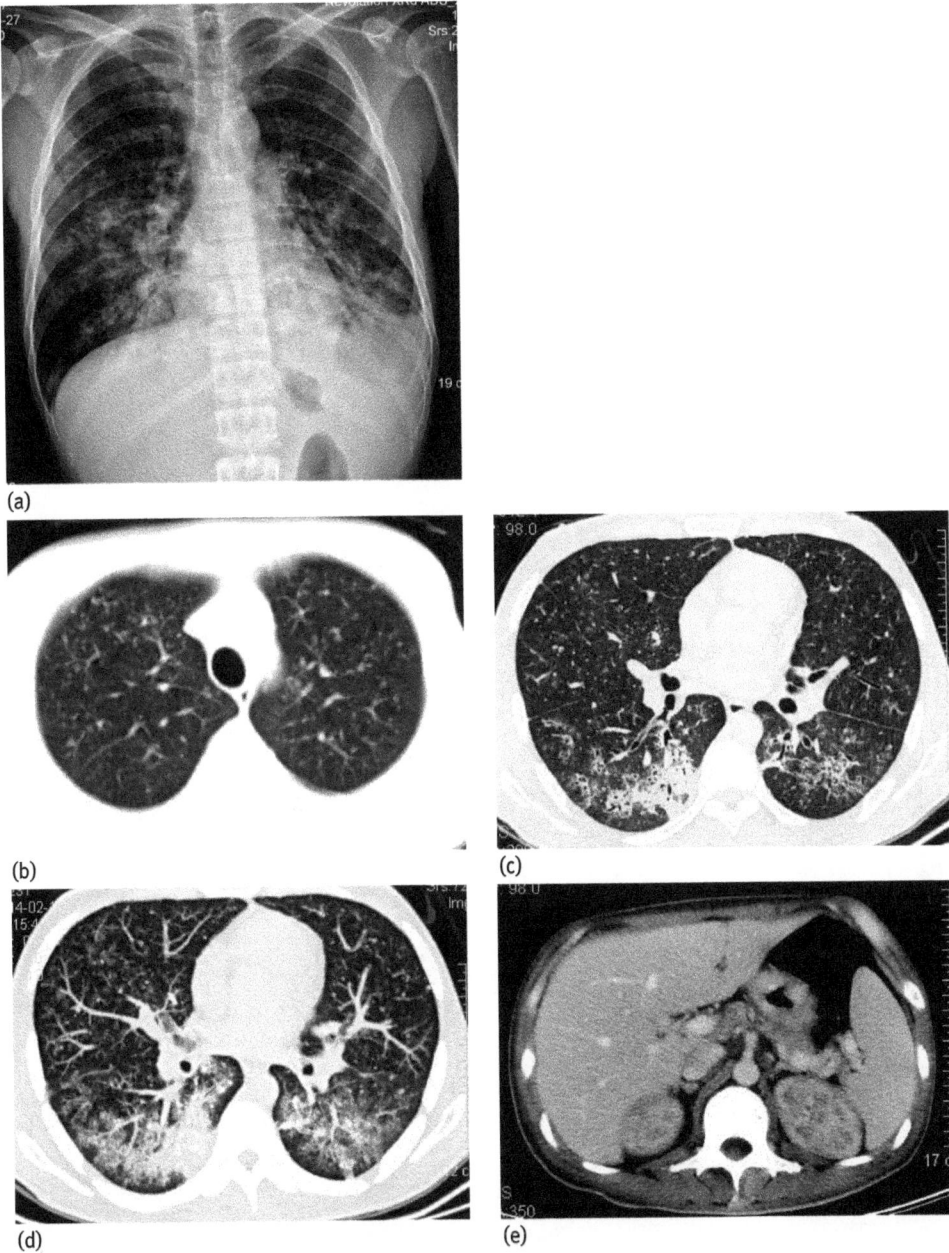

Fig. 18.12 a–e: Pulmonary mucormycosis.

The chest X-ray shows disseminated miliary lesions in the bilateral lungs combined with multiple high-density patchy shadows (a). CT and HRCT scans (b, c) show disseminated miliary lesions in the bilateral lungs combined with exudative lesions in dorsal segment of the right lower lobe and bronchiectasis in inferior lobes of the bilateral lungs. The MIP scans (d) show disseminated and random miliary lesions in the bilateral lungs combined with patchy shadows in dorsal segments of the inferior lobes of the bilateral lungs. The CT scans with mediastinal window show mild retroperitoneal lymphadenectasis, the enhanced scanning show no enhancement of the lymphadenectasis (e).

Case 18.13 (Figure 18.13 A-E) Hemolytic staphylococcus infection

The patient, a 33-year-old male, was admitted to the hospital because of recurrent fever for 4 months and cough for over 2 months, and he was then diagnosed with hemolytic staphylococcus infections by bone marrow culturing. The CD4+ cell count was 137/µl. Consequently, he was diagnosed with AIDS (C3) and hemolytic staphylococcus infections.

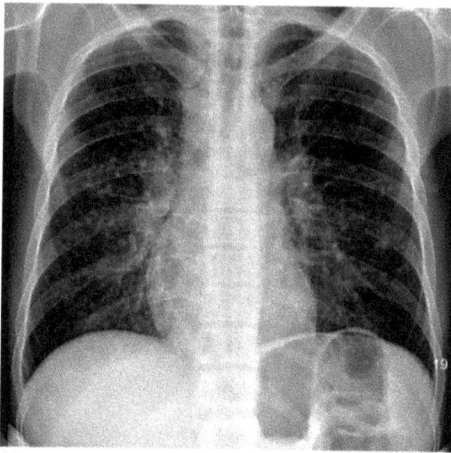

(a)

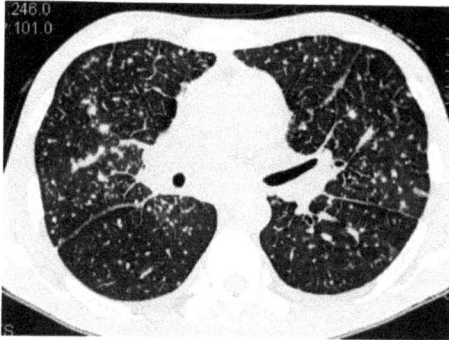

(b)

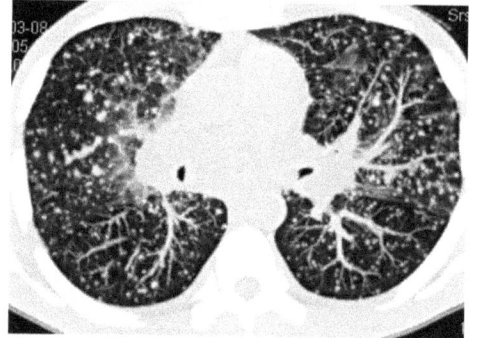

(c)

Fig. 18.13 a–e: Pulmonary hemolytic staphylococcus infection.

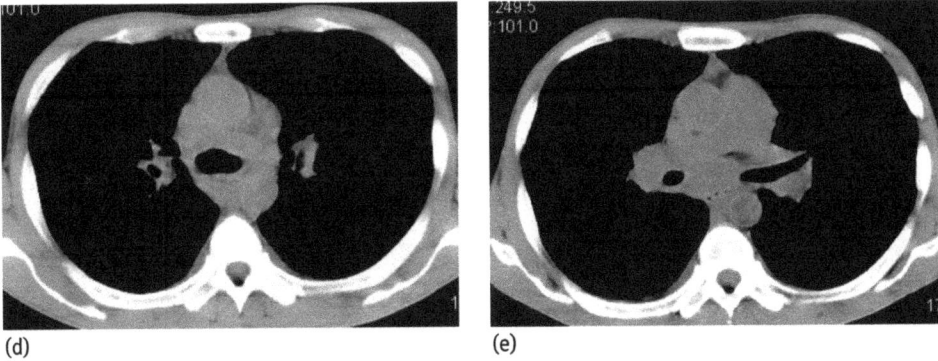

(d)   (e)

Fig. 18.13: (continuing)

The chest X-ray shows miliary lesions in the bilateral lungs (a). The HRCT and MIP scans show random miliary lesions in the bilateral lungs (b, c). The CT scans with mediastinal window (d, e) show mediastinal and hilar lymphadenectasis with slightly lower and homogeneous density accompanied with a small quantity of hydrothorax in the right thorax.

Case 18.14 (Fig. 18.14 a–e) MAC pulmonary disease

The patient, a 48-year-old female, was admitted to the hospital because of fever for over 1 month and cough for 2 weeks, and he then was diagnosed with nontuberculous mycobacterial infections which were identified as MAC infections by blood culturing. The CD4+ cell count was 2/μl. Consequently, she was diagnosed with AIDS (C3) and MAC pulmonary disease.

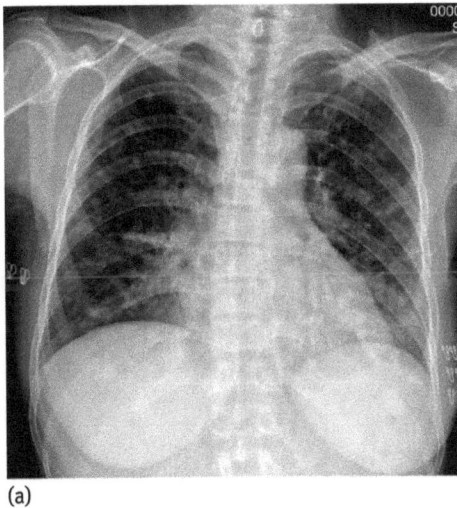

(a)

Fig. 18.14 a–e: MAC pulmonary disease.

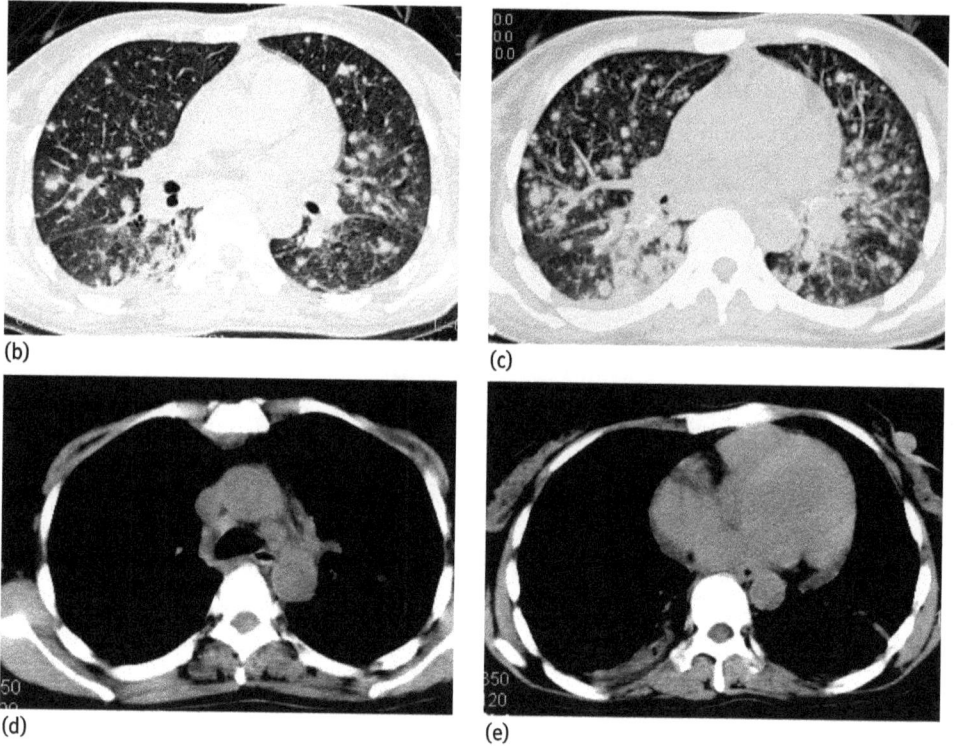

Fig. 18.14: (continuing)

The chest X-ray shows disseminated miliary lesions in the bilateral lungs (a). The HRCT and MIP scans (b, c) show disseminated and random miliary lesions in the bilateral lungs with partial nodular fusion. The CT scans with mediastinal window show multiple mediastinal lymphadenectasis accompanied with a small quantity of hydrothorax in the right thorax (d, e).

Case 18.15 (Fig. 18.15 a–e) MAC pulmonary disease

The patient, a 42-year-old male, was admitted to the hospital because of facial rash for 2 weeks, and he was then diagnosed with nontuberculous mycobacterial infections which were identified as MAC infections by bronchoalveolar lavage fluid culturing. The CD4+ cell count was 85/µl. Consequently, he was diagnosed with AIDS (C3) and MAC pulmonary disease.

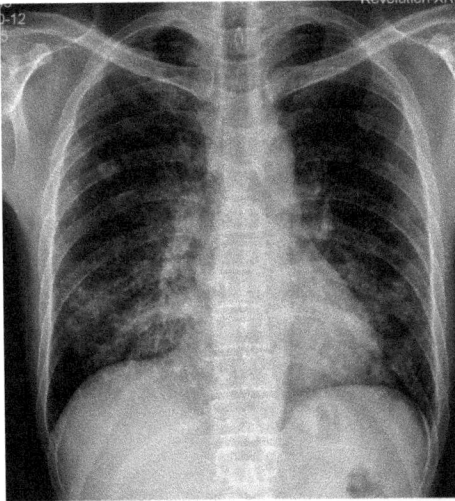

(a)

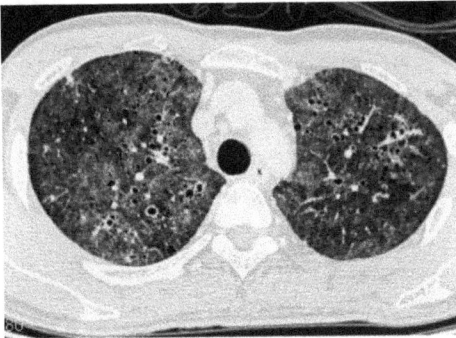

(b)

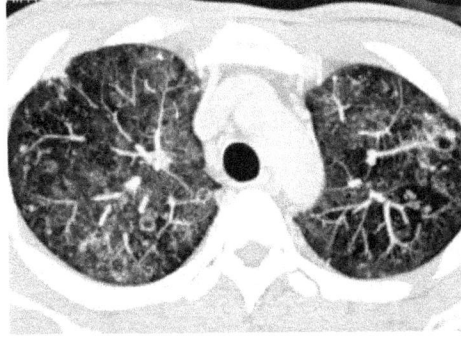

(c)

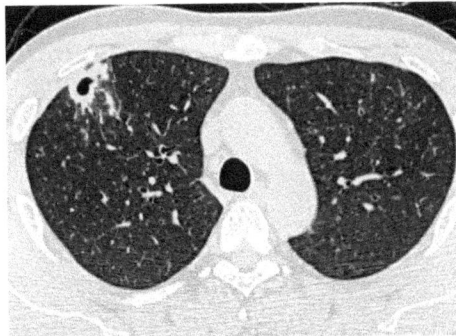

(d)

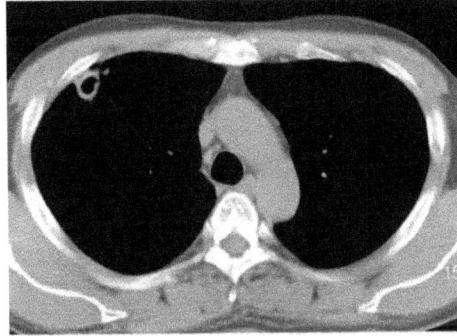

(e)

Fig. 18.15 a–e: MAC pulmonary disease.

The chest X-ray shows ground-glass changes accompanied with random miliary lesions in the bilateral lungs (a). The HRCT and MIP scans show disseminated and random miliary lesions in the bilateral lungs with ground-glass changes and bronchiectasis in the superior lobes of the bilateral lungs (b, c). The CT scans recheck

3 months after treatment show obvious absorption of the miliary lesions in the bilateral lungs and cavitation in the anterior segment of the right superior lobe (d, e).

Case 18.16 (Fig. 18.16 a–e) MAC pulmonary disease

The patient, a 37-year-old male, was admitted to the hospital because of recurrent fever and abdominal pain for over 1 month, and then he was then diagnosed with nontuberculous mycobacterial infections identified as MAC infections by blood culturing. The CD4+ cell count was 2/μl. Consequently, he was diagnosed with AIDS (C3) and MAC pulmonary disease.

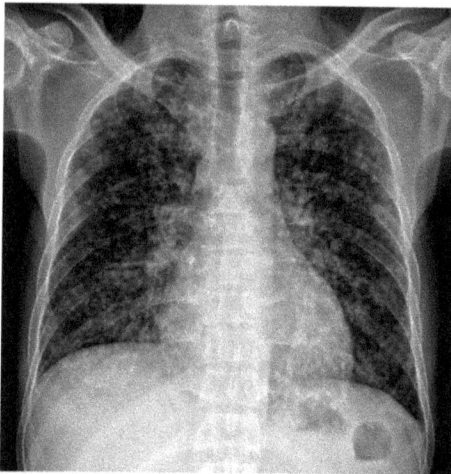

(a)

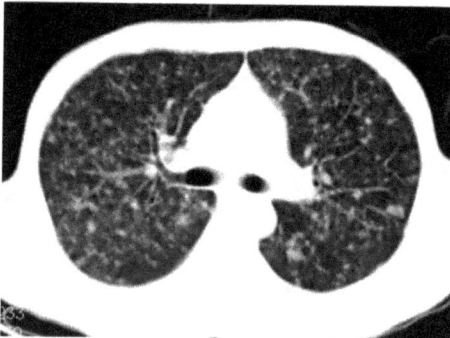

(b)

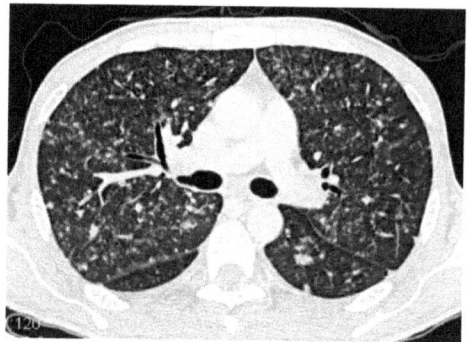

(c)

Fig. 18.16 a–e: MAC pulmonary disease.

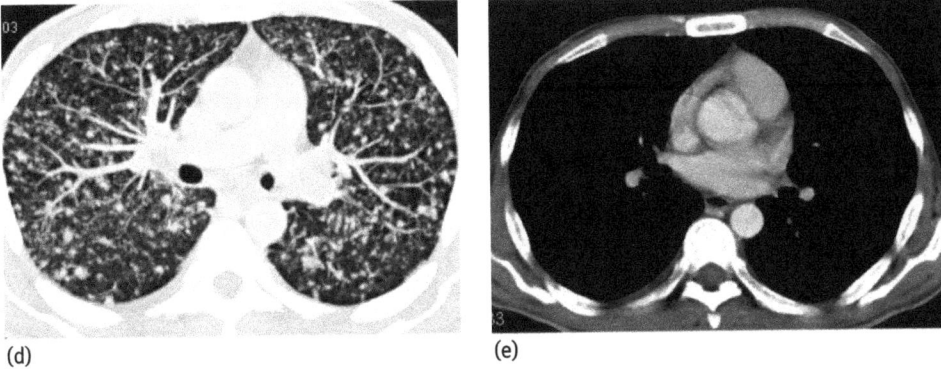

(d) (e)

Fig. 18.16: (continuing)

The chest X-ray shows ground-glass changes accompanied with random miliary lesions in the bilateral lungs with partial fusion (a). CT, HRCT and MIP scans show disseminated and random miliary lesions in the bilateral lungs with partial small nodular fusion (b–d). The CT scans with mediastinal window show a small quantity of hydrothorax in the right thorax (e).

Editors: Wanhua Guan, Qingxin Gan, Zhiping Zhang, Jinxin Liu

References

Andrianopoulos A. 2002. Control of morphogenesis in the human fungal pathogen Penicillium marneffei. Int J Med Microbiol, 292(5–6): 331–347.

Aviram G, Boiselle PM. 2004. Imaging features of bacterial respiratory infections in AIDS. Curr Opin Pulm Med, 10: 183–188.

Aviram G, Fishman JE, Sagar M. 2001. Cavitary lung disease in AIDS: etiologies and correlation with immune status. AIDS Patient Care STDS, 15(7): 353–361.

Becciolini V, Gudinchet F, Cheseaux JJ, et al. 2001. Lymphocytic interstitial pneumonia in children with AIDS: High-resolution CT findings. Eur Radiol, 11(6): 1015–1020.

Boiselle PM, Aviram G, Fishman JE. 2002. Update on lung disease in AIDS. Semin Roentgenol, 37:54–71.

Cabrera ME, Silva G, Soto A, et al. 2012. HIV-related lymphoma in a public hospital in Chile. Analysis of 55 cases. Rev Med Chil, 140(2): 243–250.

Carucci LR, Halvorsen RA. 2004. Abdominal and pelvic CT in the HIV-positive population. Abdom Imaging, 29(6): 631–642.

Castañr E, Gallardo X, Mata JM, et al. 2004. Radiologic approach to the diagnosis of infectious pulmonary diseases in patients infected with the human immunodeficiency virus. Eur J Radiol, 51(2): 114–129.

Chen BH, Liu JX, Li ZP, et al. 2008. The study of pulmonary manifestation of acquired immunodeficiency syndrome with disseminated Penicilliosis marneffei. Chin J Radiol, 42: 655–657.

Chen BH, Liu JX, Gan QX, et al. 2009. Analysis of spiral CT imaging in AIDS with pneumocystis pneumonia. Chin J CT and MRI, 7(1): 30–31.

Chen JF, Tang XP, Cai WP, et al. 2005. A clinical analysis of 12 cases of AIDS-associated Penicilliosis marneffei. Chin J Infect Dis, 23: 195–198.

Datta D, Ali SA, Henken EM, et al. 2003. Pneumocystis carinii pneumonia: the time course of clinical and radiographic improvement. Chest, 124(5): 1820–1823.

Delqado M, Sancho T,Andreu M, et al. 2000. Cavitating pneumonia in a patient infected with human immunodeficiency virus. Enferm Infec Microbiol Clin, 18: 289–290.

D'Souza GA, Sunad R, Rajagopalan N, et al. 2006. NK/T-cell lymphoma in AIDS. J Assoc Physicians India, 54: 890–892.

Edinburgh KJ, Jasmer RM, Huang L, et al. 2000. Multiple pulmonary nodules in AIDS: usefulness of CT in distinguishing among potential causes. Radiology, 214(2): 427–432.

Eisner MD,Kaplan LD,Herndier B, et al. 1996. The pulmonary manifestations of AIDS-related non-Hodgkin's lymphoma. Chest, 110(3): 729–736.

Erasmus JJ, McAdams HP, Farrell MA, et al. 1999.Pulmonary non-tuberculous mycobacterial infection: radiologic manifestation. RadioGraphics, 19: 1487–1503.

Field SK, Cowie RL. 2006. Lung disease due to the more common non-tuberculous mycobacteria. Chest, 129(6): 1653–1672.

Franquet T, Giménez A. Hidalgo A. 2004. Imaging of opportunistic fungal infections in immunocompromised patient. Eur J Radiol, 51(2): 130–138.

Franquet T, Müller NL, Giménez A, et al. 2003. Infectious pulmonary nodules in immunocompromised patients: usefulness of computed tomography in predicting their etiology. J Comput Assist Tomogr, 27(4): 461–468.

Fujiuchi S, Matsumoto H, Yamazaki Y, et al. 2003. Analysis of chest CT in patients with Mycobacterium avium complex pulmonary disease. Respiration, 70: 76–81.

Gasparetto EL, Escuissato DL, Marchiorie E, et al. 2004. High-resolution CT Findings of respiratory syncytial virus pneumonia after bone marrow transplantation. AJR, 182: 1133–1137

Geoffray A, Spehl M, Chami M, et al. 1997. Imaging of AIDS in children. J Radiol, 78(12): 1233–1243.

Goo JM, Im JG. 2002. CT of tuberculosis and non-tuberculous mycobacterial infections. Radiol Clin North Am, 40: 73–87.

Gruden JF, Huang L, Turner J, et al. 1997. High-resolution CT in the evaluation of clinically suspected Pneumocystis carinii pneumonia in AIDS patients with normal, equivocal, or nonspecific radiographic findings. AJR Am J Roentgenol, 169(4): 967–975.

Griffith DE, Aksamit T, Brown-Elliott BA, et al. 2007. An official ATS/IDSA statement: diagnosis, treatment, and prevention of nontuberculous mycobacterial diseases. Am J Respir Crit Care Med, 75: 367–416.

Gulati MS, Sarma D, Paul SB. 1999. CT appearances in abdominal tuberculosis. A pictorial essay. Clin Imaging, 23(1): 51–59.

He W, Pan JS, et al. 2004. X-ray ans CT appearance of pulmonary nontuberculosis mycobacterial infection. Chin J Radiol, 38(1): 20–25.

Hidalgo A, Falcó V, Mauleón S, et al. 2003. Accuracy of high-resolution CT in distinguishing between Pneumocystis carinii pneumonia and non-Pneumocystis carinii pneumonia in AIDS patients. Eur Radiol, 13(5): 1179–1184.

Hunt SM, Miyamoto RC, Cornelius RS, et al. 2000. Invasive fungal sinusitis in the acquired immunodeficiency syndrome. Otolaryngol Clin North Am, 33(2): 335–347.

Jasmer RM, Edinburgh KJ, Thompson A, et al. 2000. Clinical and radiographic predictors of the etiology of pulmonary nodules in HIV-infected patients. Chest, 117: 1023–1030.

Jasmer RM, Gotway MB, Creasman JM, et al. 2002. Clinical and radiographic predictors of the etiology of computed tomography-diagnosed intrathoracic lymphadenopathy in HIV-infected patients. Acquir Immune Defic Syndr, 31(3): 291–298.

Laissy JP, Cadi M, et al. 1997. Mycobacterium tuberculosis versus nontuberculous mycobacterial infection of the lung in AIDS patients: CT and HRCT patterns. J Comptu Assist Tomogr, 21(2): 312–317.

Jiang SF, Liu JX, Chen BH, et al. 2013. CT findings of cavity pulmonary diseases in patients with acquired immunodeficiency syndrome. Chin J Radiol, 47(8): 713–716.

Kedlaya I, Ing MB, Wong SS. 2001. Rhodococcus equi infections in immunocompetent hosts: case report and review. Clin Infect Dis, 1(32): E39–46.

King LJ, Padley SPG. 2002. Imaging of the thorax in AIDS. Imaging, 14: 60–76.

Koh DM, Burn PR, Mathews G, et al. 2003. Abdominal computed tomographic findings of Mycobacterium tuberculosis and Mycobacterium avium intracellulare infection in HIV seropositive patients. Can Assoc Radiol J, 54(1): 45–50.

Lacombe C, Lewin M, Monnier Cholley L, et al. 2007. Imaging of thoracic pathology in patients with AIDS. J Radiol, 88: 1145–1154.

Lagorce Pages C, Fabre A, Bruneel F, et al. 2000. Disseminated mucormycosis in AIDS. Ann Pathol, 20: 343–345.

Lee Y, Song JW, Chae EJ, et al. 2013. CT findings of pulmonary non-tuberculous mycobacterial infection in non-AIDS immunocompromised patients: A case controlled comparison with immunocompetent patients. Br J Radiol, 86: 20120209.

Li HJ, Cheng JL. 2011. AIDS complicated with intestinal lymphoma: X-ray radiology, CT scan and pathological findings. Chin Med J, 124(9): 1427–1430.

Li LH, Tang XP, Cai WP. A clinical study on 101 cases complicated with Penicilliosis Marneffei. Chin J AIDS STD, 14: 12–20.

Liu JX, Tang XP, Jiang SF, et al. 2007. The chest image appearances of penicilliosis marneffei in patients with AIDS. Chin J Radiol, 41: 239–242.

Liu JX, Tang XP, Zhang LG, et al. 2009. The imaging appearances of the pulmonary mucormycosis in patients with acquired immunodeficiency syndrome. Chin J Radiol, 43: 11–19.

Liu JX, Tang XP, Zhang LG, et al. 2010. The chest radiographic appearances of non-tuberculous mycobacterial pulmonary infection in patients with acquired immunodeficiency syndrome. Chin J Radiol, 44(9): 937–939.

Liu JX, Tang XP, Zhang LG, et al. 2011. Radilogical findings in three acquired immunodeficiency syndrome patients with Rhodococcus equi pneumonia. Chin J Radiol, 45(2): 156–158.

Liu JX, Li JF, Guan WH, et al. 2013. Differential diagnosis of high resolution CT appearances of diffuse pulmonary milliary modules in patients with acquired immunodeficiency syndrome. Chin J Radiol, 47(11): 993–996.

Lockman S, Hone N, Kenyon TA, et al. 2003. Etiology of pulmonary infections in predominantly HIV infected adults with suspected tuberculosis, Botswana. Int J Tuberculosis Lung Disease, 7(8): 714–723.

Logan PM, Finnegan MM.1998. Pulmonary complications in AIDS:CT appearances. Clin Radiol, 53: 567–573.

Luo H, Liang L.2006. Research progress in epidemiology of Penicillium marneffei. Chin J Derm Venereol, 20: 627–629.

Ma DQ. 2007. Strengthen radiological examination in diagnosis of AIDS. Chin J Radiol, 41: 225–226.

Malíková H, Míková B. 2007. Abdominal tuberculosis in CT imaging. Cas Lek Cesk, 146(6): 557–559.

Marchiori E, de Mendonca RG, Capone D, et al. 2006. Rhodococcus equi infection in acquired immunodeficiency syndrome. Computed tomography aspects. J Bras Pneumol, 32: 405–409.

Marchiori E, Gasparetto EL, Escuissato DL, et al. 2007. Pulmonary paracoccidioidomycosis and AIDS: high-resolution CT findings in five patients.J Comput Assist Tomogr, 31(4): 605–607.

Marchiori E, Muller NL, de Mendonca RG, et al. 2005. Rhodococcus equi pneumonia in AIDS: high-resolution CT findings in five patients. Br J Radiol, 78: 783–786.

Martinez S, McAdams HP, Batchu CS. 2007. The many faces of pulmonary non-tuberculous mycobacterial Infection. AJR Am J Roentgenol, 189(1): 177–186.

Mayor B, Jolidon RM, Wicky S, et al. 1995. Radiologic findings in two AIDS patients with Rhodococcus equi pneumonia. J Thorac Imaging, 10: 121–125.

McAdams HP, Rosado de Christenson M, Strollo DC, et al. 1997. Pulmonary mucormycosis: radiologic findings in 32 cases. AJR Am J Roentgenol, 168: 1541–1548.

McGuinness G, Naidich DP, Garay S, et al. 1993. AIDS associated bronchiectasis: CT features. J Comput Assist Tomogr, 17(2): 260–266.

Norton KI, Kattan M, Rao JS, et al. 2001. P(2)C(2) HIV Study Group. Chronic radiographic lung changes in children with vertically transmitted HIV-1 infection. AJR Am J Roentgenol, 176(6): 1553–1558.

Othman N, Yip CW, Intan HI, et al. 2006. An abdominal mass owing to Penicillium marneffei in an HIV-infected 7-year-old boy: Case report. Ann Trop Paediatr, 26(3): 259–262.

Padley SP, King LJ. 1999. Computed tomography of the thorax in HIV disease. Eur Radiol, 9: 1556–1569.

Panos GZ, Karydis I, Velakoulis SE, et al. 2007. Multi-skeletal Pneumocystis jiroveci (carinii) in an HIV-seropositive patient. Int J STD AIDS, 18(2): 134–137.

Pantongrag-Brown L, Krebs TL, Daly BD,et al. 1998. Frequency of abdominal CT findings in AIDS patients with M. avium complex bacteraemia. Clin Radiol, 53(11): 816–819.

Park KY, Yu JS, Yoon SW, et al. 2004. Burkitt's lymphoma representing periportal infiltrating mass on CT. Yonsei Med J, 45(4): 723–726.

Paul Saleeb, Kenneth N. Olivier. 2010. Pulmonary nontuberculous mycobacterial disease: New insights into risk factors for susceptibility, epidemiology, and approaches to management in immunocompetent and immunocompromised patients. Curr Infect Dis Rep, 12(3): 198–203.

Pompili GG, Alineri S, Arborio G, et al. 1998. Invasive aspergillosis in AIDS: findings with high-resolution computerized tomography. Radiol Med, 96(4): 325–330.

Primack SL, Müller NL. 1994. High-resolution computed tomography in acute diffuse lung disease in the immunocompromised patient. Radiol Clin North Am, 32(4): 731–744.

Pursner M, Haller JO, Berdon WE. 2000. Imaging features of Mycobacterium avium-intracellulare complex (MAC) in children with AIDS. Pediatr Radiol, 30(6): 426–429.

Raoof S, Naidich DP. 2004. Imaging of unusual diffuse lung diseases. Curr Opin Pulm Med, 10(5): 383–389.

Ray P, Antoine M, Mary-Krause M, et al. 1998. AIDS-related primary pulmonary lymphoma. Am J Respir Crit Care Med, 158(4): 1221–1229.

Rizzi EB, Schinina V, Massimo C et al. 2001. Non-Hodgkin's lymphoma of the liver in patients with AIDS: sonographic, CT, and MRI findings. J Clin Ultrasound, 29(3): 125–129.

Santiago ER, Jeremy JE, Mariano V, et al. 2003. "Crazy-paving"pattern at thin-section CT of the lungs: Radiologic-pathologic overview. RadioGraphics, 23(6): 1509–1519.

Schlossbauer T, Schmidt GP, Bogner JR, et al. 2007. Pulmonary radiological characteristics in patients with HIV infection at the time of highly active antiretroviral therapy (HAART). Eur J Med Res, 12(8): 341–346.

Scialpi M, Magli T, et al. 1994. AIDS-related lymphoma: US and CT in thoracic and abdominal manifestations. Rays, 19(2): 228–234.

Sinan T, Sheikh M, Ramadan S, et al. 2002.CT features in abdominal tuberculosis: 20 years experience. BMC Med Imaging, 2(1): 3.

Singh PN, Ranjana K, Singh YI, et al. 1999. Indigenous disseminated Penicillium marneffei infection in the state of Manipur, India: report of four autochthonous cases. J Clin Microbiol, 37(8): 2699–2702.

Solari R, De Carolis L, Canqelosi D, et al.2008.Images in medicine. Cavitary pneumonia due to Rhodococcus equi in a patient with AIDS. Medicina(B Aires), 68: 226.

Song WY, Zhao ZQ, Zhao DW, et al. 2013. Imaging findings of disseminated pulmonary tuberculosis in patients with acquired immunodeficiency syndrome. Chin J Radiol, 47(1): 13–17.

Staples CA, Kang EY, Wright JL, et al. 1995. Invasive pulmonary aspergillosis in AIDS:radiographic,CT,and pathologic findings. Radiology, 196(2): 409–414.

Suri S, Gupta S, Suri R. 1999.Computed tomography in abdominal tuberculosis. Br J Radiol, 72(853): 92–98.

Thurnher MM, Rieger A, Kleibl-Popov C, et al. 2001. Primary central nervous system lymphoma in AIDS: A wider spectrum of CT and MRI fingings. Neuroradiology, 43(1): 29–35.

Tomás Franquet, Kyung S Lee, Nestor L Müller. 2003. Thin-section CT findings in 32 immuno-compromised patients with cytomegalovirus pneumonia who do not have AIDS. AJR, 181: 1059–1063.

Tong AC, Wong M, Smith NJ. 2001. Penicillium marneffei infection presenting as oral ulcerations in a patient infected with human immunodeficiency virus. J Oral Maxillofac Surg, 59(8): 953–956.

Trojan A, Kreuzer KA, Flury R, et al. 1998. Liver changes in AIDS. Retrospective analysis of 227 autopsies of HIV-positive patients. Pathologe, 19(3): 194–200.

Tarantino L, Giorgio A, de Stefano G, et al. 2003. Disseminated mycobacterial infection in AIDS patients: abdominal US features and value of fine-needle aspiration biopsy of lymph nodes and spleen. Abdom Imaging, 28: 602–608.

Vanittanakom N, Cooper CR Jr, Fisher MC, et al. 2006. Penicillium marneffei infection and recent advances in the epidemiology and molecular biology aspects. Clin Microbiol Rev, 19: 95–110.

Vogl TJ, Hinrichs T, Jacobi V, et al. 2000. Computed tomographic appearance of pulmonary mucormycosis. Rofo, 172: 604–608.

Wicky S,Cartei F, Maryor B, et al. 1996. Radiological findings in nine AIDS patients with Rhodococcus equi pneumonia. Eur Radiol, 6: 826–830.

Wittram C, Weisbrod GL. 2002. Mycobacterium avium complex lung disease in immunocompetent patients: radiography-CT correlation. Br J Radiol, 75: 340–344.

Yeon Joo Jeong, Kyung Soo Lee, Won Jung Koh, et al. 2004. Non-tuberculous mycobacterial pulmonary infection in immunocompetent patients: Comparison of thin-section CT and histopathologic findings. Radiology, 231: 880–886.

Zhang LG, Liu JX, Jiang SF, et al. 2009. The X-ray and CT findings of the penicilliosis marneffei in children with acquired immunodeficiency syndrome. Chin J CT and MRI, 7: 27–29.

Zhang LG, Liu JX, Tang XP, et al. 2009. The abdominal CT findings of the penicilliosis marneffei in patients with acquired immunodeficiency syndrome. Chin J Radiol, 43: 369–372.

Zhang LG, Liu JX, Tang XP, et al. 2010. CT findings of abdominal tuberculosis in patients with acquired immunodeficiency syndrome. Chin J Radiol, 44(12): 1272–1275.

Zhang LG, Liu JX, Tang XP, et al. 2013. The CT findings of thoracic lymphadenopathy in patients with acquired immunodeficiency syndrome: Spectrum of disease and differential diagnosis. Chin J Radiol, 47(1): 28–33.

Zhang LG, Liu JX, Jiang SF, et al. 2013. The chest and abdominal CT findings of disseminated cryptococcosis in patients with AIDS. Chin J CT and MRI, 11(4): 38–40.

Zhao DW, Ma DQ. 2002. Imaging diagnosis of pulmonary tuberculosis in AIDS. China JMIT, 18(2): 147–148.

Zhao DW, Yuan CW, et al. 2005. Imaging findings of mediastinal tuberculous lymphadenopathy in AIDS. Chin J Radiol, 39(7): 772–775.

Zhao DW, Zhang K, Ma DQ, et al. 2002. Imaging of pneumocystis carinii pneumonia in AIDS. Chin J Radiol, 36(4): 351–353.

Zimmerli W. 2001. Pneumonia in patients with HIV infection. Ther Umsch, 58(10): 620–624.

Zinck SE, Leung AN, Frost M, et al. 2002. Pulmonary cryptococcosis: CT and pathologic findings. J Comput Assist Tomogr, 26(3): 330–334.

Zumla A, Malon P, Henderson J, et al. 2000. Impact of HIV infection on tuberculosis. Post grad Med J, 76(3): 259–268.

Index

www.ingramcontent.com/pod-product-compliance
Lightning Source LLC
Chambersburg PA
CBHW050037220326

41599CB00040B/7188